10th Anniversary of *Biomedicines*—Advances in Multiple Sclerosis

10th Anniversary of *Biomedicines*—Advances in Multiple Sclerosis

Guest Editor

Víctor M. Rivera

MDPI

Basel • Beijing • Wuhan • Barcelona • Belgrade • Novi Sad • Cluj • Manchester

Guest Editor
Víctor M. Rivera
Department of Neurology
Baylor College of Medicine
Houston
USA

Editorial Office
MDPI AG
Grosspeteranlage 5
4052 Basel, Switzerland

This is a reprint of the Special Issue, published open access by the journal *Biomedicines* (ISSN 2227-9059), freely accessible at: https://www.mdpi.com/journal/biomedicines/special_issues/10th_MS.

For citation purposes, cite each article independently as indicated on the article page online and as indicated below:

Lastname, A.A.; Lastname, B.B. Article Title. *Journal Name* **Year**, *Volume Number*, Page Range.

ISBN 978-3-7258-5481-3 (Hbk)
ISBN 978-3-7258-5482-0 (PDF)
https://doi.org/10.3390/books978-3-7258-5482-0

Contents

About the Editor

Víctor M. Rivera

Victor M. Rivera, MD, FAAN, is a Distinguished Emeritus Professor of Neurology at Baylor College of Medicine and an Emeritus/Honorary Neurologist at Houston Methodist Hospital in Houston, Texas, USA. He is a Senior Member and Fellow of the American Academy of Neurology, as well as a Founder of the Mexican Academy of Neurology and the Latin American Committee for Treatment and Research in MS (LACTRIMS), and he is Chancellor of that organization. Prof. Rivera is an advisor for the Central American and Caribbean Forum for MS (FOCEM). He is the Founder and inaugural Director of the Maxine Mesinger Multiple Sclerosis Comprehensive Care Center & Clinic at the Baylor College of Medicine in Houston, Texas. Prof. Rivera has been recognized with unprecedented Lifetime Achievement Awards by both the Consortium of MS Centers (CMSC) and the National MS Society (US) and received recognition as one of the 2022 Giants in MS from the CMSC in the Global Impact Category.

biomedicines

MDPI

Editorial

Advances in Multiple Sclerosis

Victor M. Rivera

Department of Neurology, Baylor College of Medicine, One Baylor Plaza, Houston, TX 77030, USA;
vrivera@bcm.edu; Tel.: +1-832-407-0668

1. Introduction

Multiple sclerosis (MS) is the most common demyelinating and inflammatory disease of the CNS; it has a global distribution with increasing prevalence [1]. MS affects individuals of most ethnicities [2], placing a substantial regional socioeconomic burden in a vast range of geographic areas [3]. This disease poses numerous challenges for individuals, including the need to cope with the still unidentified aspects involved in its mechanistic processes, including a multifactorial etiological complex influenced by environmental epigenetic factors [4], as well as the immune and inflammatory molecular mechanisms involved in the development of the disease [5]. With the evolution of knowledge in this field, some of the elements discovered may eventually be helpful as diagnostic markers, and some have the potential to be translated into therapeutic targets. In recent decades, studies on MS have been carried out in many branches of neuroscience. Epidemiologically, this disease is observed in the highest frequency in the northern- and southern-most areas of the world: Canada, US, Scandinavia, the British Islands, most of Europe, New Zealand and Australia. An inheritable genetic factor is recognized to comprise at least one-third of the complex MS etiological make-up, identified as the HLA-DRB1 * 15:01 [6]. The current theory explaining the world-wide dissemination of this disease, including the Americas, the Middle and Far East, is the European genetic risk factor, passed on throughout history though military invasions, migration and other historical and socio-political phenomena [7,8]. While the causality of MS is multifactorial, autoimmunity is the main driver behind its mechanisms [9]; it is involved in the initiation of the characteristic, erroneous, autoimmune cascade, a response of the innate immune system to an antigen, followed by the participation of the adaptive immune system. The latter phase is essentially responsible for the structural damage recognized in the disease, inflammation, demyelination and neurodegeneration, caused by cellular and humoral factors. Pathological alterations are not restricted to white matter but are also present in the gray matter of the CNS, including abnormalities in synapses and synaptic networks. These abnormalities have also been observed in animal models of MS in research laboratories. A critical molecular step in the pathogenesis of this disorder is the traffic of activated immune cells through the blood–brain barrier (BBB), particularly their deleterious effect on the CNS. Some of the aforementioned elements of the disease have been discussed in previous works [10]. The neurological clinical manifestations are extremely varied, establishing MS as one of the most symptomatic diseases in human pathology. The current clinical classification considers several dynamic varieties conditioned by the activity of the disease, whether this manifests clinically (exacerbation, acute relapse, increased EDSS) or as MR imaging behavior (T1 lesions enhancing post-infusion of contrast material, appearance of a new T2 or enlargement of a previous T2 lesion). The identified clinical varieties, i.e., relapsing/remitting disease, and secondary progressive or primary progressive MS, may

 https://doi.org/10.3390/biomedicines13020266

transform into a worse form of the disease, subject to factors associated with its activity [11]. The nomenclature of the MS clinical classification continues to evolve. At present, the term "Clinically Isolated Syndrome" generally refers to the first event, or the initiation of the relapsing/remitting form of the disease (if the rest of the diagnostic criteria are met). New concepts such as Progression Independent of Relapse (PIRA) and Relapse-Associated Worsening (RAW) are recognized in clinical situations, and are most likely to be incorporated in future classificatory proposals. Undetected inflammation, a chronic low-level inflammatory process occurring in the CNS, is identified as the underlying pathology of PIRA, most likely being reflected clinically as a form of secondary progressive MS [12]. The diagnosis of MS becomes more challenging as our understanding of this disease increases in complexity. To assist in diagnostic accuracy and prevent misdiagnosis, diverse diagnostic criteria have been established. In the modern era, different versions of the so-called McDonald Criteria have been produced by different international panels, starting in 2001. Each version has incorporated updated knowledge on this condition through MRI findings, as well as laboratory and clinical endeavors. The most recent version of the McDonald Criteria, created in 2017 [13], will be replaced by the 2024 version, which is to be officially published and implemented in 2025. The development of therapeutic molecules for MS over the last three decades has exceeded that of available treatments for any other neurological disease. All approved MS therapies have demonstrated significant effects in controlled trials, including reductions in annualized relapse rates and in the progression of the disease, as well as improvements in MRI activity. The large variety of therapies, including interferons, glatiramer acetate, teriflunomide, fumarates, S1P1 receptor modulators, cladribine, and the monoclonal antibodies antiα4-integrin, antiCD20 and antiCD52, have been classified as being of high, moderate or modest efficacy, adhering to the guidelines provided by the Association of British Neurologists (ABN 2015 guidelines), according to their average relapse reduction [14]. This classification helps practitioners in selecting the appropriate therapy when considering the degree of clinical and MRI aggressiveness presented by the case.

An Overview of Published Articles. This Special Issue addresses *Advances in Multiple Sclerosis*, celebrating the 10th Anniversary of *Biomedicines*, and consists of nine articles covering a broad range of themes that will be briefly discussed in the following paragraphs. The purpose of this Special Issue is to highlight these studies and encourage readers to engage with this ever-relevant topic. El-Samad et al. [15] studied the role of glutamate excitotoxicity in MS pathogenesis, particularly early changes at the photoreceptor synapses, related to the visual system. Using quantitative and qualitative immunofluorescence microscopy and Western blotting, this study analyzed whether the EAAT5 glutamate transporter could be involved in the structure alterations and function of glutamatergic photoreceptor ribbon synapses in an EAE mouse model of MS. The data showed that EAAT5 was strongly reduced at the photoreceptor synapses of EAE retinas in comparison with photoreceptor synapses of the control retinas, and Western blot analyses demonstrated decreased EAAT5 expression in EAE retinas. The authors encourage future investigations to be conducted, in order to further elucidate the precise mechanisms involved. Coagulation components have been shown to provide immunomodulatory and proinflammatory effects in the CNS, resulting in inflammation and degeneration. Whether patients with MS exhibit an overrepresentation of polymorphisms implicated in coagulation and if these genes are associated with disease progression and disability were studied by Hadjiagapiou et al. [16]. The cardiovascular disease (CVD) strip assay performed, analyzing 11 genetic polymorphisms associated with thrombosis and CVD in MS patients and controls, showed that PAI-1 5G/5G homozygosity was more frequently observed in MS patients (OR:6.33 (95% CI: 1.32–30.24); $p = 0.016$). Advanced neurological disability ($p = 0.03$) and disease worsening ($p = 0.02$) were demonstrated in carriers of the HPA-1a/1b polymorphism. These findings suggest that MS may be linked to thrombophilia-related polymorphisms, hence warranting further investigation. The review article by Kee et al. [17] discusses the role of meningeal tertiary lymphoid structures (TLS) or B-cell follicles, and compartmentalized inflammation (trapped inflammatory cells) in the form of organized clusters of immune cells in the connective tissue spaces of the vasculature and leptomeninges behind an intact BBB. These pathophysiological processes are associated with the most severe clinical forms of MS: PIRA and primary progressive MS. The contributors to this review feel that TLS could represent an important marker of disease activity, as well as a therapeutic target for mitigating the most severe outcomes of disease. Huss et al. [18] performed a prospective study investigating the composition of the gut microbiota in MS patients, the presence of the *Clostridium perfrigens* epsilon toxin in serum, and the influence of some disease-modifying therapies (DMT) on epsilon toxin levels and on microbiota. The MS cohort in this study comprised patients with relapsing/remitting disease treated with the therapeutic molecules teriflunomide and fingolimod, and the monoclonal antibodies natalizumab and ocrelizumab. Untreated patients were also included. Neither epsilon toxin nor antibodies against it were detected. No significant differences in the relative abundance of fecal microbiota in the gut microbiota of MS patients receiving DMT were observed. This study did not show evidence supporting the hypothesis of a causal relationship between the *Clostridium perfringens* epsilon toxin and MS. Neurogenic lower urinary tract dysfunction (NLUTD) is common among MS patients regardless of the clinical type and duration of disease. While uroflowmetry (UF) is performed by some authors instead of urodynamics (UD), the inter-rater reliability concerning diagnosis and therapy based on UF remains challenging. Jaekel et al. [19] prospectively studied 92 people with MS (PwMS), classified using the diagnostic criteria of 'normal findings', 'detrusor overactivity', 'detrusor underactivity', 'detrusor -sphincter dyssynergia", and 'bladder outlet obstruction'. Four raters assessed the diagnostic criteria, which were applied to a possible treatment scheme that included 'no treatment', 'catheter placement', 'alpha-blockers', 'detrusor-attenuating medication', botulinum toxin', neuromodulation', and 'physiotherapy/biofeedback'. The authors noted the high influence of the individual raters (kappa rating for diagnosis = normal findings; kappa rating for therapy = botulinum toxin), and that UD remains the gold standard for the diagnosis of NLUTD in PwMS. Reverchon et al. [20] utilized three MS groups, acute relapsing patients (ARMS), natalizumab-treated (NTZ), and control subjects, to study the serotonin receptor 5-HT7 expressed on circulating lymphocytes and evaluated the effects of its activation on cytokine production with peripheral blood mononuclear cell (PBMC) cultures. The researchers found a significant increase in the 5-HT7 surface expression on T lymphocytes and on the different CD4 + T cell subsets exclusively in NTZ-treated patients. These findings strengthen the evidence that 5-HT7 may play a role in the immune-protective mechanisms of NTZ in MS disease. This work constitutes the first study on the receptor 5-HT7activating naïve T cells and influencing the inflammatory response in MS persons treated with NTZ, a humanized monoclonal antibody against the cell adhesion molecule α4-integrin. In the pathologic MS microenvironment, α4-integrin facilitates the traffic of immune cells from the peripheral circulation into the CNS. NTZ inhibits this process. The research study by Geβner et al. [21] demonstrated the importance of detecting subtle motor deficits in people with MS below the clinical threshold, in the early stages of the disease, utilizing complex motor functions. These methods have potential use as baselines and as assessments throughout the course of the disease. The study evaluated the countermovement jump (CMJ), a high-challenge task in the form of a maximal vertical bipedal jump (three maximal CMJs) on a force plate, in 99 PwMS and 33 healthy controls (HCs). These cohorts did not differ significantly in age, disease duration, body mass index (BMI) or EDSS. PwMS demonstrated significantly decreased CMJ performance in terms of kinetic, temporal and performance parameters ($p < 0.05$). The authors encourage longitudinal studies to be performed to evaluate whether the CMJ can be used to measure disease progression. In another study [22] by Geβner et al., the authors expanded their evaluations of the CMJ in association with age, sex and BMI, utilizing 164 PwMS and 98 HCs, within a cross-sectional design. All participants performed three maximal CMJs on a force plate. Analysis of the dynamic components of the CMJ showed the most significant effects of sex on flight time ($\eta^2 = 0.23$), jump height ($\eta^2 = 0.23$), and positive power ($\eta^2 = 0.13$). PwMS showed significantly lower CMJ performance compared to HCs in middle-aged (31–49-year-old) individuals, with normal weight to overweight and in both women and men. The researchers concluded that age, sex, and BMI are associated with muscle mechanical function in PwMS and HCs, and emphasize the value of integrating the CMJ into the diagnostic assessment of people with early MS and in developing individualized neurorehabilitative therapy. The article by Moore et al. [23], investigating the MS healthcare disparities among ethnic minorities, including Hispanic and Black populations in the United States, addresses a sociological concern shared by those in countries with a high prevalence of the disease: increasing frequencies of MS among minorities, and by extension, increasing frequencies affecting new migrants as well. This review emphasizes the current understanding about the patterns of disease presentation, genetic considerations, response to treatment, and future directions of inquiry, subsequently proposing practical methods with which to overcome these challenges.

2. Conclusions

This Special Issue, Advances in Multiple Sclerosis, provides the reader with a varied collection of articles conveying very recent discoveries related to genetic markers and the contribution of coagulation factors to the multifactorial etiology of MS; the lack of confirmation of a relationship between the *Clostridium perfringens* epsilon toxin and this disease is also highlighted. The utilization of uroflowmetry in the evaluation of neurogenic lower tract dysfunction (a rather common problem in people with MS regardless of age or clinical type), and the challenges posed by interrater variability, are discussed in a well-designed study addressing these questions. Tertiary Lymphoid Structures constitute the meningeal sites of compartmental inflammation in the CNS, and the pathophysiological path for progressive forms of MS. An original study demonstrated the T-lymphocyte receptor 5-HT7 may play a role in the immune-protective mechanism of the high-efficacy monoclonal antibody natalizumab. One study reports that the CMJ detects subtle motor deficits below the clinical threshold in MS, and another paper from the same laboratory describes neuromuscular and muscle mechanical function, as assessed by the CMJ, associated with age, sex and BMI. Concerns about the health disparities affecting minorities, particularly Hispanic and Black populations in the US, are studied, with future directions being suggested by another group of authors. Thus, an invaluable, comprehensive review of these findings is presented in this Special Issue.

Funding: This research received no external funding.

Institutional Review Board Statement: Not applicable.

Informed Consent Statement: Not applicable.

Acknowledgments: As Guest Editor of the Special Issue **"Advances in Multiple Sclerosis-10th Anniversary of Biomedicines"**, I would like to express my deep appreciation to all authors whose valuable work was published in this issue, thus contributing to the success of this edition.

Conflicts of Interest: The author declares no conflicts of interest.

References

1. Multiple Sclerosis International Federation-Atlas of MS-3rd Edition. Available online: https://www.msif.org (accessed on 30 September 2024).
2. Rosati, G. The prevalence of Multiple Sclerosis in the world: An update. *Neurol. Sci.* **2001**, *22*, 117–139. [CrossRef]
3. Simoens, S. Societal economic burden of multiple sclerosis and cost-effectiveness of disease-modifying-therapies. *Front. Neurol.* **2022**, *13*, 1015256. [CrossRef]
4. Pakpoor, J.; Schmierer, K.; Cuzick, J.; Giovannoni, G.; Dobson, R. Estimated and projected burden of multiple sclerosis attributable to smoking and childhood and adolescent high-body mass index: A comparable risk management. *Int. J. Epid.* **2021**, *49*, 2051–2057. [CrossRef]
5. Gracias, M.; Cassacia, P. Epigenetic mechanisms in multiple sclerosis. *Rev. Esp. Escler. Mult.* **2018**, *6*, 25–35.
6. Hollenbach, J.A.; Oksenberg, J.R. The immunogenetics of Multiple Sclerosis: A Comprehensive Review. *J. Autoimmun.* **2015**, *64*, 13–25. [CrossRef] [PubMed]
7. Beecham, A.; Amezcua, L.; Chinea, A.; Manrique, C.; Rubi, C.; Isobe, N.; Lund, B.; Santaniello, A.; Beecham, G.; Burchard, E.; et al. The genetic diversity of multiple Sclerosis risk among Hispanic and African American populations living in the United States. *Mult. Scler.* **2019**, *26*, 1329–1339. [CrossRef] [PubMed]
8. Correa, E.; Paredes, V.; Martínez, B. Prevalence of multiple sclerosis in Latin America and its relationship with European migration. *Mult. Scler. J. Exp. Transl. Clin.* **2016**, *2*, 20555217316666407. [CrossRef]
9. Barkhane, Z.; Elmadi, J.; Kumar, L.S.; Pugalenthi, L.S.; Ahmad, M.; Reddy, S. Multiple Sclerosis and Autoimmunity: A Veiled Relationship. *Cureus* **2022**, *14*, e24294. [CrossRef]
10. Rivera, V.M. Editorial of Special Issue "Multiple Sclerosis: Diagnosis and Treatment II". *Biomedicines* **2021**, *9*, 1605. [CrossRef]
11. Lublin, F.D. New multiple sclerosis phenotypic classification. *Eur. Neurol.* **2014**, *72* (Suppl. S1), 1–5. [CrossRef]
12. Giovannoni, G.; Popescu, V.; Wuerfel, J.; Hellwig, K.; Iacobaeus, E.; Jensen, M.B.; García-Domínguez, J.M.; Sousa, L.; De Rossi, N.; Hupperts, R.; et al. Smouldering multiple sclerosis: The "real MS". *Ther. Adv. Neurol. Dis.* **2022**, *15*, 17562864211066751. [CrossRef] [PubMed]
13. Thompson, A.; Banwell, B.L.; Barkhof, F.; Carroll, W.; Coetzee, T.; Comi, G.; Correale, J.; Fazekas, F.; Filippi, M.; Freedman, M.S.; et al. Diagnpsis of multiple sclerosis: 2017 revisions of the McDonald criteria. *Lancet Neurol.* **2018**, *17*, 162–173. [CrossRef]
14. A Samjoo, I.; Worthington, E.; Drudge, C.; Zhao, M.; Cameron, C.; A Häring, D.; Stoneman, D.; Klotz, L.; Adlard, N. Efficacy classification of modern therapies in multiple sclerosis. *J. Comp. Eff. Res.* **2021**, *10*, 495–507. [CrossRef] [PubMed]
15. El-Samad, A.; Jaffal, J.; Ibrahim, D.R.; Schwarz, K.; Schmitz, F. Decreased expression of the EAAT5 glutamate transporter at photoreceptor synapses in early, pre-clinical experimental autoimmune encephalomyelitis, a mouse model of multiple sclerosis. *Biomedicines* **2024**, *12*, 2545. [CrossRef] [PubMed]
16. Hadjiagapiou, M.S.; Krasias, G.; Deeba, E.; Kallis, G.; Papaloizou, A.; Costeas, P.; Christodoulou, C.; Pantzaris, M.; Lambrianides, A. Genetic Markers for Thrombophilia and Cardiovascular Disease Associated with Multiple Sclerosis. *Biomedicines* **2022**, *10*, 2665. [CrossRef] [PubMed]
17. Kee, R.; Naughton, M.; McDonnell, G.V.; Howell, O.W.; Fitzgerald, D.C. A Review of Compartmentalized Inflammation and Tertiary Lymphoid Structures in the Pathophysiology of Multiple Sclerosis. *Biomedicines* **2022**, *10*, 2604. [CrossRef] [PubMed]
18. Huss, A.; Bachhuber, F.; Feraudet-Tarisse, C.; Hiergeist, A.; Tumani, H. Multiple Sclerosis and *Clostridium perfringens* Epsilon Toxin: Is There a Relationship? *Biomedicines* **2024**, *12*, 1392. [CrossRef] [PubMed]
19. Jaekel, A.K.; Rieger, J.; Butscher, A.-L.; Mohr, S.; Schindler, O.; Queissert, F.; Hoffmann, A.; Schmidt, P.; Kirschner-Hermanns, R.; Knüpfer, S.C. Diagnosis and Treatment Recommendations—Interrater Reliability of Uroflowmetry in People with Multiple Sclerosis. *Biomedicines* **2024**, *12*, 1598. [CrossRef]
20. Reverchon, F.; Guillard, C.; Mollet, L.; Auzou, P.; Gosset, D.; Madouri, F.; Valéry, A.; Menuet, A.; Ozsancak, C.; Pallix-Guyot, M.; et al. Lymphocyte Serotonin 5-HT7 Receptor is Dysregulated in Natalizumab-Treated Multiple Sclerosis Patients. *Biomedicines* **2022**, *10*, 2418. [CrossRef] [PubMed]
21. Geβner, A.; Stölzer-Hutsch, H.; Trentzsch, K.; Schriefer, D.; Ziemssen, T. Countermovement Jumps Detect Subtle Motor Deficits in People with Multiple Sclerosis below the Clinical Threshold. *Biomedicines* **2023**, *11*, 774. [CrossRef]
22. Geβner, A.; Hartmann, M.; Trentzsch, K.; Stölzer-Hutsch, H.; Schriefer, D.; Ziemssen, T. The Association of Age, Sex, and BMI on Lower Limb Neuromuscular and Muscle Mechanical Function in People with Multiple Sclerosis. *Biomedicines* **2024**, *12*, 971. [CrossRef] [PubMed]
23. Moore, M.Z.; Pérez, C.A.; Hutton, G.J.; Patel, H.; Cuascut, F.X. Health Disparities in Multiple Sclerosis among Hispanics and Black populations in the United States. *Biomedicines* **2023**, *11*, 1227. [CrossRef] [PubMed]

biomedicines

MDPI

Article

T Lymphocyte Serotonin 5-HT$_7$ Receptor Is Dysregulated in Natalizumab-Treated Multiple Sclerosis Patients

Flora Reverchon [1,*], Colleen Guillard [2], Lucile Mollet [2], Pascal Auzou [3], David Gosset [2], Fahima Madouri [2], Antoine Valéry [4], Arnaud Menuet [1], Canan Ozsancak [3], Maud Pallix-Guyot [3,†] and Séverine Morisset-Lopez [2,†]

1 UMR7355, Experimental and Molecular Immunology and Neurogenetics, CNRS and University of Orléans, 45071 Orleans, France
2 UPR4301, Center for Molecular Biophysics, CNRS, 45071 Orleans, France
3 Neurology Department, Regional Hospital Orleans, 45100 Orleans, France
4 Medical Information Department, Regional Hospital Orleans, 45100 Orleans, France
* Correspondence: flora.reverchon@cnrs-orleans.fr; Tel.: +33-0238257974
† These authors contributed equally to this work.

Abstract: Serotonin (5-HT) is known as a potent immune cell modulator in autoimmune diseases and should be protective in the pathogenesis of multiple sclerosis (MS). Nevertheless, there is limited knowledge about receptors involved in 5-HT effects as well as induced mechanisms. Among 5-HT receptors, the 5-HT$_7$ receptor is able to activate naïve T cells and influence the inflammatory response; however, its involvement in the disease has never been studied so far. In this study, we collected blood sample from three groups: acute relapsing MS patients (ARMS), natalizumab-treated MS patients (NTZ), and control subjects. We investigated the 5-HT$_7$ expression on circulating lymphocytes and evaluated the effects of its activation on cytokine production with peripheral blood mononuclear cell (PBMC) cultures. We found a significant increase in the 5-HT$_7$ surface expression on T lymphocytes and on the different CD4$^+$ T cell subsets exclusively in NTZ-treated patients. We also showed that the selective agonist 5-carboxamidotryptamine (5-CT)-induced 5-HT$_7$R activation significantly promotes the production of IL-10, a potent immunosuppressive cytokine in PBMCs. This study provides for the first time a dysregulation of 5-HT$_7$ expression in NTZ-MS patients and its ability to promote IL-10 release, suggesting its protective role. These findings strengthen the evidence that 5-HT$_7$ may play a role in the immuno-protective mechanisms of NTZ in MS disease and could be considered as an interesting therapeutic target in MS.

Keywords: serotonin; 5-HT$_7$ receptor; multiple sclerosis; natalizumab treatment; T lymphocyte (T-cell); PBMCs (peripheral blood mononuclear cells); interleukin-10 (IL-10)

1. Introduction

The neurotransmitter serotonin (5-HT) acts primarily by binding to its G-protein-coupled receptors divided into seven subfamilies (5-HT$_1$ to 5-HT$_7$, except the 5-HT$_3$, which is a ligand-gated ion channel) whose expression extends to several organs such as the lungs, intestine, liver, and both the peripheral and central nervous systems (CNS). This broad serotonin system representation allows 5-HT to influence many physiological functions with specific effects to the activated 5-HT receptor and the targeted cell type [1]. Moreover, 5-HT is able to modulate the immune response, both innate and adaptive, through its receptors expressed on the surface of immune cells, including neutrophils, eosinophils, monocytes, macrophages, dendritic cells, mast cells, and natural killer cells [2]. The chemoattractant properties of 5-HT are mediated by 5-HTR$_{1A}$ and 5-HTR$_{2A}$ pathways on human mast cells and eosinophils, respectively. Moreover, it has been demonstrated that 5-HT depletion using parachlorophenylalanine limits the priming adaptative immune cells by blocking T cell activation by macrophages [2].

Thus, 5-HT was shown to play an immune-modulatory role in the pathogenesis of autoimmune diseases such as multiple sclerosis (MS) [3], without understanding precisely the molecular events involved.

MS is a chronic, immune-mediated, inflammatory, and demyelinating disease of the CNS, with immune cell reactivity against the myelin sheath of neuronal axons. The invasion of lymphocytes is correlated with cytokine activity in the CNS, with disease activity associated to higher expression of inflammatory cytokines such as IFN-γ, IL-1β, IL-17, IL-22, and TNF [4]. A major involvement of $CD8^+$ and $CD4^+$ T infiltrated cells has been demonstrated in the MS pathogenesis and inflammatory relapses, associated with deleterious pro-inflammatory roles of $CD4^+$ T_H1 and $CD4^+$ T_H17 T cell subpopulations [4]. This immunological imbalance seems to be modified by exogenous 5-HT in favor of an immunomodulatory response by regulatory $CD4^+$ T cells (Treg) [5]. Much attention has been devoted to identifying the 5-HT receptors and signaling pathways involved. Recent studies demonstrated the anti-inflammatory role of 5-HT_{1A} and 5-HT_{2B} receptors on the $CD4^+$ T cell surfaces in MS [6,7]. Nevertheless, the mechanisms by which 5-HT modifies autoimmune responses remain poorly understood [3,8].

Among the 5-HT receptors, the most recently discovered, the 5-HT_7 receptor, seems to be an interesting candidate in the CNS. Indeed it has been shown to regulate important pathophysiological processes and has become a promising target in the treatment of CNS disorders such as sleep disorders, migraine, neuropathic pain, or neuro-psychiatric disorders [9,10]. Moreover, the 5-HT_7 receptor presence on the surface of innate and adaptive immune cells [2] suggests its role in immune-mediated disorders [1]. The activation of 5-HT_7 receptor induced by 5-HT endogenous signal has been shown to promote T-cell activation and proliferation [11], as well as the regulation of cytokine releases such as TNF-α and IFN-γ [1]. More recently, the 5-HT_7 receptor has been shown to be expressed on the surface of accumulated Treg cells in the mouse brain after ischemic stroke. In this context, the 5-HT_7 receptor could participate in the moderating and neuroprotective roles of Treg cells [11]. Therefore, on the basis of its therapeutic potential, modulation of 5-HT_7 activity has been the focus of numerous drug discovery programs, and several 5-HT_7-specific ligands have been successfully developed during the past two decades [12]. Among them, the LP-44, a specific 5-HT_7 agonist, was shown to modulate the inflammatory response by inhibiting the inflammatory cytokine releases such as TNF-α, whereas the antagonist SB-269970 reduced it [1].

Despite increasing data reporting 5-HT_7 receptor involvement in T-cell activation and inflammation, its actual expression level in different inflammatory pathological conditions has not been extensively reported. Taking into account that 5-HT is able to modulate T-cell behavior in MS [5], our study focused on the 5-HT_7 expression and its functions in three groups: acute relapse MS patients (ARMS) in the course of an acute inflammation, natalizumab-treated MS patients (NTZ) with a stable clinical state, and healthy subjects. We investigated the 5-HT_7 receptor expression on the main subsets of peripheral lymphocyte by flow cytometry. We were interested in the possible correlation between the immune response in the MS context (with or without NTZ treatment) and the 5-HT_7 receptor expression and/or function. For this purpose, we analyzed the *Htr7* gene activity in peripheral blood mononuclear cells (PBMCs) in the three groups. Then, 5-HT_7 receptor was activated in PBMCs cultures, and we performed immunoassays to access its possible effects on immune function.

2. Materials and Methods

2.1. Standard Protocol Approvals and Subject Characterization

This study was carried out in accordance with the protocol validated by the Ethics Committee EST IV from Strasbourg in France. Trial registration at clinicaltrials.gov is NCT04546698. All written informed consent forms followed the ethical guidelines that the 1964 Declaration of Helsinki had set. MS patients were diagnosed according to the 2018 revised McDonald criteria [13] and were recruited from the neurology unit of the "Centre

Hospitalier Régional d'Orléans". Healthy subjects were recruited from the "Établissement Français du Sang" (Orléans, France). Starting with blood samples, the study design is summarized in Figure 1. Samples from MS patients with acute relapse were obtained during an inflammatory phase before any treatment to limit relapse. Natalizumab-treated MS patients were cured for at least 6 months, and blood samples were obtained at the end of one cycle of natalizumab (4-week cycle) and before the next infusion. They were clinically stable with normal MRI scans and a minimum of 6 months of treatment. The following demographic and clinical characteristics were evaluated in every case: age, sex, disease duration, MS group (ARMS: acute relapsing MS, NTZ: natalizumab-treated MS), disability scores (EDSS: Expanded Disability Status Scale), and treatment with selective serotonin recapture inhibitors. Healthy controls were matched for age and sex, as displayed in Table 1.

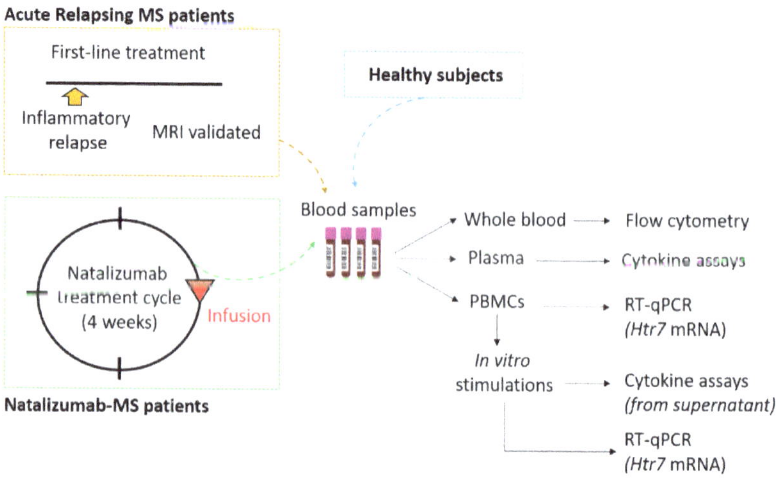

Figure 1. Experimental design and analyses performed. Abbreviations: PBMCs: peripheral blood mononuclear cells; RT: reverse transcription; qPCR: quantitative polymerase chain reaction; mRNA: messenger ribonucleic acid; *Htr7*: serotonin 5-HT$_7$ receptor gene.

Table 1. Clinical characteristics of MS patients and healthy subjects.

Clinical Characteristics	Natalizumab Treated MS Patients (n = 30)	Acute Relapsing MS Patients (n = 18)	Healthy Subjects (n = 30)
Age, y, mean (SEM)	37.8 (1.86)	34.1 (2.13)	39.2 (1.57)
Female, n (%)	25 (83)	13 (81)	25 (83)
MS symptom onset, y (SEM)	8.6 (1.24)	5.4 (1.03)	/
EDSS score, mean (SEM)	2.3 (0.40)	2.8 (0.50)	/
SSRI treatment, n (%)	7 (23)	1 (6)	/
Natalizumab infusions, n (SEM)	49 (7.55)	/	/

Abbreviations: MS: multiple sclerosis; EDSS: Expanded Disability Status Scale; SSRI: selective serotonin recapture inhibitor; /: not applicable.

2.2. *Analysis of 5-HT$_7$ Receptor Expression on Lymphocyte Surface*

5-HT$_7$ receptor expression level was evaluated from whole blood using flow cytometry. We performed three tubes per patient corresponding to unlabeled blood cells, Fluorescence Minus One (FMO) controls, and cells labeled for the 5-HT$_7$ receptor. All staining reactions were performed at room temperature for 30 min in the dark. Briefly, cells were first stained with specific primary antibody (Ab) for 5-HT$_7$ receptor (13830-1-AP, Proteintech,

Manchester, Europe). This first step concerns only labeled cells. The rest of the protocol concerns labeled cells and the FMO control. Then, cells were washed with Stain Buffer (554657, BD Biosciences, Paris, France), followed by centrifugation at 1500 rpm for 5 min. Secondary Ab specific to the primary (ab150077, abcam, Cambridge, England) was incubated. Leucocytes were then washed and stained using a combination of the following fluorochrome-conjugated Ab (BD Biosciences®), diluted in Brilliant Stain Buffer (563794): CD45-BV510 (563204, 1/200), CD19-BV786 (563325, 1/200), CD3-APC-H7 (560171, 1/200), CD8-PerCp-Cy5 (565310, 1/200), CD4-APC (566915, 1/200), CXCR3-BV711 (563156, 1/200), CCR4-BV421 (562579, 1/200), CCR6-PE (551773, 1/50), CD25-PE-CF594 (562403, 1/200), CD127-PE-Cy7 (560822, 1/200). Red blood cells were then lysed (349202, BD Biosciences) at room temperature for 10 min in the dark. Finally, cells were fixed (339860, BD Biosciences) at 4 °C for >30 min in the dark, washed, and re-suspended in Stain Buffer. Flow cytometry analyses were performed on LSR Fortessa X-20 flow cytometer (Becton Dickinson). Gating strategy was set up according to FMO control for all antibodies. One hundred thousand $CD4^+$ cells were recorded in order to have a sufficient regulatory T (Treg) cell number, representing the minority subpopulation. Final analysis and graphical output were performed using FlowJo software version 10 (Tree Star, Ashland, OR, USA).

2.3. Isolation and Stimulation of Peripheral Blood Mononuclear Cells

Peripheral blood mononuclear cells (PBMCs) from 30 healthy controls, 30 natalizumab-treated MS patients, and 18 acute relapsing MS patients were isolated from blood samples collected in EDTA tubes using Ficoll density gradient centrifugation (11753219, Fisher Scientific, Massachusetts, United States) at 2000 rpm for 20 min. PBMCs were then quickly re-suspended in 1X PBS and washed twice with centrifugations at 1400 rpm for 7 min.

PBMCs were incubated in RPMI 1640 (GIBCO, Life Technologies, Pleasanton, CA, USA) supplemented with 1% L-glutamine, 1% pyruvate sodium, 1% penicillin–streptomycin, 1% MEM non-essential amino acids solution, and 10% heat-inactivated fetal calf serum (FCS) in 24-wellsplate at 37 °C overnight. PBMCs (2×10^6 cells/well) were then stimulated with lipopolysaccharides (LPS, 100 ng/mL)-(L2630, Sigma-Aldrich, Saint-Quentin Fallavier, France) or 5-carboxamidotryptamine (5-CT, 10 μM)-(0458, TOCRIS) for 4 h at 37 °C. PBMCs and supernatants were collected at the end of stimulation and stored at −80 °C for RNA extractions and cytokine assays.

2.4. Cytokine Assays in Plasma Samples and PBMC Supernatants

Plasma was collected from patient's whole blood after centrifugation at room temperature for 5 min at 1500 rpm and stored at −80 °C until the assays. ELISA (R&D systems) quantified human IL-17 (DY317-05), IL-1β (DY201-05), IFN-γ (DY285B-05), IL-10 (DY217B-05), and IL-4 (DY204-05) assays in plasmas and PBMCs supernatants, according to the manufacturer's instructions.

2.5. Analysis of 5-HT_7 Receptor Transcription Level

RNA was collected and extracted using a miRNeasy Mini Kit according to the manufacturer's instructions (Qiagen, Hilden, Germany) from PBMCs. RNA integrity and quality were controlled with Agilent RNA 6000 Nano Chips kit® (5067-1511, Agilent, Santa Clara, CA, USA). Reverse transcription was performed with SYBR® Premix Ex Taq™ (Takara, Kusatsu, Japan), and cDNA was subjected to quantitative real-time PCR using primers for *Htr7* (#QT00012481, Qiagen) and ONEGreen® Fast qPCR Premix (Ozyme, Saint Cyr l'Ecole, France). Relative RNA expression was normalized to *Hprt1* and *Gapdh* expressions (Qiagen), and raw data were analyzed by the $2^{\Delta\Delta Ct}$ method [14].

2.6. Statistical Analysis

All graphic data are presented as mean ± SEM. Statistical analyses were performed with R software using, according to data distribution, either one factor within subject ANOVA with Tukey contrasts for post hoc comparisons or the Kruskal–Wallis test and pairwise Wilcoxon test with Holm–Sidak p-value adjustment. Statistical differences were considered significant when $p < 0.05$, with asterisks denoting the degree of significance (* $p < 0.05$; ** $p < 0.01$; *** $p < 0.001$). The graphical representations were performed with GraphPad Prism 9.0 software.

3. Results

3.1. High Surface Expression of 5-HT$_7$ Receptor on T Cells in Natalizumab-Treated MS Patients

The neuroprotective role of serotonin [3] is associated with its ability to modulate the inflammatory response of lymphocytes [6] involved in MS disease course [15], but the knowledge of the receptors involved is limited. Moreover, several studies reported an important activation of immune cells in peripheral blood from MS patients, including changes in surface phenotype [16].

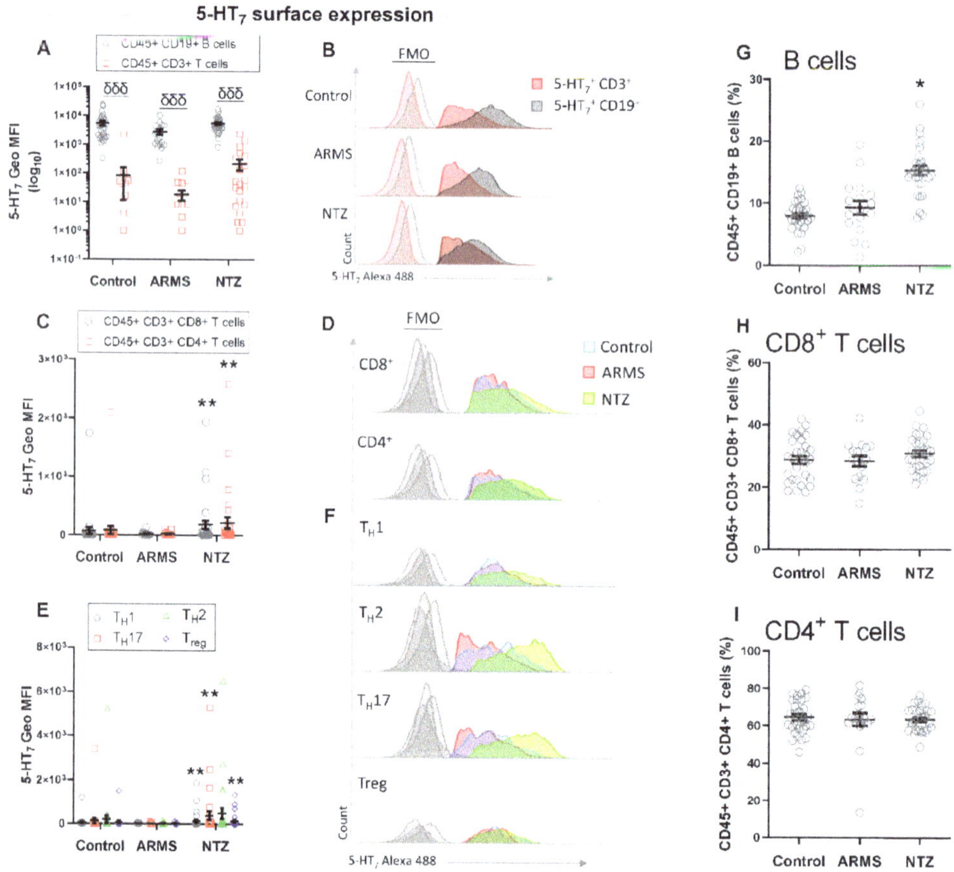

Figure 2. 5-HT$_7$ expression level on the surface of circulating lymphocytes from control, ARMS, and NTZ patients. Geometric mean fluorescence intensity (Geo MFI) of 5-HT$_7$ surface expression and histogram representation of the cytometry analysis on CD45$^+$ CD19$^+$ B and CD45$^+$ CD3$^+$ T lymphocytes (**A**,**B**), on CD3$^+$ CD8$^+$ and CD3$^+$ CD4$^+$ T cells (**C**,**D**), and CD4$^+$ T cell subsets (**E**,**F**). Proportions of circulating cells analyzed by flow cytometry are shown for B cells (**G**), CD8$^+$ (**H**), and CD4$^+$ T cells (**I**) from control, ARMS, and NTZ patients. Results are given as mean ± SEM. B cells compared with T cells for each group. *: compare with control. δδδ $p < 0.001$; * $p < 0.05$; ** $p < 0.01$.

Therefore, we investigated the surface expression levels of 5-HT$_7$ on different lymphocyte populations from whole blood samples. We found that the 5-HT$_7$ expression was significantly higher on the surface of CD19$^+$ B lymphocytes than on CD^{3+} T lymphocytes for all three groups ($p < 0.001$, Figure 2A,B). When compared to their control counterparts, ARMS samples did not show any significant differences, while NTZ patients' cells displayed a significant increase in the 5-HT$_7$ surface expression on CD3$^+$ CD8$^+$ and CD3$^+$ CD4$^+$ T cells ($p < 0.01$, Figure 2C,D), as well as on the CD4$^+$ T cell subsets CD4$^+$ CD183$^+$ T$_H$1, CD4$^+$ CD196$^+$ T$_H$17, CD4$^+$ CD194$^+$ T$_H$2, and CD4$^+$ CD25 (high) CD12$_7$ (low) Treg ($p < 0.01$, Figure 2E,F). Next, we investigated the circulating T and B lymphocyte proportions that are supposed to be modified under natalizumab treatment, which induces compartmentalization of immune cells at the periphery [17]. We found significantly more circulating CD19$^+$ B lymphocytes in the NTZ MS patients ($p < 0.05$, Figure 2G), while CD3$^+$ T cells were unchanged (Figure 2H,I).

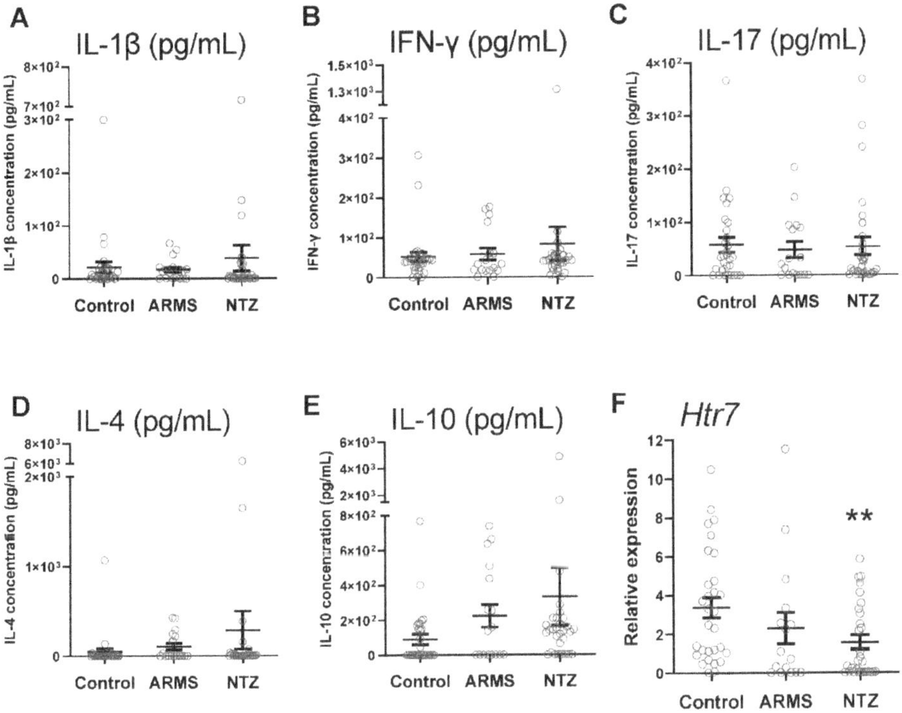

Figure 3. Plasma immunological context and *Htr7* gene expression in PBMCs from control, ARMS, and NTZ patients. Cytokines assays: IL-1β (**A**), IFN-γ (**B**), IL-17 (**C**), IL-4 (**D**), and IL-10 (**E**) from plasma samples of control, ARMS, and NTZ patients. *Htr7* was analyzed by RT-qPCR. The relative expression of *Htr7* mRNA levels, normalized to Gapdh and Hprt1 of control subjects, is shown (**F**). Results are given as mean ± SEM. ** $p < 0.01$ compared with control.

3.2. Decreased 5-HT$_7$ Receptor Gene Activity in the Absence of a Peripheral Inflammatory Context in Natalizumab-MS Patients

The gene expression level is to be considered when its protein is modified in order to better understand the intracellular mechanisms involved. In the context of stress protocols performed on rat lymphocytes, it was observed that there was an increase in the number of 5-HT$_7$-receptor-positive lymphocytes, correlated with an increased activity of the gene. The authors suggest a potential role for the receptor in stress response mechanisms involving the lymphocytes [16]. Considering our findings of increased 5-HT$_7$ receptor expression on the surface of T cells in NTZ patients, we were interested in *Htr7* gene expression level within PBMCs and a possible link with the peripheral inflammatory context by measuring some plasma cytokine levels as well as in the peripheral cytokine context in the three groups.

We assessed on one hand the peripheral inflammatory context by cytokine assays from plasma samples and on the other hand the transcriptional level of the receptor in PBMCs. We found no IL-1β, IFN-γ, IL-17, IL-4, and IL-10 level differences between the three groups (Figure 3A–E), while the 5-HT_7 was transcribed at significantly lower levels in PBMCs of NTZ patients compared to ARMS patients and healthy subjects ($p < 0.01$, Figure 3F).

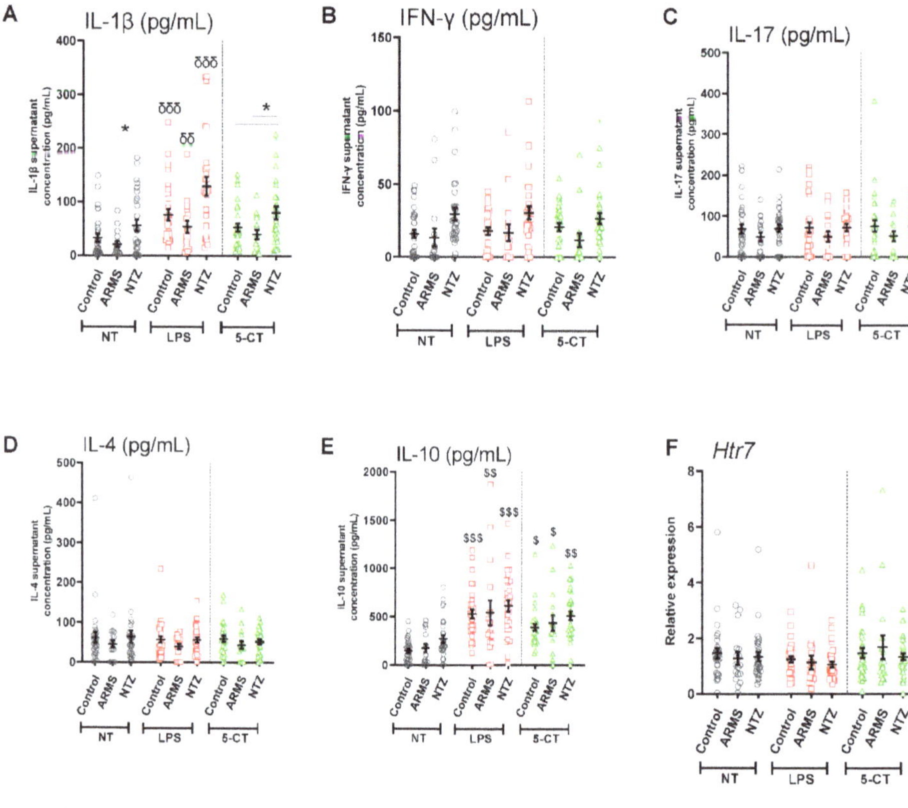

Figure 4. Effects of 5-HT_7 receptor agonist 5-CT on PBMC cytokine releases compared to LPS stimulation. Cytokines assays: IL-1β (**A**), IFN-γ (**B**), IL-17 (**C**), IL-4 (**D**), and IL-10 (**E**) were performed from PBMC supernatants of control, ARMS, and NTZ patients. *Htr7* was analyzed by RT-qPCR. The relative expression of *Htr7* mRNA levels, normalized to *Gapdh* and *Hprt1* of non-treated PBMCs from the control, is shown (**F**). Results are given as mean ± SEM. *: compare the values under the bars. \$: compare with the respective non-treated (NT) condition. Compare with both NT and 5-CT conditions. $^{*}\ p < 0.05$; $^{\$}\ p < 0.05$; $^{\$\$}\ p < 0.01$; $^{\$\$\$}\ p < 0.001$; $^{\delta\delta}\ p < 0.01$; $^{\delta\delta\delta}\ p < 0.001$.

3.3. 5-HT_7 Activation Promoted IL-10 Release from PBMCs under Physiological and Pathological Conditions

To evaluate their intrinsic cytokine secretion capacity, isolated PBMCs from patients and controls were cultured outside their in vivo immunological context and maintained in vitro with an identical culture medium. Indeed, clinical and animal studies demonstrated cellular reactivity in MS, particularly that of T and B lymphocytes as well as monocytes, which is involved in the pathogenesis [18,19]. First, without any stimulation, we observed a significantly higher basal IL-1β release in the NTZ patients ($p < 0.05$), compared to the two other groups, suggesting a different activation state of NTZ PBMCs cells. Then, to determine how pathological conditions may influence the ability of PBMCs to respond to exogenous stimulation, we performed *LPS* in vitro stimulation as a positive control. As expected, we found that LPS stimulation significantly promoted the pro-inflammatory IL-1 β release in all three groups compared with the 5-CT stimulation and the untreated basal condition ($p < 0.01$, $p < 0.001$; Figure 4A). Conversely, we observed no response of LPS to induce IFN-γ, IL-17, and IL-4 productions (Figure 4B–D), and we reported a significant increase in the anti-inflammatory IL-10 release by PBMCs after LPS stimulation from all three groups compared to the basal condition ($p < 0.01$, $p < 0.001$, Figure 4E). Then, we stimulated PBMCs with the 5-HT_7 receptor agonist 5-CT to determine the role of 5-HT_7 receptor in PBMC cytokine release and whether these 5-HT_7 functions could be altered in MS patients. Interestingly, 5-CT did not modify IL-1β, IFN-γ, IL-17, and IL-4 production in any group (Figure 4A–D), while it induced a specific and significant IL-10 release by PBMCs in all three groups ($p < 0.05$, $p < 0.01$; Figure 4E). Then, we evaluated the 5-HT_7 transcriptional level under both LPS and 5-CT conditions and we did not find any significant differences for all groups (Figure 4F).

4. Discussion

Previous studies demonstrated that 5-HT influences the chronic deleterious inflammation in MS [20]. Supported by the MS animal model, i.e., experimental autoimmune encephalomyelitis (EAE), clinical data showed the beneficial effects of selective serotonin reuptake inhibitors on MS pathogenesis [21]. The 5-HT_7 receptor has been described to be expressed at the surface of lymphocytes [11] and thus may be an important player of the inflammation regulation in MS mediated by lymphocytes. Nevertheless, no studies have distinguished the receptor expression on the surface of B cells versus T cells, with the two subsets having very distinct roles in the MS pathogenesis.

For the first time, we showed a higher surface expression of the 5-HT_7 receptor on the B cells compared to the T cells for all three groups, thereby meaning this expression appears to be independent of the disease and treatment. This large B cell expression suggests that the 5-HT_7 receptor may play a relevant physiological role on this particular lymphocyte subset. When focusing on T lymphocytes, we found that 5-HT_7 receptor expression was significantly higher on the surface of $CD4^+$ and $CD8^+$ T cells in NTZ patients compared to ARMS patients and healthy subjects. Romme Christensen et al., demonstrated that immune cells in peripheral blood from progressive MS patients presented a higher level of activation with increased frequencies of $ICOS^+$ T_{FH} cells and changes in surface phenotype with a larger quantity of IL-23 receptor expression on $(IL23R)^+CD4^+$ T cell surface [22]. Analysis of T_H1, T_H17, T_H2, and Treg $CD4^+$ T lymphocyte subpopulations confirmed the 5-HT_7 receptor overexpression on their surface exclusively in NTZ patients. Natalizumab treatment blocks the lymphocyte infiltration toward the tissues, including CNS, resulting in changes in blood lymphocyte composition [17] with increased circulating T-cell reactivity [23,24]. Börnsen et al., provided evidence that the NTZ treatment not only alters the percentage of circulating leukocytes but may promote a direct pro-inflammatory effect on PBMCs [25]. Indeed, VLA-4 antigen binding occurring with the NTZ treatment provides a co-stimulatory signal to the cells, promoting their activation and accumulation in the periphery [26]. On the basis of these results, we show that the 5-HT_7 receptor was overexpressed on the surface of probably reactive T cells in NTZ patients.

Interestingly, Urbina et al., showed that 5-HT_7 overexpression on the surface of isolated rat $CD4^+$ and $CD8^+$ T cells after concanavalin A activation suggests a 5-HT_7 protective role in the inflammatory context [16]. In order to understand whether the 5-HT_7 overexpression in NTZ patients was also associated with an inflammatory context, we investigated the peripheral immunological response. We assayed five cytokines in the patient's plasma; IL-1β, IFN-γ, and IL-17 as biomarkers of pro-inflammatory response; and IL-10 and IL-4 as anti-inflammatory response. We found no difference in the cytokine production in whole plasma samples between the three groups. A study performed on the cerebrospinal fluid

(CSF) of MS patients demonstrated a systemic inflammatory response correlated with aberrant lymphocyte activation [22]. This suggests that the method we used to measure cytokine production was not sensitive enough to detect slight variations between groups. Alternatively, our results suggest that CSF is preferable to plasma for cytokine assays in neuro-inflammatory diseases such as MS [27].

The study by Urbina et al., proposed a link between 5-HT_7 overexpression on activated isolated rat $CD4^+$ and $CD8^+$ T cells and a significantly increased *Htr7* gene activity [16]. In contrast, our results showed a significant decrease in *Htr7* gene activity specifically in PBMCs isolated from NTZ-treated patients compared to ARMS patients and healthy subjects. Previously, Albayrak et al., investigated the *Htr7* gene activity in carrageenan-induced inflammatory context in rats and showed that 5-HT_7 receptor activation by agonist leads to a decrease in gene activity associated with reduction of serum TNF-α, IL-1β, and IL-6 levels [28]. These results suggested a protective mechanism through 5-HT_7 desensitization with an *Htr7* gene activity downregulation that is common among G-protein coupled receptors [29]. Thus, for the first time, our study showed *Htr7* gene downregulation specifically in NTZ patients whose 5-HT_7 receptor expression on the activated T lymphocyte surfaces was much higher than that of ARMS patients and healthy subjects. Only one study has investigated desensitization by internalization of the three human 5-HT_7 receptor isoforms and discussed the pattern of receptor trafficking in response to agonists [30]. Guthrie et al., provided evidence that the surface 5-HT_7(d) isoform receptor are constitutively internalized in the absence of agonists, while the majority of 5-HT_7(a) and 5-HT_7(b) isoforms remain on the surface. Comprehensive investigations will be required to identify the 5-HT_7-receptor-mediated intracellular pathways involved in the negative *Htr7* gene activity.

The 5-HT_7 receptor has been shown to modulate the production of pro- and anti-inflammatory cytokines in different contexts. The receptor promotes the IL-1β release by dendritic cells, while it reduces TNF-α and IL-6 in liver chronic injury [1]. Nevertheless, no data have been provided regarding its role on the leukocyte-mediated immunological response in MS. In isolated PBMCs cultures, we first showed a significantly higher IL-1β release from NTZ patients' PBMCs in the absence of exogenous stimulation, suggesting a basal inflammation state. Indeed, animal and clinical studies have demonstrated cellular activity in MS and particularly of B and T lymphocytes, which are involved in the pathogenesis [17,18]. In addition, it has been demonstrated that there is an immune cell proportion altered in the CSF of MS patients that is associated with inflammatory mediators such as IL-1β [31]. Then, we showed the ability of these cells to respond to in vitro positive control LPS stimulation with a massive release of both IL-1β pro-inflammatory and IL-10 anti-inflammatory cytokines to counterbalance the response.

Furthermore, we showed that the 5-HT_7 receptor agonist 5-CT resulted in a significant increase in the anti-inflammatory IL-10 release in all three groups. Interestingly, in contrast to the LPS effect, stimulation by 5-CT did not significantly influence the IL-1β release compared to non-treated conditions, suggesting that the 5-HT_7 receptor is not involved in this pro-inflammatory pathway mediated by IL-1β. Several recent studies provide evidence of the 5-HT_7 receptor anti-inflammatory effect with a protective role by decreasing the pro-inflammatory cytokine release as TNF-α or by limiting cell apoptosis [1,21,22]. Moreover, it has been shown that the 5-HT_7 receptor is associated with macrophage M2 polarization, characterized as protective cells in an inflammatory context [20]. A recent review describes the known protective roles of 5-HT_7 receptors in neurodegenerative diseases that are associated with reduction of oxidative stress, synaptic remodeling, and immunomodulation [32]. All these reports support our results and the 5-HT_7 receptor ability to modulate immune function in MS and beyond. Our in vitro results show that the release of IFN-γ, IL-17, or IL-4 was not induced by LPS, nor by 5-CT in all three groups, suggesting that 5-HT_7-receptor-mediated signaling pathways are not directly involved in these cytokine releases. Moreover, in the two stimulation conditions, LPS or 5-CT had no effect on the *Htr7* gene activity for the three groups, suggesting an absence of in vitro regulation in our experimental conditions. Further experiments would be required to understand the *Htr7* gene regulation and the signaling pathways involved in PBMC cultured cells. Indeed, it seems that the incubation time of the 5-HT$_7$ agonist could be an important factor in this regulation. Thus, it was shown that the 5-HT$_7$ receptor agonist LP-44 does not induce any modification of *Htr7* gene activity after 2 h of stimulation; however, increases it after 4 h and conversely decreases it at 6 h [21,33].

The influence of natalizumab treatment on the 5-HT$_7$ receptor requires further investigation. Indeed, NTZ patients' samples were collected at the end of a 4-week cycle and before the next one. The dysregulation of 5-HT$_7$ expression could also be associated with a rebound disease activity after termination of NTZ treatment [23]. In addition, the 5-HT$_7$ level expression on the T lymphocyte populations and the *Htr7* gene activity observed during an inflammatory attack in the ARMS group were similar to those of the healthy subjects. We cannot exclude the fact that the tissue cellular infiltration contributed to masking significant results obtained on the periphery. It would be interesting to perform further analyses in this group outside of an inflammatory phase. Moreover in future studies on the understanding of 5-HT$_7$ receptor in MS, its heterodimeric form with 5-HT$_{1A}$ [34] will be an important element to consider. Indeed, as shown by our 5-HT$_7$ receptor results, the 5-HT$_{1A}$ receptor is overexpressed on the T cell surfaces in an EAE model and is also associated with an anti-inflammatory role [7]. The involvement of the receptor present on the surface of monocytes will also be a point of clarification, as in the review by Melnikov et al., including the sometimes conflicting roles of the receptor depending on the cell type [20]. In fact, the alterations of innate immunity found in the peripheral blood [22] and in the CSF [31] of MS patients are evidence that further study is needed to determine the 5HT7 receptor involvement on the surface of innate immune cells.

To conclude, this study shows for the first time that the 5-HT$_7$ receptor specifically is upregulated on the surface of CD8$^+$ T cells and CD4$^+$ T cell subpopulations in clinical stable MS patients treated with NTZ for at least 6 months. In these patients, we observed an *Htr7* gene expression downregulation that could be linked to G-protein-coupled receptors' protective mechanism, even though signaling pathways have not yet been elucidated. Furthermore, common to all three groups, an increase in IL-10 release was evidenced, produced by in vitro 5-CT-treated PBMCs. This suggests an anti-inflammatory effect of 5-HT$_7$ receptor through IL-10 release. Moreover, IL-10 release has been shown to be elevated in serum after first NTZ infusion, associated with beneficial effects of treatment [35]. Thus, our study suggests that reactive T cells [17,18], which are peripherally blocked by NTZ treatment, overexpress the 5-HT$_7$ receptor and may promote IL-10 release, which the system needs to restore immunological balance. Altogether, our findings provide the first evidence for 5-HT$_7$ implication in MS patients under NTZ treatment.

Author Contributions: Conceptualization, F.R. and M.P.-G.; methodology, F.R., C.G., L.M., F.M., D.G. and M.P.-G.; software, F.R. and A.V.; validation, F.R., P.A., C.O., M.P.-G. and S.M.-L.; formal analysis, F.R.; investigation, F.R. and C.G.; writing—original draft preparation, F.R.; writing—review and editing, F.R., L.M., P.A., A.M. and S.M.-L.; funding acquisition, S.M.-L. All authors have read and agreed to the published version of the manuscript.

Funding: This research was funded by University of Orleans, CNRS, and also a Region grant (Centre Val-de Loire) APR-IR NeuroMabster for S.M.-L. A FRM grant funded the post-doctoral salary of F.R.

Institutional Review Board Statement: The study was conducted in accordance with the Declaration of Helsinki and approved by the Ethics Committee EST IV from Strasbourg in France (March 2020). Trial registration at clinicaltrials.gov is NCT04546698.

Informed Consent Statement: Informed consent was obtained from all subjects involved in the study. Written informed consent was obtained from the patients to publish this paper.

Data Availability Statement: Data is contained within the article.

Acknowledgments: We are grateful to all the members of the neurology department of the Regional Hospital Center of Orleans and the PRIMMO platform for their help in including patients, and also to the patients for donating their samples. Thanks to Chloé Robin from the Center for Molecular Biophysics (CNRS UPR4301, Orleans) for the access to the culture room. Thanks also to MotivHealth for recruiting Colleen Guillard, and SFR FED 4226 for its financial support for the publication.

Conflicts of Interest: The authors declare no conflict of interest. The funders had no role in the design of the study; in the collection, analyses, or interpretation of data; in the writing of the manuscript; or in the decision to publish the results.

References

1. Quintero-Villegas, A.; Valdés-Ferrer, S.I. Role of 5-HT7 receptors in the immune system in health and disease. *Mol. Med.* **2019**, *26*. [CrossRef]
2. Shajib, M.S.; Khan, W.I. The role of serotonin and its receptors in activation of immune responses and inflammation. *Acta Physiol.* **2015**, *213*, 561–574. [CrossRef]
3. San Hernandez, A.M.; Singh, C.; Valero, D.J.; Nisar, J.; Ramirez, J.I.T.; Kothari, K.K.; Isola, S.; Gordon, D.K. Multiple Sclerosis and Serotonin: Potential Therapeutic Applications. *Cureus* **2020**, *12*, e11293. [CrossRef]
4. Pegoretti, V.; Swanson, K.A.; Bethea, J.R.; Probert, L.; Eisel, U.L.M.; Fischer, R. Inflammation and Oxidative Stress in Multiple Sclerosis: Consequences for Therapy Development. *Oxid. Med. Cell Longev.* **2020**, *2020*, 7191080. [CrossRef] [PubMed]
5. Bell, L.; Lenhart, A.; Rosenwald, A.; Monoranu, C.M.; Berberich-Siebelt, F. Lymphoid Aggregates in the CNS of Progressive Multiple Sclerosis Patients Lack Regulatory T Cells. *Front. Immunol.* **2019**, *10*, 3090. [CrossRef]
6. Sacramento, P.M.; Monteiro, C.; Dias, A.S.O.; Kasahara, T.M.; Ferreira, T.B.; Hygino, J.; Wing, A.C.; Andrade, R.M.; Rueda, F.; Sales, M.C.; et al. Serotonin decreases the production of Th1/Th17 cytokines and elevates the frequency of regulatory CD4+ T-cell subsets in multiple sclerosis patients. *Eur. J. Immunol.* **2018**, *48*, 1376–1388. [CrossRef]
7. Hernández-Torres, G.; Enríquez-Palacios, E.; Mecha, M.; Feliú, A.; Rueda-Zubiaurre, A.; Angelina, A.; Martín-Cruz, L.; Martín-Fontecha, M.; Palomares, O.; Guaza, C.; et al. Development of a Fluorescent Bodipy Probe for Visualization of the Serotonin 5-HT1A Receptor in Native Cells of the Immune System. *Bioconjug. Chem.* **2018**, *29*, 2021–2027. [CrossRef]
8. Sviridova, A.; Rogovskii, V.; Kudrin, V.; Pashenkov, M.; Boyko, A.; Melnikov, M. The role of 5-HT2B-receptors in fluoxetine-mediated modulation of Th17- and Th1-cells in multiple sclerosis. *J. Neuroimmunol.* **2021**, *356*, 577608. [CrossRef] [PubMed]
9. Wan, M.; Ding, L.; Wang, D.; Han, J.; Gao, P. Serotonin: A Potent Immune Cell Modulator in Autoimmune Diseases. *Front. Immunol.* **2020**, *11*, 186. [CrossRef]
10. Glass, J.D.; Grossman, G.H.; Farnbauch, L.; Di Nardo, L. Midbrain Raphe Modulation of Nonphotic Circadian Clock Resetting and 5-HT Release in the Mammalian Suprachiasmatic Nucleus. *J. Neurosci.* **2003**, *23*, 7451–7460. [CrossRef]
11. León-Ponte, M.; Ahern, G.P.; O'Connell, P.J. Serotonin provides an accessory signal to enhance T-cell activation by signaling through the 5-HT7 receptor. *Blood* **2007**, *109*, 3139–3146. [CrossRef]
12. Ito, M.; Komai, K.; Mise-Omata, S.; Iizuka-Koga, M.; Noguchi, Y.; Kondo, T.; Sakai, R.; Matsuo, K.; Nakayama, T.; Yoshie, O.; et al. Brain regulatory T cells suppress astrogliosis and potentiate neurological recovery. *Nature* **2019**, *565*, 246–250. [CrossRef] [PubMed]
13. Thompson, A.J.; Banwell, B.L.; Barkhof, F.; Carroll, W.M.; Coetzee, T.; Comi, G.; Correale, J.; Fazekas, F.; Filippi, M.; Freedman, M.S.; et al. Diagnosis of multiple sclerosis: 2017 revisions of the McDonald criteria. *Lancet Neurol.* **2018**, *17*, 162–173. [CrossRef]
14. Bustin, S.A.; Benes, V.; Garson, J.A.; Hellemans, J.; Huggett, J.; Kubista, M.; Mueller, R.; Nolan, T.; Pfaffl, M.W.; Shipley, G.L.; et al. The MIQE guidelines: Minimum information for publication of quantitative real-time PCR experiments. *Clin. Chem.* **2009**, *55*, 611–622. [CrossRef] [PubMed]
15. van Langelaar, J.; Rijvers, L.; Smolders, J.; van Luijn, M.M. B and T Cells Driving Multiple Sclerosis: Identity, Mechanisms and Potential Triggers. *Front. Immunol.* **2020**, *11*, 760. [CrossRef] [PubMed]
16. Urbina, M.; Arroyo, R.; Lima, L. 5-HT7 receptors and tryptophan hydroxylase in lymphocytes of rats: Mitogen activation, physical restraint or treatment with reserpine. *Neuroimmunomodulation* **2014**, *21*, 240–249. [CrossRef] [PubMed]
17. Carotenuto, A.; Scalia, G.; Ausiello, F.; Moccia, M.; Russo, C.V.; Saccà, F.; De Rosa, A.; Criscuolo, C.; Del Vecchio, L.; Morra, V.B.; et al. CD4/CD8 ratio during natalizumab treatment in multiple sclerosis patients. *J. Neuroimmunol.* **2017**, *309*, 47–50. [CrossRef]
18. Van Kaer, L.; Postoak, J.L.; Wang, C.; Yang, G.; Wu, L. Innate, innate-like and adaptive lymphocytes in the pathogenesis of MS and EAE. *Cell Mol. Immunol.* **2019**, *16*, 531–539. [CrossRef]
19. González-Oria, M.C.; Márquez-Coello, M.; Girón-Ortega, J.A.; Argente, J.; Moya, M.; Girón-González, J.-A. Monocyte and Lymphocyte Activation and Regulation in Multiple Sclerosis Patients. Therapy Effects. *J. Neuroimmune Pharmacol.* **2019**, *14*, 413–422. [CrossRef] [PubMed]
20. Melnikov, M.; Sviridova, A.; Rogovskii, V.; Oleskin, A.; Boziki, M.; Bakirtzis, C.; Kesidou, E.; Grigoriadis, N.; Boyko, A. Serotoninergic system targeting in multiple sclerosis: The prospective for pathogenetic therapy. *Mult. Scler. Relat. Disord.* **2021**, *51*, 102888. [CrossRef]
21. Bhat, R.; Mahapatra, S.; Axtell, R.C.; Steinman, L. Amelioration of ongoing experimental autoimmune encephalomyelitis with fluoxetine. *J. Neuroimmunol.* **2017**, *313*, 77–81. [CrossRef]
22. Romme Christensen, J.; Börnsen, L.; Ratzer, R.; Piehl, F.; Khademi, M.; Olsson, T.; Sorensen, P.S.; Sellebjerg, F. Systemic inflammation in progressive multiple sclerosis involves follicular T-helper, Th17- and activated B-cells and correlates with progression. *PLoS ONE* **2013**, *8*, e57820. [CrossRef] [PubMed]

23. Kivisäkk, P.; Healy, B.C.; Viglietta, V.; Quintana, F.J.; Hootstein, M.A.; Weiner, H.L.; Khoury, S.J. Natalizumab treatment is associated with peripheral sequestration of proinflammatory T cells. *Neurology* **2009**, *72*, 1922–1930. [CrossRef] [PubMed]
24. Mellergård, J.; Edström, M.; Jenmalm, M.C.; Dahle, C.; Vrethem, M.; Ernerudh, J. Increased B cell and cytotoxic NK cell proportions and increased T cell responsiveness in blood of natalizumab-treated multiple sclerosis patients. *PLoS ONE* **2013**, *8*, e81685. [CrossRef]
25. Börnsen, L.; Christensen, J.R.; Ratzer, R.; Oturai, A.B.; Sørensen, P.S.; Søndergaard, H.B.; Sellebjerg, F. Effect of natalizumab on circulating CD4+ T-cells in multiple sclerosis. *PLoS ONE* **2012**, *7*, e47578. [CrossRef] [PubMed]
26. Frisullo, G.; Iorio, R.; Plantone, D.; Marti, A.; Nociti, V.; Patanella, A.K.; Batocchi, A.P. CD4+T-bet+, CD4+pSTAT3+ and CD8+T-bet+ T cells accumulate in peripheral blood during NZB treatment. *Mult. Scler.* **2011**, *17*, 556–566. [CrossRef]
27. Lepennetier, G.; Hracsko, Z.; Unger, M.; Van Griensven, M.; Grummel, V.; Krumbholz, M.; Berthele, A.; Hemmer, B.; Kowarik, M.C. Cytokine and immune cell profiling in the cerebrospinal fluid of patients with neuro-inflammatory diseases. *J. Neuroinflammation* **2019**, *16*, 219. [CrossRef]
28. Albayrak, A.; Halici, Z.; Cadirci, E.; Polat, B.; Karakus, E.; Bayir, Y.; Unal, D.; Atasoy, M.; Dogrul, A. Inflammation and peripheral 5-HT7 receptors: The role of 5-HT7 receptors in carrageenan induced inflammation in rats. *Eur. J. Pharmacol.* **2013**, *715*, 270–279. [CrossRef]
29. Luttrell, L.M.; Lefkowitz, R.J. The role of beta-arrestins in the termination and transduction of G-protein-coupled receptor signals. *J. Cell Sci.* **2002**, *115*, 455–465. [CrossRef]
30. Guthrie, C.R.; Murray, A.T.; Franklin, A.A.; Hamblin, M.W. Differential agonist-mediated internalization of the human 5-hydroxytryptamine 7 receptor isoforms. *J. Pharmacol. Exp. Ther.* **2005**, *313*, 1003–1010. [CrossRef]
31. Li, Z.; Liu, Y.; Jia, A.; Cui, Y.; Feng, J. Cerebrospinal fluid cells immune landscape in multiple sclerosis. *J. Transl. Med.* **2021**, *19*, 125. [CrossRef]
32. Quintero-Villegas, A.; Valdés-Ferrer, S.I. Central nervous system effects of 5-HT7 receptors: A potential target for neurodegenerative diseases. *Mol. Med.* **2022**, *28*, 70. [CrossRef]
33. Ayaz, G.; Halici, Z.; Albayrak, A.; Karakus, E.; Cadirci, E. Evaluation of 5-HT7 Receptor Trafficking on In Vivo and In Vitro Model of Lipopolysaccharide (LPS)-Induced Inflammatory Cell Injury in Rats and LPS-Treated A549 Cells. *Biochem. Genet.* **2017**, *55*, 34–47. [CrossRef]
34. Renner, U.; Zeug, A.; Woehler, A.; Niebert, M.; Dityatev, A.; Dityateva, G.; Gorinski, N.; Guseva, D.; Abdel-Galil, D.; Frohlich, M.; et al. Heterodimerization of serotonin receptors 5-HT1A and 5-HT7 differentially regulates receptor signalling and trafficking. *J. Cell Sci.* **2012**, *125*, 2486–2499. [CrossRef]
35. Ramos-Cejudo, J.; Oreja-Guevara, C.; Stark Aroeira, L.; Rodriguez de Antonio, L.; Chamorro, B.; Diez-Tejedor, E. Treatment with Natalizumab in Relapsing–Remitting Multiple Sclerosis Patients Induces Changes in Inflammatory Mechanism. *J. Clin. Immunol.* **2011**, *31*, 623–631. [CrossRef]

biomedicines

MDPI

Review

A Review of Compartmentalised Inflammation and Tertiary Lymphoid Structures in the Pathophysiology of Multiple Sclerosis

Rachael Kee [1,2,*], Michelle Naughton [1], Gavin V. McDonnell [2], Owain W. Howell [3] and Denise C. Fitzgerald [1]

1 Wellcome-Wolfson Institute for Experimental Medicine, Queen's University Belfast, Belfast BT9 7BL, UK
2 Department of Neurology, Royal Victoria Hospital, Belfast BT12 6BA, UK
3 Institute of Life Sciences, Swansea University, Wales SA2 8QA, UK
* Correspondence: rkee03@qub.ac.uk

Abstract: Multiple sclerosis (MS) is a chronic, immune-mediated, demyelinating disease of the central nervous system (CNS). The most common form of MS is a relapsing–remitting disease characterised by acute episodes of demyelination associated with the breakdown of the blood–brain barrier (BBB). In the relapsing–remitting phase there is often relative recovery (remission) from relapses characterised clinically by complete or partial resolution of neurological symptoms. In the later and progressive stages of the disease process, accrual of neurological disability occurs in a pathological process independent of acute episodes of demyelination and is accompanied by a trapped or compartmentalised inflammatory response, most notable in the connective tissue spaces of the vasculature and leptomeninges occurring behind an intact BBB. This review focuses on compartmentalised inflammation in MS and in particular, what we know about meningeal tertiary lymphoid structures (TLS; also called B cell follicles) which are organised clusters of immune cells, associated with more severe and progressive forms of MS. Meningeal inflammation and TLS could represent an important fluid or imaging marker of disease activity, whose therapeutic abrogation might be necessary to stop the most severe outcomes of disease.

Keywords: multiple sclerosis; progressive multiple sclerosis; nervous system; compartmentalised inflammation; meningeal inflammation; tertiary lymphoid structures; disease modifying therapy

1. Introduction

Multiple sclerosis (MS) is a chronic, immune-mediated, demyelinating disease of the central nervous system (CNS) [1]. Relapsing-remitting MS (RRMS) is the most common form of the disease. Patients with RRMS experience episodic relapses, characterised by neurological signs and symptoms which wax and wane. Relapses are caused by acute inflammatory demyelinating attacks in the CNS after which follows a period of remission where there is either incomplete or complete clinical recovery. A significant proportion of people with RRMS will go on to develop secondary progressive MS (SPMS) that is characterised by accumulation of irreversible disability [1–4]. A smaller number of patients are diagnosed with primary progressive MS (PPMS) characterised by a continual accrual of disability from symptom onset. In the progressive disease stages, accrual of neurological disability occurs in a pathological process independent of relapses and is accompanied by a trapped or compartmentalised inflammatory response, most notable in the connective tissue spaces of the vasculature and leptomeninges. Recent studies suggest that the incidence of MS is increasing [5,6]. Most people with MS are diagnosed between 20–40 years of age and so this demyelinating disease has huge personal and economic costs [7]. Whilst disease-modifying treatments (DMTs) for RRMS have improved patient outcomes over the past 20 years, effective treatments for those entering progressive disease stages are lacking [8]. Fundamental to establishing effective treatments targeted at progressive stages of MS is increasing our understanding of these pathological mechanisms.

This review focuses on compartmentalised inflammation in MS and in particular, what we know about meningeal tertiary lymphoid structures (TLS; also called B cell follicles) which are organised clusters of immune cells, associated with more severe and progressive forms of MS. Meningeal inflammation and TLS could represent an important fluid or imaging marker of disease activity, whose therapeutic abrogation might be necessary to stop the most severe outcomes of disease.

2. Compartmentalised Inflammation and Tertiary Lymphoid Structures in Multiple Sclerosis

In early histological studies of post-mortem MS tissue and mouse models of CNS inflammatory demyelination called Experimental Autoimmune Encephalomyelitis (EAE), pockets of immune cells in distinct areas such as perivascular and periventricular spaces were observed [9–11]. Extensive inflammatory infiltrates within the leptomeninges and perivascular spaces were described in a cohort of post-mortem MS cases that had active demyelination [9]. In a further study of post-mortem tissue, lymphatic-like channels were identified in perivascular spaces of chronic MS lesions [10]. This lymphatic tissue appeared to have similar features to that of the antibody-producing regions of lymph nodes. Leptomeningeal infiltrates were also observed within the spinal cord of a chronic relapsing EAE mouse model [11].

Over the past couple of decades our knowledge of inflammatory infiltrates within CNS compartments and their relevance in the pathophysiology of MS has continued to expand. Pathological hallmarks of early MS and RRMS are active white matter lesions accompanied by a breakdown of the blood–brain barrier (BBB) [12]. In the later disease stages and in progressive MS, inactive, smoldering (slow expansion of pre-existing demyelinated lesions) or shadow (remyelinated) white matter lesions are most commonly observed, with the findings of active white matter lesions relatively rare [13]. In the progressive disease stages evidence of BBB disruption is also rare and inflammation becomes compartmentalised behind an intact or repaired BBB [14]. Focal areas of inflammation can be observed within the meninges of progressive MS cases [15]. Within the meninges, these clusters of immune cells can exist as simple groupings of B and T cells to more organised cellular aggregates reminiscent of secondary lymphoid organs (SLOs). Secondary lymphoid organs include lymph nodes, spleen, Peyer's patches, bronchus-associated lymphoid tissue (BALT) and mucosa-associated lymphoid tissue (MALT) and are involved in surveying self and foreign antigens to determine if an adaptive immune response should be initiated [16,17]. When clusters of immune cells gather in ectopic, non-lymphoid sites and demonstrate a more organised assemblage similar to SLOs, they are termed tertiary lymphoid structures [18–20]. Within the literature there are interchangeable terms such as ectopic lymphoid organs, ectopic lymphoid tissue, lymphoid-like structures and B cell follicles used to describe these organised cell clusters. For the purpose of this review, we will refer to these structures as tertiary lymphoid structures (TLS).

TLS have been identified in both post-mortem MS cases (Table 1) and mouse models of MS [15,21–31]. In post-mortem tissue, TLS have been identified in the meninges of the cerebral hemispheres, particularly within the deep sulci, cerebellum, brain stem and spinal cord [15,23,25,32,33]. Tertiary lymphoid structures are not unique to MS and have been identified in other immune-mediated conditions, infections and cancers [18]. In some disease processes the presence of TLS is associated with a favourable prognosis and in others, a more severe disease course occurs. In immune-mediated conditions, TLS tend to be found at sites of chronic inflammation and are associated with a more severe disease course [18]. Useful insights have been gained from studies in rheumatoid arthritis (RA) were the identification of TLS within synovial fluid of patients can be used to help inform treatment response and disease prognostication. It was identified in these studies that patients with RA, who had TLS, tended to have a greater disease severity and a poorer response to anti-tumour necrosis family (TNF)-α therapy [34,35].

Table 1. Summary of human TLS studies.

Study	Cases	TLS Identified	Findings	Location of TLS
Serafini et al., 2004 [25]	SPMS n = 3 PPMS n = 2 RRMS n = 1 Control (non-neurological disease) n = 1 Post-mortem FFPE and fixed frozen tissue	2 SPMS cases had TLS. 0 TLS identified in PPMS and RRMS	TLS consisted of CD3$^+$ T cells, CD35$^+$ cells, CXCL13$^+$ cells, Ki67$^+$ nuclei. Plasma cells were identified in periphery of follicle.	In TLS+ cases, inflammatory infiltrates found around blood vessels in cerebral leptomeninges. B cells accumulated perivascularly in chronic inactive lesions and in subarachnoid space.
Magliozzi et al., 2007 [15]	SPMS n = 29 PPMS n = 7 Controls n = 3 Post-mortem FFPE and snap frozen tissue	PPMS: 0 TLS cases, 3 cases demonstrated moderate meningeal inflammation SPMS: TLS cases n = 12	IHC staining identified inflammatory infiltrate of CD3$^+$ T cells, CD20$^+$ B cells, CD138$^+$ or Ig$^-$ plasmablasts/plasma cells, CD68$^+$ macrophages. TLS had evidence of CD35$^+$ and CXCL13$^+$ cells, Ki67$^+$ B cells and Ig$^+$ plasmablasts/plasma cells.	TLS observed in frontal, temporal, parietal lobes and cingulate gyrus. 1 TLS identified in brainstem. TLS always found adjacent to subpial lesions and along depth of cerebral sulci. TLS cases associated were with more severe grey matter pathology.
Serafini et al., 2007 [36]	MS n = 22 Other inflammatory neurological conditions n = 7 Non-neurological controls n = 2 Alzheimers n = 1 Non EBV related lymphoblastic leukaemia n = 1 Post-mortem FFPE and fixed frozen tissue	B follicles consisting of CD20$^+$ B cells, clustered around network of stromal/FDCs that expressed CXCL13. Furthermore, contained cells expressing AID and caspase-3. Cells expressing anti-apoptotic molecule bcl-2 also observed.	ISH staining for EBER transcripts on 8 MS cases with B follicles identified EBER$^+$ cells within meninges, with maximal enrichment in follicles (n = 15), perivascular cuffs of acute (n = 4) and chronic active (n = 15) WM lesions. 70–90% of EBER$^+$ cells identified as CD20$^+$ B cells. The highest percentage of B cells expressing EBERs were detected inside and around ectopic B cell follicles suggesting that these structures may originate from the expansion of EBV infected B cells. Ectopic B cell follicles contained numerous LMP1$^+$ but no EBNA2$^+$ cells. A high frequency of BFRF1$^+$ cells was observed inside and around all intrameningeal B cell follicles analysed indicating that these structures represent main sites of viral reactivation. Double immunostainings showed that BFRF1 immunoreactivity was present in a substantial proportion of intrameningeal B cells and plasma cells (30–55%) but was much stronger in plasma cells than in B cells.	B follicles observed in cerebral meninges.
Kooi et al., 2009 [37]	PPMS n = 7 Progressive relapsing n = 1 SPMS n = 12 MS subtype not determined n = 8 Controls n = 6 Post-mortem FFPE tissue	0 TLS cases	Meninges from chronic MS patients contained more CD3$^+$ T cells, CD68$^+$ macrophages, DC-SIGN dendritic cells than controls. There were fewer CD20$^+$ B cells and CD138$^+$ plasma cells were seen occasionally in chronic MS meninges versus controls. Meningeal inflammation was not found to be associated with adjacent subpial demyelination.	TLS not observed in this cohort

Table 1. *Cont.*

Study	Cases	TLS Identified	Findings	Location of TLS
Willis et al., 2009 [38]	23 FFPE tissue specimens from 12 MS cases with confirmed B cell infiltrates and 12 fixed frozen MS cases with meningeal tissue were examined for EBV by ISH. 17 snap frozen MS lesions with confirmed B cell infiltrate from 5 cases and 12 snap frozen MS tissue containing meninges from 12 cases were examined for EBV by rt-PCR.	B cell aggregates identified in 3/12 cases within brain parenchyma 4/12 cases had a loose B cell infiltrate within the meninges.	In tissue specimens each containing white matter lesions (n = 23), EBV was examined by ISH - all were negative for the EBV transcript EBER. Subset of cases further examined with IHC for expression of EBV latent proteins and found to be negative for LMP1 and EBNA2. RT-PCR was used to detect genomic EBV or EBER1. Neither detected from 17 snap frozen specimens from 5 MS cases. All examined tissue specimens had CD20$^+$ B cells detected.	B cell aggregates in brain parenchyma
Frischer et al., 2009 [39]	67 MS Cases - 9 acute (died within 1 year disease onset) - 5 RRMS - 35 SPMS - 13 PPMS - 5 benign - 28 non neurological disease controls FFPE post-mortem tissue	Follicle structures identified in meninges in 15/67 cases	In SPMS and PPMS cases, follicles were only present in cases with active progressive disease. Active demyelination and neurodegeneration was only observed in cases with pronounced inflammation in the brain.	Infiltrates of CD3$^+$ T cells, CD20$^+$ B cells and Ig$^+$ plasma cells identified in meninges. B cells and plasma cells noted to predominantly accumulate in the perivascular spaces and the meninges.
Peferoen et al., 2010 [40]	Screened 632 CNS specimens from 94 MS cases (Netherlands Brain Bank) 12 blocks from 12 cases used in Serafini et al. JEM 2007 (UK MS Society Brain Bank). Post-mortem FFPE tissue used for EBER ISH (as per supplementary material)	Screening of 11 patients (76 blocks) did not identify B follicles as defined by the presence of CXCL13 or podoplanin. 60 blocks from 16 patients had evidence of prominent B cell infiltrates but ectopic/lymphoid follicles not observed. All UK samples negative for EBV encoded RNA technique. IHC for BZLF1, BMRF1, BFRF3 and BLLF1 + LMP1 also performed.	B cell rich areas screened for EBV encoded RNA and EBV viral lytic (BZLF1, BMRF1, BFRF3, BLLF1) and latent (LMP1) proteins. Nuclear EBV encoded RNA was found in only one tissue specimen from a single MS case. All others negative. RT-PCR to search for EBV genomes and encoded RNAs in 5 tissue blocks containing B cell rich areas did not detect EBV DNA or RNA. Single sample (EBV encoded RNA Negative) was positive for multiple EBV lytic cycle markers (BZLF1, BMRF1, BLLF1). All samples screened from UK MS Society Brain Bank cohort were negative for EBV encoded RNA and EBV lytic and latent proteins.	TLS not observed in this cohort
Magliozzi et al., 2010 [22]	SPMS n = 37 Controls (no neurological disease) n = 14 Non-MS neurological inflammatory diseases n = 9 Post-mortem FFPE, snap frozen and fixed frozen.	SPMS: TLS cases n = 20 TB meningitis: TLS cases n = 1 Luetic meningitis: TLS cases n = 1	TLS demonsrtated Ki67$^+$CD20$^+$ B cells, CD35$^+$ and CXCL13$^+$ stromal cells/FDCs, Ig$^+$ plasmablasts. Lacked GCs.	Frontal, temporal, parietal, occipital lobes examined. CD20$^+$ B cells detected along and in depth of some sulci of frontal, temporal, parietal lobes-in particular cingulate and precentral gyrus. TLS always adjacent to subpial lesions.

Table 1. *Cont.*

Study	Cases	TLS Identified	Findings	Location of TLS
Torkildsen et al., 2010 [41]	Microarray analysis of 6 MS and 8 controls (no neurological disease) Post-mortem FFPE and snap frozen. For qPCR validation–5 additional MS and 4 controls used.	No CD20⁺ B cell follicles detected in meninges. CD3⁺ cells found in meninges and active lesions. Small number of CD20⁺ B cells in meninges and cortex.	572 probes were identified as differentially expressed between MS samples and controls: 296 downregulated and 276 upregulated in MS. 33 of 276 upregulated genes mapped to molecular function Ig. A total of 83 Ig-related probes showed detectable expression among the MS and control samples, targeting 67 unique genes. Almost half of all Ig-related genes present show a significant upregulation in cortical samples of MS patients compared with controls. qPCR on RNA samples with primers specifically targeting the transcripts of the EBV lytic protein BZLF1 and the latent proteins LMP1 and 2 and EBNA1 and 2 showed no signs of latent or lytic EBV infections in any of the MS or control samples.	CD20⁺ B cell follicles not detected in meninges.
Serafini et al., 2010 [42]	SPMS n = 9 (Post-mortem snap or fixed frozen) Non-neurological controls n = 3 (Post mortem FFPE or snap frozen)	Ectopic B follicles (n = 12) identified in 8 out of 9 MS cases.	In all MS brain specimens analysed, LMP-2A (EBV encoded latent membrane protein) immunoreactivity localised to surface of many lymphocytes within perivascular cuffs of active and chronic active WMLs, meningeal immune infiltrates and B cell follicles. Double immunofluorescence staining showed majority of LMP-2A⁺ cells were CD20⁺ B cells. 80–90% of B cells within meningeal follicles were CD27⁺ antigen experienced cells. 2 MS cases had evidence of BAFF⁺ cells in sparse meningeal infiltrates and B cell follicles. In B cell follicles BAFF⁺ cells co-localised with CD20⁺ B cells and the percentage of B cells expressing BAFF ranged between 10% and 50%. Within the B cell follicles, LMP-2A⁺ cells expressing BAFF ranged between 15% and 90%. BAFF was rarely detected in meningeal iba-1 positive microglia/macrophages.	B cell follicles were detected in meninges.
Howell et al., 2011 [23]	SPMS n = 123 Post-mortem FFPE or fixed frozen.	107/123 (87%) at least one sample with moderate inflammatory meningeal infiltrate. 64/123 (52%) substantial ('++') perivascular or meningeal inflammatory infiltrate. 49/123 (40%) had evidence of TLS	TLS+ cases had a 6 fold increase in total grey matter lesion area. There was a greater meningeal inflammatory infiltrate. TLS+ cases presented at earlier ages and entered progressive stages sooner.	TLS predominantly found in deep cerebral sulci–cingulate, insula, temporal and frontal gyri. Always in close association with subpial lesions.

Table 1. *Cont.*

Study	Cases	TLS Identified	Findings	Location of TLS
Lucchinetti et al., 2011 [43]	Brain biopsy samples with sufficient cortex available n = 138. FFPE tissue. 43/138 cases had meningeal tissue available. 13/43 cases with meningeal tissue were excluded due to surgical haemorrhage.	TLS not specifically looked for.	15/43 cases with meningeal tissue had evidence of cortical demyelination. Diffuse meningeal inflammation was associated with cortical demyelination, particularly subpial lesions.	IHC staining showed the presence of perivascular meningeal infiltrates containing $CD3^+$ T cells and $CD20^+$ B cells.
Lovato et al., 2011 [44]	Post-mortem (half of samples FFPE and half snap frozen) 11 MS cases - 7 SPMS - 3 chronic progressive - 1 RRMS CSF obtained from 1 case post-mortem.	Meningeal B cell aggregates identified in a subset of MS cases with CD20 IHC analysis. Number of cases with meningeal B cell aggregates not stated.	This study characterised B cell repertoires from meningeal B cell aggregates and the corresponding parenchymal infiltrates from brain tissue. Observed similar features of antigen experience in B cell clones. The relative clonal expansion of B cells in meningeal aggregates was 24% and in parenchymal infiltrates 28%. Mutation frequency in Immunoglobulin (Ig) variable region heavy chain (VH) sequences similar in both areas. ~90% IgG isotype and remainder IgM. This is in contrast to the IgG/IgM ratio of 15:85 expected in peripheral blood of healthy controls.	B cell aggregates identified in meninges.
Choi et al., 2012 [24]	PPMS n = 26 Controls n = 6 326 frozen blocks (50 fixed and 276 snap frozen) and 416 paraffin-embedded blocks from 26 PPMS cases 24 FFPE blocks from control cases were examined.	0 TLS	8/26 cases had substantial ('++') meningeal and perivascular immune cell aggregates. Meningeal inflammation was evident in this cohort of PPMS cases. A greater extent of meningeal inflammation was associated with greater neurite loss and more severe MS disease.	8 cases with substantial meningeal immune cell aggregates had evidence of $CD3^+$ T cells and $CD20^+$ B cells. Other defining features of TLS; $Ki67^+$ and $CD20^+$ double positive cells and $CD35^+$ cells were not observed in these aggregates.
Magliozzi et al., 2013 [45]	181 brain tissue blocks (cerebral cortex) from 44 SPMS cases - 26 Follicle positive (F+) - 18 Follicle negative (F-) 17 frozen tissue blocks from cerebral hemisphere of 11 follicle positive SPMS cases	F+ cases with infiltrated cortical lesions had $CD20^+$ B cells and Ig^+ plasmablasts/plasma cells. 11/26 subpial cortical lesions contained dense perivascular immune infiltrates. 0/18 F- cases contained infiltrated cortical lesions.	ISH for EBER demonstrated EBER positive cells in 3/3 intracortical perivascular infiltrates analysed. EBER positive cells also detected in adjacent inflamed meninges and in WMLs. EBER signals typically nuclear. Perivascular cells showing nuclear reactivity for BZLF1 (early EBV lytic stage) were detected in all infiltrated active cortical lesions (n = 4) but not in chronic active cortical lesion. BZLF1-positive cells were also detected in the meninges adjacent to the infiltrated cortical lesions. BFRF1 immunoreactivity was expressed in a substantial proportion of Ig^+ plasmablasts/plasma cells in the cortical perivascular cuffs, the adjacent meninges and in WMLs.	Follicle+ cases had a higher frequency of active WMLs and a higher frequency of active and chronic active cortical lesions. Perivascular immune infiltrates in cortex typically formed around small venules in layers II and III.

Table 1. *Cont.*

Study	Cases	TLS Identified	Findings	Location of TLS
Howell et al., 2015 [46]	SPMS n = 27 (Subset of cases previously characterised [23] with known TLS (n = 12) and TLS negative (n = 15) Non-neurological controls n = 11 Post-mortem FFPE	0 TLS in cerebellar blocks examined. One forebrain TLS+ case had evidence of substantial meningeal infiltration (+++) within the cerebellum however unable to further analyse due to loss of the area of interest in subsequent tissue sections.	This study investigated the extent of meningeal inflammation within the cerebellum of a previously characterised cohort of TLS+ and TLS- SPMS cases. Cases that were known to have TLS in the forebrain meninges had evidence of mild-moderate ('−' and '++') meningeal immune cell infiltrate within the cerebellum. Inflammation of the meninges was associated with more extensive cerebellar GM demyelination.	TLS not observed within this cohort of cerebellar tissue.
Serafini et al., 2016 [47]	SPMS n = 15 (29 cerebral tissue blocks examined) PFA-fixed frozen snap-frozen sections Controls: fixed-frozen and snap-frozen human adult lymph nodes (1 abdominal and 2 hilo-pulmonary lymph nodes) and 1 snap frozen tonsil	TLS n = 5	TLS contained $CD35^+$ stromal cells RORγt immunoreactivity was mainly nuclear and observed in 6 SPMS cases (5 TLS+ and 1 TLS-). This was almost exclusively localised to meninges. $ROR\gamma t^+$ cells found in the periphery of 12 out of 18 TLS, generally clustering in areas enriched with $CD3^+$ T cells.	Located in meninges.
Bevan et al., 2018 [33]	Short MS disease duration n = 12 Progressive MS n = 21 Non diseased controls n = 11 Other neurological inflammatory disease controls n = 6 Post-mortem FFPE	4 out of 12 cases in short disease duration cohort had evidence of TLS.	TLS+ cases had evidence of increased meningeal $CD68^+$ macrophages, $CD3^+$ T cells and $CD20^+$ B cells. TLS comprised $CD8^+$ cytotoxic T cells, B cells co-expressing PCNA and leukocytes expressing transcripts of CXCL13.	TLS were associated with subpial GML. TLS+ cases had extensive neurodegeneration and elevated parenchymal microglia/macrophage activation.
Hassani et al., 2018 [48]	MS n = 101 Non-MS control n = 21 Other neurological controls n = 9 Post-mortem FFPE	Minimal-moderate meningeal infiltration observed. Negligible lymphoid aggregates in examined sections.	This study investigated for the presence of EBV in MS brain tissue detecting EBV by PCR and EBER ISH. 47/101 cases were positive for EBV in meninges. EBER ISH showed EBV positive cells in 83/101 MS cases–80/101 EBV+ cells detected in brain parenchyma and 60/101 EBV+ cells detected in meninges. 5/21 non-MS neurological controls had evidence of EBV+ cells. Double staining IHC performed on 18 EBV heavily infected cases identified 11/18 and 7/18 cases were found to be double positive for EBV/GFAP and EBV/Iba-1 respectively.	
Bell et al., 2019 [49]	11 PPMS 22 SPMS 2 PD 13 healthy controls Post-mortem FFPE	11/22 SPMS cases TLS+ 0/11 PPMS cases had TLS	$CD20^+$ B cells, $CD35^+$ cells, $CD138^+$ plasma cells and CXCR5 expression on lymphocytes detected in TLS. Investigated for evidence of GC function; 4/38 TLS positive for Bcl-6 but all expressed CXCR5 (homing receptor for GCs) Investigated for evidence of regulatory T cells within TLS-FOXP3$^+$ cells not detected within follicles and almost completely absent in tissue section.	75% of chronic active lesion brain and 88% of chronic active lesion spinal cord cases had evidence of $CD3^+$ T cell and/or $CD20^+$ B cell infiltrates.

Table 1. *Cont.*

Study	Cases	TLS Identified	Findings	Location of TLS
Reali et al., 2020 [32]	22 SPMS 5 non neurological controls Spinal cord meninges from 11 TLS+ cerebral cases 11 TLS- cerebral cases Post-mortem fixed-frozen.	TLS were observed in 3/11 spinal cord meninges that had known cerebral TLS.	TLS comprised $CD20^+$ B cells, $CD35^+$ FDCs, $CD3^+$ T cells, $CD8^+$ T cells, $Ki67^+$ B cells and Ig^+ plasma cells. Cases that had TLS within spinal cord meninges had more $CD20^+$ B cells in comparison to TLS- cases (3-fold higher in number in the TLS+ SPMS cases). $CD4^+$ T cells were found to be more numerous within meninges, grey and white matter perivascular cuffs in TLS+ cases. There was a trend towards greater areas of demyelinated white and grey matter in TLS+ cases ($p = 0.052$). The density of meningeal B cells in TLS+ SPMS correlated with the extent of axon loss in the lateral corticospinal tract, dorsal column and combined spinal cord tracts axons.	Spinal cord meninges.

Abbreviations: MS, multiple sclerosis; SPMS, secondary progressive MS; PPMS, primary progressive MS; RRMS, relapsing–remitting MS; FFPE, formalin-fixed paraffin embedded; TLS, tertiary lymphoid structure; IHC, immunohistochemistry; EBV, Epstein–Barr virus; AID, activation-induced cytidine deaminase; WM, white matter; EBER, Epstein-Barr encoding region; EBNA, Epstein-Barr nuclear antigen; FDC, follicular dendritic cell; ISH, *in situ* hybridisation; LMP, latency membrane protein; rt-PCR, reverse transcription-polymerase chain reaction; CNS, central nervous system; RNA, ribonucleic acid; DNA, deoxyribonucleic acid; TB, tuberculosis; GC, germinal centre; qPCR, quantitative polymerase chain reaction; WML, white matter lesion; BAFF, B-cell activating factor; GML, grey matter lesion; GM, grey matter; PCNA, proliferating cell nuclear antigen; GFAP, glial fibrillary acidic protein.

In post-mortem MS studies, TLS were initially observed in SPMS cases [15]. More recently however TLS have also been identified in early MS [33,43]. It is difficult to ascertain the incidence of TLS in MS. TLS have been observed in up to 54% of post-mortem SPMS cases however these are selected cohorts [22]. The incidence of TLS in early MS cases is unknown and due to the rarity of short disease duration post-mortem MS cases, will be difficult to establish.

In MS it is often difficult to predict which patients will develop a more active or progressive disease course, particularly at early stages when patients are first facing treatment decisions. Furthermore, predicting patient response to DMTs is challenging. Whilst it is not feasible to study TLS in vivo in humans at this point, we can gain an understanding of TLS composition, formation and function from mouse models of MS and post-mortem studies. A better understanding of TLS in MS will be essential to inform studies investigating biomarkers and therapeutic targets in progressive MS and aggressive disease courses. Given that the meninges appear to be the primary site of TLS in MS it is important to gain an understanding of how immune cells traffic within the meninges and enter/exit to peripheral and CNS compartments.

2.1. The Meninges; Vascular Channels and Lymphatic Networks

The meninges consist of three layers; the dura, arachnoid and pia mater, that envelope the cortex. The subarachnoid space lies between the arachnoid and pial layers and contains cerebrospinal fluid (CSF). Produced by the choroid plexus, CSF circulates through the ventricular system and subarachnoid space and has important functions for mechanical protection of the CNS and cerebral autoregulation. The blood-CSF barrier also has an important role in the transport of immune cells and molecules, and is responsible for the removal of waste products from the CNS [50].

The CNS was once thought to be an immune-privileged site however, we now know that immune cells can traffic within the meninges and through the CSF, providing surveillance for foreign antigens. Indeed the meninges harbour a diverse range of immune cells with distinct populations between the brain parenchyma, lymphatic system and even between the different meningeal layers, providing an important interface between the periphery and CNS parenchyma [51–54]. The meninges can therefore serve as a site for coordinating adaptive immune responses and orchestrating homeostatic and neuroinflammatory responses [55].

The dura and leptomeninges (arachnoid and pia mater) comprise distinct vascular compartments. The dura mater consists of vast arterial, venous and capillary networks, which lack tight junctions and includes large venous sinuses (the sagittal and transverse sinuses), which drain blood from the cerebral veins into the systemic circulation [54]. The pial vascular network has connections into the CNS parenchyma. Unlike the dural vasculature, pial blood vessels have tight junctions, selectively transporting molecules and immune cells into and out of the CSF and parenchyma [54].

The CNS was generally described as devoid of lymphatic vessels however CNS lymphatics were described in the late 18th century [56]. There has been renewed interest in the CNS lymphatic network with several recent studies identifying meningeal lymphatic vessels within the dura [57,58]. This dural lymphatic network appears to be an important site for the movement of molecules, immune cells, interstitial fluid and CSF from the CNS to the periphery [57,59]. Evidence from experimental animal models suggest that the dural sinuses are a critical site for immune surveillance. In the healthy state, CNS antigens from the CSF have been found to gather in the dural sinuses where antigen presenting cells interact with circulating T cells [60]. Furthermore T cells appear to be able to traffic from the circulation into the meningeal lymphatic vessels and then drain into the deep cervical lymph nodes (cLN) [57,58,61].

Interestingly, in a mouse model of EAE, removing the deep cLNs was associated with a reduction in EAE severity [62]. In a recent study, again using a mouse model of EAE, meningeal T cells were observed to drain to deep cLNs in a CCR7-dependent manner [59]. Furthermore this study observed that when the meningeal lymphatic system was reduced, this resulted in a reduced inflammatory response and less severe pathology [59]. These studies suggest that CNS draining lymph nodes could be a site for antigen presentation and lymphocyte activation and that the meninges are an important site for this inflammatory process.

In a study investigating immune cell trafficking into the CNS, a mouse model was used to label bone marrow-derived cells (neutrophils) in the skull and tibia [63]. This study identified distinct vascular channels within the skull bone and found these to be directly connected to the vasculature of the dura mater [63]. Furthermore, when CNS inflammation was induced in a mouse model of ischaemic stroke and aseptic meningoencephalitis, neutrophils originating from the skull bone marrow, migrated to the inflamed sites and were far more numerous than neutrophils originating from the tibial bone marrow in both these mouse models. Interestingly the authors also imaged portions of skull bones from 3 patients that underwent craniectomy and identified similar channels within the inner skull cortex connecting to marrow cavities [63].

By characterising the phenotype of meningeal B cells in young and aged mice, single cell RNA sequencing (scRNA-seq) and B cell receptor sequencing (BCR-seq) data identified that a large proportion of dural B cells were in early stages of B cell development [64]. This was in contrast to blood, where very few early B cell markers were identified making it unlikely that dural B cells were derived from the systemic circulation [64]. The authors of this study also found evidence of vascular channels within the skull and using a CD19 reporter mouse, identified that IgM^- B cells migrated through these vascular channels from the skull bone marrow to the meninges [64].

These studies challenge previously accepted concepts about immune cell migration in the CNS and suggest that perhaps cellular migration and recruitment to inflamed sites, is occurring independent of the systemic circulation. Understanding the meningeal vascular and lymphatic networks and their connections to the periphery will likely give us important clues about immune cell trafficking and potential sites of CNS antigen presentation to T cells. However, our understanding of immune processes in these networks is limited in MS and further studies will be required if we are to understand this important aspect of immunoreactivity in diseased states.

Understanding how cells and molecules traffic to and from the meningeal compartment will be important for our ability to detect and monitor the meningeal inflammatory microenvironment in MS. Increasing our knowledge of the vascular and lymphatic networks connecting through the meninges and CNS parenchyma and how these relate to, or reflect, the peripheral lymphatics and vasculature, will be important in our search for serum or CSF biomarkers for disease prognostication.

2.2. Composition of Tertiary Lymphoid Structures

Most of our initial understanding of the composition, formation and functional mechanisms of TLS arose from studies investigating SLOs [18–20,65–67]. Tertiary lymphoid structures are often defined by features of SLOs [18]. Secondary lymphoid organs consist of distinct B and T cell zones, germinal centres (GCs), follicular dendritic cells (FDCs), reticular networks comprising fibroblastic reticular cells (FRCs) and high endothelial venules (HEVs).

The composition of TLS in other immune-mediated diseases and cancers often show similarities to that of SLOs [18,65]. In contrast, the composition of cellular clusters in MS can range from aggregates of B cells, aggregates of B and T cells, to more organised structures reflective of SLOs (Figure 1). The more organised structures are often defined as TLS in MS if there is evidence of B cells, T cells, FDCs and cell proliferation within the cluster [23]. However, post-mortem studies have shown heterogeneity of cellular organisation within TLS in MS and this heterogeneity has also been demonstrated in several mouse models of EAE [15,21,28].

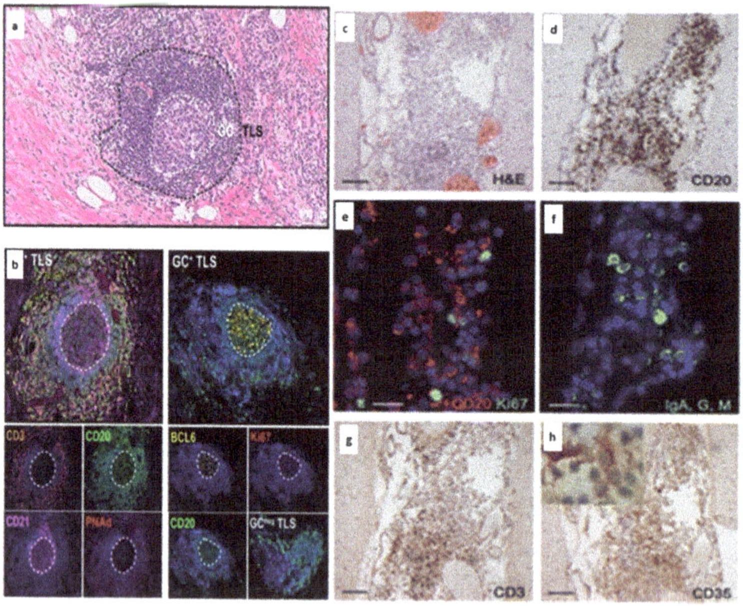

Figure 1. Tertiary lymphoid structures in cancer and multiple sclerosis [23,68]. Tertiary lymphoid structures (TLS) in pancreatic cancer demonstrate features reminiscent of secondary lymphoid organs with evidence of germinal centres (**a**), distinct B and T cell zones and PNAd^{+} high endothelial venules (**b**). BCL6^{+} cells indicate germinal centre reactions and cells undergoing proliferation (Ki67^{+}) are concentrated in the germinal centre (**b**). In comparison, meningeal TLS in MS typically demonstrate a loose aggregate of CD20^{+} B cells (**d**) interspersed with proliferating (CD20^{+}Ki67^{+}) B cells (**e**), immunoglobulin A, G, M^{+} plasma cells/plasmablasts (**f**), CD3^{+} T cells (**g**) and CD35^{+} follicular dendritic cells (**h**). Permissions: (**a**,**b**) Gunderson AJ et al. (2021) Germinal center reactions in tertiary lymphoid structures associate with neoantigen burden, humoral immunity and long-term survivorship in pancreatic cancer, OncoImmunology, 10:1, DOI: 10.1080/2162402X.2021.1900635 by permission of Taylor & Francis Ltd. www.tandfonline.com. Accessed on 18 July 2022. (**c**–**h**) Howell OW et al. Meningeal inflammation is widespread and linked to cortical pathology in multiple sclerosis. Brain 2011 134; 2755–2771 by permission of Oxford University Press. Accessed on 5 July 2022.

In EAE, with disease progression into chronic stages, B cell aggregates show evidence of developing into more organised structures reminiscent of SLOs [30]. In post-mortem SPMS studies TLS can contain CD3^{+} T cells, CD20^{+} B cells, CD138^{+} plasma cells and CD68^{+} macrophages within the meninges [25]. Follicular dendritic cells play an important role in the cellular organisation and B cell recruitment into TLS. The prominent B cell chemoattractant CXCL13 is produced by FDCs and binds to the CXCR5 receptor expressed on a subset of T helper cells [69–71]. In post-mortem SPMS cases, FDCs expressing CXCL13 within TLS have been observed [25].

B cell activating factor (BAFF), a member of the TNF family, also has a critical role in B cell development, proliferation and survival [72,73]. In SJL mice, levels of CXCL13 and BAFF mRNA expression were elevated in relapsing–remitting and chronic-relapsing EAE [21]. This was accompanied by the formation of organised lymphoid structures within the meninges, some of which contained CD35^{+} and M1-expressing FDCs [21]. In further studies using SJL mice and MBP-PLP fusion protein (MP4)-induced EAE, FDCs have also been observed and appear to co-localise with B cell aggregates [28,30]. In human MS studies BAFF mRNA levels in monocytes and BAFF receptor mRNA levels in B and T cells have been found to be increased in comparison to healthy controls [74]. An upregulation of BAFF expression in both acute and chronic MS lesions has also been observed in a post-mortem study [75]. In this study, BAFF expression co-localised with astrocytes suggesting they were the pre-dominant cell type producing BAFF and highlights the key role of resident cells in coordinating recruitment and retention of lymphocytes to the CSF-filled spaces.

Another feature of SLOs are reticular fibres which provide a structural collagen support network to trap and traffic lymphocytes [65]. In two studies using SJL mice immunised with $PLP_{139\text{-}151}$, FRCs and the formation of reticular networks within the meninges was observed [21,31]. Reticular networks have also been observed in TLS in other mouse models of EAE, sometimes encapsulating the entire immune cell aggregate [29,30]. These reticular networks are not always observed or as well formed in TLS in post-mortem cases [25].

To facilitate the trafficking of lymphocytes, SLOs develop HEVs. These vascular networks are not a frequent finding within TLS observed in EAE. In a mouse model of MP4-induced EAE, HEVs have been observed however this is not a consistent finding in other mouse models [29,30]. In a cohort of post-mortem SPMS cases, HEVs were not observed within TLS [25]. Perhaps the good vascular networks that exist within the meningeal compartment or differing adhesion molecules expressed on meningeal blood vessels may explain this lack of HEVs.

Another important feature of SLOs is the presence of GCs. Within SLOs, GCs are the sites in which B cells undergo somatic hypermutation and clonal expansion to produce memory B cells and plasma cells [18]. In other immune-mediated conditions, GCs have been observed within TLS and appear to maintain the autoimmune response [76,77]. Both in mouse models of EAE and post-mortem MS cases, proliferating B cells and plasma cells have been observed, suggesting the presence of GCs [21,25,29]. Whilst there is evidence of some germinal centre features within TLS in post-mortem MS cases, this is not a conclusive finding across all observed TLS [25].

2.3. What Drives the Formation of Tertiary Lymphoid Structures?

The formation of TLS appears to share similarities to that of SLOs [65,78–80]. SLO development involves members of the TNF-lymphotoxin (LT) family [17,65]. Interactions between $CD45^+CD4^+CD3^-$ lymphoid-tissue initiator (LTi) cells-a group 3 innate lymphoid cell (ILC) population, and tissue resident stromal organiser cells results in the production of cytokines and chemokines involved in B and T cell recruitment [16,17,65,79,80]. The LT heterotrimeric complex, $LT\alpha_1\beta_2$, is expressed on the surface of embryonic LTi cells, B cells, natural killer cells and activated T cells. $LT\alpha_1\beta_2$ binds to the $LT\beta$ receptor ($LT\beta R$) which is expressed on stromal cells, dendritic cells and macrophages. This binding induces the expression of chemokines such as CCL19, CCL21 and CXCL13, which recruit and organise T and B cells within TLS [65,80,81]. The interaction between LTi cells and stromal organiser cells also promotes the development of HEVs, which facilitate lymphocyte trafficking in SLOs [17,79,81].

The initiating cell(s) and signalling pathways for TLS development in MS are unclear. Mouse models investigating the formation of TLS in EAE indicate that Th17 cells may play a significant role in the initiation of TLS. Following the adoptive transfer of Th17 cells into C57BL/6 mice, TLS formation was observed in 16 of 22 recipients during EAE [29]. In contrast, TLS formation was not observed following the adoptive transfer of Th2 and Th9 cells, and in only one of seven Th1 cell-recipient mice, despite development of disease in the majority of cases. This suggests Th17 cells are playing a pivotal role in TLS formation. Further evidence that Th17 cells have an initiating role in TLS development was demonstrated in a MP4-induced EAE mouse model [82]. In this mouse model, B cell aggregate formation is observed. The study found that there was an absence of $CD3^-CD5^-CD4^+ROR\gamma t^+$ LTi cells however $CD3^+CD5^+CD4^+ROR\gamma t^+$ Th17 cells were observed in the cerebellum of mice with EAE. Th17 cells were observed at peak of disease and again during the chronic stages but this time at higher frequencies. Th17 cells were also observed in close association with

TLS formation in another study using a MP4-induced EAE mouse model, although the functional role of Th17 cells was not investigated in this study [30].

In a study of post-mortem tissue from SPMS patients, there was also a suggestion that Th17 cells and group 3 ILCs play a role in TLS formation [47]. The authors identified retinoic acid receptor-related orphan receptor-γt (RORγt)$^+$ cells within, or in close proximity to, the majority of identified B-cell aggregates. Most of the RORγt$^+$ cells co-expressed CD3 and a minority were CD3 negative, suggesting these cells could represent Th17 cells and group 3 ILCs respectively.

Similarities exist between Th17 and LTi cells. Both cells express RORγt and $LT\alpha_1\beta_2$ and produce IL-17 and IL-22 [83,84]. For the initiation of TLS in MS, Th17 cells may adopt a similar role to that of the LTi cell in SLO formation. IL-27, which inhibits Th17 cells and EAE [85–88], has also been shown to inhibit TLS formation in a mouse model of inflammatory arthritis [89]. It would be interesting to determine whether a similar inhibitory effect of IL-27 on TLS development would be observed in a mouse model of EAE harbouring TLS.

The LT signalling pathway also appears to be implicated in TLS formation in EAE. The SJL-proteolipid protein$_{139\text{-}151}$ (PLP$_{139\text{-}151}$)-immunised mouse model develops a relapsing–remitting clinical disease course somewhat similar to RRMS. A study using this model demonstrated an upregulation of LTβ and LTβR gene expression in the CNS at EAE onset and during subsequent relapses [28]. In addition, the authors found that blocking of the LTβR resulted in a reduced inflammatory infiltrate, reduced B cell aggregation within the meninges and TLS were not observed in those cases. Further evidence that LTβR signalling supports the accumulation of B cells within TLS was demonstrated in another EAE study using SJL mice [31]. Furthermore, the authors reported that following the adoptive transfer of Th17 cells, LTβ expression was required to propagate inflammation and disease.

Germinal centre-derived memory B cells are the primary site of latent Epstein–Barr virus (EBV) infection [90,91]. There is evidence that TLS in MS can be a reservoir of latent EBV with some studies showing that meningeal B cell follicles can harbour latent EBV transcripts (EBV-encoded small nuclear mRNA) and EBV latent membrane protein LMP-2A [36,42]. The persistence of latent EBV in meningeal B cells could be a factor in the propagation and expansion of TLS in MS. This is interesting particularly given the recent study from Bjornevik et al. demonstrating EBV as a clear risk factor for the development of MS, with a 32-fold increase in MS risk following EBV seroconversion [92].

The factors required for TLS formation and ongoing maintenance are complex and likely involve multiple cell signalling pathways. Investigating mechanisms of TLS formation in human MS tissue is challenging, however if we can gain a better understanding of TLS cellular composition, particularly during different disease phases, we may gain better insights of potential immune signals required for TLS development and maintenance.

2.4. *Potential Function of Tertiary Lymphoid Structures*

2.4.1. Could TLS Be a Site for B Cell Maturation and Immunoglobulin Synthesis?

The presence of oligoclonal bands (OCBs) in CSF is a common feature in MS, being present in over 95% of cases [93]. The detection of OCBs is included as part of the diagnostic criteria for MS [94]. Alongside the presence of OCBs, the findings of somatically hypermutated and clonally expanded B cells in the CSF of MS patients suggest there is an antigen-driven immune component to disease pathogenesis [95–99]. Whether these B cells undergo expansion and maturation within the meningeal compartment or are recruited into the CNS from the periphery, or potentially both, is unclear.

Germinal centres within SLOs such as the spleen and lymph nodes, are sites of B cell maturation and production of antibody-secreting plasma cells in the periphery. In response to the presentation of antigen, B cells within the GC proliferate, initially within the dark zone where they undergo somatic hypermutation. GC B cells differentiate into centroblasts and centroctyes. Proliferating centroblasts are involved in immunoglobulin class switching and during this process express activation-induced cytidine deaminase

(AICD). This leads to affinity maturation and the differentiation of GC B cells into memory B cells and long-lived plasma cells [100–102].

In autoimmune diseases such as Sjogren's syndrome (SS), rheumatoid arthritis, Hashiomoto's thyroiditis (HT) and Graves' disease (GD), TLS exhibiting GCs are thought to contribute to the production of autoantibodies. Tertiary lymphoid structures demonstrating cardinal features of GCs with distinct dark and light zones, HEVs, dendritic cells and mantle zones have been identified in thyroid glands of patients with HT and GD [77]. Higher levels of serum autoantibodies, anti-thyroperoxidase (TPO) in HT and anti-thyroid stimulating hormone receptor (TSH-R) in GD are associated with patients who have TLS. Similarly in SS, patients who have TLS in salivary glands (the affected organ in SS) have been found to have significantly higher levels of anti-Ro and anti-La autoantibodies [103]. This suggests that GCs within TLS are playing a role in the production of pathogenic autoantibodies. Further evidence of GC function is the identification of populations of clonally expanded B cells and hypermutation of the immunoglobulin V genes in salivary glands in SS [104] and the expression of AICD in TLS found in synovial fluid of rheumatoid arthritis patients [105] indicating somatic hypermutation of Ig genes is occurring. Plasma cells producing the pathogenic antibody anti-citrullinated protein (ACPA) have been identified in close proximity to TLS in RA further implicating TLS GCs as a source of autoantigen [105].

Could meningeal TLS in MS therefore serve as a site for the production of clonally expanded B cells and IgG synthesis? In the CSF of MS patients, immunoglobulins are often class-switched and have signs of affinity maturation which would suggest that GC reactions are occurring within the CNS compartment [95,98,106]. In some post-mortem SPMS cases, TLS have demonstrated features of GCs comprising FDCs, proliferating B cells and plasma cells [25] however it is unclear whether these TLS demonstrate all typical features of GCs including the distinct dark and light zones and further studies investigating this are needed. In the post-mortem MS TLS studies reviewed here (Table 1), the presence of CSF OCBs was not available in the included data. Given CSF OCBs are detected in >90% of MS patients, it is unlikely that OCB production is dependent on TLS however there could be a distinct pattern of OCB antibodies in TLS+ cases which may provide important clues on disease pathogenesis.

Investigating the functional role of TLS in MS is difficult in humans. Animal models of MS may help us to address key mechanistic questions of GC formation and function. In some mouse models of MS, lymphoid aggregates with evidence of GCs have been identified. The proliferation marker Ki67, $CD138^+$ plasma cells and AICD have been observed in TLS in MP4-induced EAE [30]. One study did not observe GC-like reactions in early EAE although difficulty with CD138 staining may have led to an underestimation [27]. More recently, in a MOG-induced EAE rat model, lymphoid structures closely resembling SLOs with distinct T and B cell zones and HEVs were observed in the meninges [107]. These animal models may help advance our understanding of how TLS form, are maintained, their functional role(s) and how they are potentially affected by treatments. However, it is important to note the limitations of EAE models. The most commonly used model of MOG_{35-55}-induced EAE usually features acute onset of ascending clinical signs from tail tip to limbs caused by a high number of concurrent, rapidly developing spinal cord, optic nerve and brain lesions. There is little clinical recovery in this model with persistent neurological impairment from the initial acute events. It is also important to note that EAE studies routinely use female, young adult rodents with limited follow-up time relative to the life-long nature of MS after diagnosis which affects both sexes. Thus, notwithstanding the considerably usefulness of EAE model in the development of current DMTs for MS, the models fall short of representing the full spectrum of neuropathological processes in MS.

Whether meningeal TLS are the sites GC reactions and production of antibody secreting plasma cells in MS remains to be determined. It will also be important to establish if GCs can form within TLS in early disease stages or if are they restricted to TLS in a more chronic inflammatory environment. The lack of capacity to detect or study TLS in living patients is a key limitation in understanding the pathological importance of these structures and developing an approach to tackle this limitation would be a major advance for both clinical and research purposes.

2.4.2. Could TLS Propagate Subpial Neuroinflammation and Contribute to Progression in MS?

Evidence from post-mortem studies demonstrates that cases with TLS had a more severe MS disease course, entering progressive stages sooner and acquiring disability at faster rates [25,28,32]. A hallmark of the progressive stage of MS is the accumulating neurodegeneration and cortical demyelinating pathology, which is related to the extent of overlying inflammation nested in the meninges [22,23,108]. Inflammatory cortical demyelination is also observed in early MS and correlates with a worse disease outcome [43].

We also know from post-mortem studies, that cases with TLS have a greater degree of inflammatory infiltrate within the meninges, which correlates with a larger number and area of cortical demyelinating lesions [15,24,25,25]. TLS are often, but not always, found overlying subpial cortical lesions and there is a relative grade of inflammation extending from the subpial surface to the subcortical white matter, suggesting TLS are involved in the propagation of neuroinflammation [15].

In post-mortem MS tissue, higher degrees of meningeal inflammation are also associated with increased gene and protein expression of TNF-α and interferon (IFN)-γ. These expression levels are further increased in cases that have TLS [109]. Furthermore in post-mortem TLS cases there is upregulation of TNF receptor 1 (TNFR1) and genes involved in the TNF/TNFR1 necroptotic signalling pathway and downregulation of caspase-8 dependent apoptosis [110,111]. These studies indicate that TNF signalling is being directed towards TNFR1 necroptotic cell death and that this is potentially being influenced by cytokine release from meningeal inflammatory cells. In a rat model of chronic meningeal inflammation, introduction of TNF-α and IFN-γ into the CSF resulted in meningeal inflammation and cortical neurodegeneration, increased neuronal expression of TNFR1 and activation of necroptotic signalling pathways [111,112]. This demonstrates that in this animal model, meningeal inflammation and a cytotoxic milieu can lead directly to subpial demyelination and substantial neurodegeneration in a pattern similar to that observed in progressive MS.

2.4.3. Identifying which Patients Have Higher Degrees of Meningeal Inflammation and a High Likelihood of TLS

Identifying which patients have higher degrees of meningeal inflammation and TLS could help predict disease course, inform therapeutic strategies and assess response to DMTs. The difficulty is how we identify such patients. Given the close proximity of the pial meningeal layer to the subarachnoid space, investigating CSF immune profiles could provide important clues for the meningeal inflammatory microenvironment.

Indeed, there does appear to be distinct CSF profiles in MS cases. In a study seeking to identify CSF biomarkers of intrathecal inflammation, CSF profiles of MS, other inflammatory neurological disease (OIND) and non-inflammatory neurological disease (NIND) were investigated [113]. Raised CSF levels of IL-8 and IL-12p40 were found to distinguish MS cases from the OIND group, furthermore CSF IL-12p40 levels were distinct between the PPMS and RRMS groups. This study highlighted that distinct CSF profiles exist between neurological inflammatory diseases and between different subtypes of MS. An investigation of CSF profiles in post-mortem MS cases with known TLS, reported an increased expression of inflammatory cytokines such as IFN-γ and TNF-α and chemokines/cytokines related to lymphoid neogenesis, such as CXCL13, CXCL10, IL-6 and IL-10 [114]. In a clinical study investigating CSF profiles and magnetic resonance imaging (MRI) in a cohort of treatment-naïve RRMS patients, after a four year follow up period it was found that patients who experienced evidence of disease activity had higher CSF levels of CXCL13, CXCL12, IFN-γ, TNF, sCD163, LIGHT and APRIL at time of diagnosis [115]. Furthermore, there was a strong correlation between CXCL13 CSF levels and the development of new cortical lesions on MRI, indicating that CSF profiles could be useful to distinguish patients at greater risk of cortical lesion accumulation. The immune signatures of TLS and inflammatory profiles in CSF could therefore potentially predict more progressive and severe forms of MS if found at elevated levels in early disease.

MRI is the gold standard imaging technique to aid diagnosis in MS and specific radiological criteria are included in the McDonald 2017 diagnostic criteria [68,94]. The detection and monitoring of white matter brain and spinal cord MS lesions with MRI can inform treatments decisions and help assess response to DMTs [116]. It is difficult to detect grey matter lesions (GMLs) using conventional MRI techniques routinely available in the clinic. Given the association between extent of grey matter demyelination and progression in MS and the findings of TLS overlying subpial GM, the ability to detect GMLs on MRI could help stratify patients and monitor progressive phases of MS non-invasively.

In recent years, advances in MRI techniques and ultra high field 7 T MRI has improved our ability to detect GMLs and in particular subpial demyelination [117–122]. Several MRI studies have investigated the presence of leptomeningeal contrast enhancement (LMCE) as a potential marker for leptomeningeal inflammation in MS. On 3 T and 7 T MRI, LMCE has been identified in cohorts of RRMS, SPMS and PPMS cases and appears to correlate with subpial demyelination and overlying areas of meningeal inflammatory cells [123–126] but not TLS per se. The highest prevalence of LMCE appears to be in progressive MS were it has been detected in 33–85.7% of cases on 3 T MRI [123,126]. In their study using 3 T MRI, Zivadinov et al. reported a persistence of LMCE in 50% of cases (after a 5 year follow up period) and multiple LMCE foci were more likely to be observed in SPMS [126]. However, findings from a 7 T MRI study suggested a different prevalence and persistence pattern of LMCE with no difference observed between RRMS and progressive MS groups and LMCE persisted in ~70–85% of patients after 2 years [127], although a shorter follow up period and using more sensitive MRI may account for these differences. The presence of LMCE is associated with increased GM volume loss, a faster rate of GM atrophy, longer disease duration and increased disability in MS [123–126]. Some studies suggest that LMCE is not affected by the use of DMTs [123,126–129]. In two studies using anti-CD20 therapies, the administration of intrathecal rituximab and intravenous ocrelizumab did not reduce the appearance of LMCE [130,131]. In summary, these studies suggest that LMCE may reflect inflammation and disturbance to the blood-CSF barriers within the meningeal compartment, particularly in progressive cases where chronic inflammation tends to persist within the leptomeninges and MRI could be used to monitor treatment response or lack of.

However, caution does still need to be applied in the interpretation of LMCE as this can be seen in other neuroinflammatory, infective and neoplastic conditions [93]. A further caveat is that most neurology clinics only have access to 1.5 T or 3 T MRI scanners where the detection of LMCE is difficult. At present the utility of 7 T MRI is largely confined to research. The increasing use of advanced MRI techniques within clinical trial settings however will hopefully further expand our ability to detect radiological features of GMLs and LMCE and eventually pave a way for routine clinical use. Alongside CSF analysis, the use of MRI will be vital to help better predict which patients are more likely to enter progressive disease stages and assess treatment response.

3. Therapeutic Strategies Targeting Meningeal Inflammation and TLS

Alongside observational studies, evidence from clinical trials has shown that anti-CD20, B cell depleting therapies, reduce relapse rates in patients with RRMS and slow disease progression in PPMS and SPMS [132–135]. Given that B cells are a predominant cell type within TLS and that TLS associate with more severe and progressive forms of MS, could targeting these structures with B cell therapies, slow or halt progression?

In a mouse model of EAE that develops immune cell aggregates reminiscent of TLS, anti-CD20 treatment was administered prior to EAE onset and after EAE onset to investigate whether anti-CD20 treatment could prevent formation of TLS or change the disease course. Treatment with anti-CD20 resulted in depletion of B cells within the peripheral blood and lymph nodes, however meningeal lymphoid structures still developed. Furthermore, the authors observed that administering anti-CD20 treatment after EAE onset did not affect the clinical course of spontaneous chronic EAE. Anti-CD20 treatment however did influence B cell composition of TLS, with reduced numbers of B220^{+} B cells and increased numbers of MPO^{+} neutrophils [136].

Similarly in the opticospinal encephalomyelitis (OSE) mouse, anti-CD20 treatment administered after disease onset depleted B cells peripherally, however B cell aggregates were still observed in spinal cord meninges, and no effect was observed on disease progression [137]. The effects of anti-CD19 CAR-T cell administration was investigated and it was found that whilst there was reduction in TLS formation, paradoxically, the progressive disease course was exacerbated. These studies suggest that depleting peripheral B cell populations alone will be insufficient to reduce or stop TLS formation and may not alter the progressive disease course. These studies highlight our lack of understanding of TLS and the need for caution when directly or indirectly targeting these structures with therapeutic interventions.

Interestingly the DMT siponimod, which is licenced for SPMS, was found to reduce the formation of meningeal lymphoid structures in a mouse model of EAE [138]. It was observed that when siponimod was administered prior to EAE onset, formation of TLS was reduced. Similarly, when siponimod was administered at peak of disease, there was a reduction in TLS in comparison to the vehicle treated control mice. Siponimod is a sphingosine 1-phosphate receptor (S1PR) 1,5 modulator which traps B and T lymphocytes within lymph nodes, thus reducing both B and T cells in the peripheral circulation. Siponimod is also known to cross the BBB and therefore may also have a direct effect on meningeal inflammation [139]. Future post-mortem studies of tissue from individuals that have been treated with siponimod and B cell-depleting DMTs may provide insight to the effect of these interventions on either the development, or the persistence, of these structures in the CNS.

Another interesting therapeutic target is Bruton's tyrosine kinase (BTK). BTK is an enzyme of the B cell receptor signalling pathway, which if inhibited, reduces B cell proliferation [140]. Multiple BTK inhibitors have been developed and are currently in clinical use for a number of immune-mediated and lymphoproliferative disorders [141]. In vivo studies suggest BTK inhibitors reduce meningeal inflammation. In a mouse model which demonstrates meningeal inflammation, MRI with post-contrast imaging observed that treatment with the BTK inhibitor evobrutinib, reduced meningeal contrast enhancement in comparison to controls [142]. In RRMS patients, a placebo-controlled phase 2 trial of evobrutinib demonstrated that patients receiving evobrutinib had fewer enhancing lesions on MRI [143]. Whilst no significant difference was observed in annualised relapse rate (ARR) or expanded disability status scale (EDSS), there was a relatively short follow-up period. BTK inhibitors therefore could have therapeutic potential in progressive MS, potentially via targeting B cells outside and as well as within the CNS, and further clinical trial data are eagerly awaited.

4. Conclusions

There is clear evidence that patients who have TLS have a more severe MS disease course, however our understanding of the functional role of TLS and the reason for the heterogeneity observed in meningeal inflammation is lacking. Given the heterogeneity of TLS in MS, future research should investigate the cellular composition of TLS, exploring B and T cell subset analysis in the different disease stages. Increasing our understanding of the composition of TLS and determining if there are distinctions in the immune profiles of TLS in different disease stages, may provide further insights into how these structures develop, how they could be contributing towards chronic inflammation in MS and how they could be targeted therapeutically. Investigating a post-mortem cohort treated with MS DMTs, with different mechanisms of actions, such as natalizumab (selective binding of $\alpha_4\beta_1$-integrin), ocrelizumab, ofatumumab and rituximab (anti-CD20 monoclonal antibodies), fingolimod and siponimod could also reveal further insights into TLS formation and potential alterations that may occur to TLS structures following treatment.

Whilst our knowledge of inflammation within the meningeal compartment and TLS in MS has increased dramatically over the past two decades, it is important to continue advancing our knowledge of TLS and the contribution TLS have on progressive pathogenic mechanisms. If we can better understand TLS immune signatures and bioactivity, we can inform future studies searching for prognostic markers and the development of therapeutic targets that will slow or halt progression in MS.

Author Contributions: Conceptualization, R.K., M.N., O.W.H. and D.C.F.; writing—original draft preparation, R.K. and O.W.H.; writing—review and editing, R.K., M.N., G.V.M., O.W.H. and D.C.F.; supervision, D.C.F. All authors have read and agreed to the published version of the manuscript.

Funding: This work was supported by HSC R&D Division, Public Health Agency [EAT/5496/18] (to R.K.) and Wellcome Trust Grant [110138/Z/15/Z] (to D.C.F.).

Institutional Review Board Statement: Not applicable.

Informed Consent Statement: Not applicable.

Data Availability Statement: Not applicable.

Conflicts of Interest: D.C.F. has received collaborative research funding from, and served as a consultant for, Sangamo Inc. The other authors declare no conflict of interest. The funders had no role in the design of the study; in the collection, analyses, or interpretation of data; in the writing of the manuscript, or in the decision to publish the results.

References

1. Reich, D.S.; Lucchinetti, C.F.; Calabresi, P.A. Multiple sclerosis. *N. Engl. J. Med.* **2018**, *378*, 169–180. [CrossRef]
2. Koch, M.; Kingwell, E.; Rieckmann, P.; Tremlett, H.; Adams, D.; Craig, D.; Daly, L.; Devonshire, V.; Hashimoto, S.; Hrebicek, O.; et al. The natural history of secondary progressive multiple sclerosis. *J. Neurol. Neurosurg. Psychiatry* **2010**, *81*, 1039–1043. [CrossRef]
3. Debouverie, M.; Pittion-Vouyovitch, S.; Louis, S.; Guillemin, F. Natural history of multiple sclerosis in a population-based cohort. *Eur. J. Neurol.* **2008**, *15*, 916–921. [CrossRef]
4. Confavreux, C.; Vukusic, S.; Moreau, T.; Adeleine, P. Relapses and progression of disability in multiple sclerosis. *N. Engl. J. Med.* **2000**, *343*, 1430–1438. [CrossRef]
5. Koch-Henriksen, N.; Thygesen, L.C.; Stenager, E.; Laursen, B.; Magyari, M. Incidence of MS has increased markedly over six decades in Denmark particularly with late onset and in women. *Neurology* **2018**, *90*, e1954–e1963. [CrossRef]
6. Wallin, M.T.; Culpepper, W.J.; Nichols, E.; Bhutta, Z.A.; Gebrehiwot, T.T.; Hay, S.I.; Khalil, I.A.; Krohn, K.J.; Liang, X.; Naghavi, M.; et al. Global, regional, and national burden of multiple sclerosis 1990–2016: A systematic analysis for the Global Burden of Disease Study 2016. *Lancet Neurol.* **2019**, *18*, 269–285. [CrossRef]
7. Castelo-Branco, A.; Landfeldt, E.; Svedbom, A.; Löfroth, E.; Kavaliunas, A.; Hillert, J. Clinical course of multiple sclerosis and labour-force absenteeism: A longitudinal population-based study. *Eur. J. Neurol.* **2019**, *26*, 603–609. [CrossRef]
8. Feinstein, A.; Freeman, J.; Lo, A.C. Treatment of progressive multiple sclerosis: What works, what does not, and what is needed. *Lancet Neurol.* **2015**, *14*, 194–207. [CrossRef]
9. Guseo, A.; Jellinger, K. The significance of perivascular infiltrations in multiple sclerosis. *J. Neurol.* **1975**, *211*, 51–60. [CrossRef] [PubMed]
10. Prineas, J.W. Multiple sclerosis: Presence of lymphatic capillaries and lymphoid tissue in the brain and spinal cord. *Science* **1979**, *203*, 1123–1125. [CrossRef]
11. Raine, C.S.; Mokhtarian, F.; McFarlin, D.E. Adoptively transferred chronic relapsing experimental autoimmune encephalomyelitis in the mouse. Neuropathologic analysis. *Lab. Investig.* **1984**, *51*, 534–546.
12. Kirk, J.; Plumb, J.; Mirakhur, M.; McQuaid, S. Tight junctional abnormality in multiple sclerosis white matter affects all calibres of vessel and is associated with blood-brain barrier leakage and active demyelination. *J. Pathol.* **2003**, *201*, 319–327. [CrossRef]
13. Frischer, J.M.; Weigand, S.D.; Guo, Y.; Kale, N.; Parisi, J.E.; Pirko, I.; Mandrekar, J.; Bramow, S.; Metz, I.; Brück, W.; et al. Clinical and pathological insights into the dynamic nature of the white matter multiple sclerosis plaque. *Ann. Neurol.* **2015**, *78*, 710–721. [CrossRef]
14. Hochmeister, S.; Grundtner, R.; Bauer, J.; Engelhardt, B.; Lyck, R.; Gordon, G.; Korosec, T.; Kutzelnigg, A.; Berger, J.J.; Bradl, M.; et al. Dysferlin is a new marker for leaky brain blood vessels in multiple sclerosis. *J. Neuropathol. Exp. Neurol.* **2006**, *65*, 855–865. [CrossRef]

15. Magliozzi, R.; Howell, O.; Vora, A.; Serafini, B.; Nicholas, R.; Puopolo, M.; Reynolds, R.; Aloisi, F. Meningeal B-cell follicles in secondary progressive multiple sclerosis associate with early onset of disease and severe cortical pathology. *Brain* **2007**, *130*, 1089–1104. [CrossRef]
16. Van de Pavert, S.A.; Mebius, R.E. New insights into the development of lymphoid tissues. *Nat. Rev. Immunol.* **2010**, *10*, 664–674. [CrossRef]
17. Drayton, D.L.; Liao, S.; Mounzer, R.H.; Ruddle, N.H. Lymphoid organ development: From ontogeny to neogenesis. *Nat. Immunol.* **2006**, *7*, 344–353. [CrossRef]
18. Pitzalis, C.; Jones, G.W.; Bombardieri, M.; Jones, S.A. Ectopic lymphoid-like structures in infection, cancer and autoimmunity. *Nat. Rev. Immunol.* **2014**, *14*, 447–462. [CrossRef]
19. Mitsdoerffer, M.; Peters, A. Tertiary Lymphoid Organs in Central Nervous System Autoimmunity. *Front. Immunol.* **2016**, *7*, 451. [CrossRef]
20. Pikor, N.B.; Prat, A.; Bar-Or, A.; Gommerman, J.L.; Reynolds, R. Meningeal Tertiary Lymphoid Tissues and Multiple Sclerosis: A Gathering Place for Diverse Types of Immune Cells during CNS Autoimmunity. *Front. Immunol.* **2016**, *6*, 657. [CrossRef]
21. Magliozzi, R.; Columba-Cabezas, S.; Serafini, B.A.F.; Magliozzi, R.; Columba-Cabezas, S.; Serafini, B.; Aloisi, F. Intracerebral expression of CXCL13 and BAFF is accompanied by formation of lymphoid follicle-like structures in the meninges of mice with relapsing experimental autoimmune encephalomyelitis. *J. Neuroimmunol.* **2004**, *148*, 11–23. [CrossRef]
22. Magliozzi, R.; Howell, O.W.; Reeves, C.; Roncaroli, F.; Nicholas, R.; Serafini, B.; Aloisi, F.; Reynolds, R. A Gradient of neuronal loss and meningeal inflammation in multiple sclerosis. *Ann. Neurol.* **2010**, *68*, 477–493. [CrossRef]
23. Howell, O.W.; Reeves, C.A.; Nicholas, R.; Carassiti, D.; Radotra, B.; Gentleman, S.M.; Serafini, B.; Aloisi, F.; Roncaroli, F.; Magliozzi, R.; et al. Meningeal inflammation is widespread and linked to cortical pathology in multiple sclerosis. *Brain* **2011**, *134*, 2755–2771. [CrossRef]
24. Choi, S.R.; Howell, O.W.; Carassiti, D.; Magliozzi, R.; Gveric, D.; Muraro, P.A.; Nicholas, R.; Roncaroli, F.R.R.; Choi, S.R.; Howell, O.W.; et al. Meningeal inflammation plays a role in the pathology of primary progressive multiple sclerosis. *Brain* **2012**, *135*, 2925–2937. [CrossRef]
25. Serafini, B.; Rosicarelli, B.; Magliozzi, R.; Stigliano, E.; Aloisi, F. Detection of ectopic B-cell follicles with germinal centers in the meninges of patients with secondary progressive multiple sclerosis. *Brain Pathol.* **2004**, *14*, 164–174. [CrossRef]
26. Haider, L.; Zrzavy, T.; Hametner, S.; Hoftberger, R.; Bagnato, F.; Grabner, G.; Trattnig, S.; Pfeifenbring, S.; Bruck, W.; Lassmann, H. The topograpy of demyelination and neurodegeneration in the multiple sclerosis brain. *Brain* **2016**, *139*, 807–815. [CrossRef]
27. Parker Harp, C.R.; Archambault, A.S.; Cheung, M.; Williams, J.W.; Czepielewski, R.S.; Duncker, P.C.; Kilgore, A.J.; Miller, A.T.; Segal, B.M.; Kim, A.H.J.; et al. Neutrophils promote VLA-4–dependent B cell antigen presentation and accumulation within the meninges during neuroinflammation. *Proc. Natl. Acad. Sci. USA* **2019**, *116*, 201909098. [CrossRef]
28. Columba-Cabezas, S.; Griguoli, M.; Rosicarelli, B.; Magliozzi, R.; Ria, F.; Serafini, B.; Aloisi, F. Suppression of established experimental autoimmune encephalomyelitis and formation of meningeal lymphoid follicles by lymphotoxin β receptor-Ig fusion protein. *J. Neuroimmunol.* **2006**, *179*, 76–86. [CrossRef]
29. Peters, A.; Pitcher, L.A.; Sullivan, J.M.; Mitsdoerffer, M.; Acton, S.E.; Franz, B.; Wucherpfennig, K.; Turley, S.; Carroll, M.C.; Sobel, R.A.; et al. Th17 Cells Induce Ectopic Lymphoid Follicles in Central Nervous System Tissue Inflammation. *Immunity* **2011**, *35*, 986–996. [CrossRef]
30. Kuerten, S.; Schickel, A.; Kerkloh, C.; Recks, M.S.; Addicks, K.; Ruddle, N.H.; Lehmann, P. V Tertiary lymphoid organ development coincides with determinant spreading of the myelin-specific T cell response. *Acta Neuropathol.* **2012**, *124*, 861–873. [CrossRef]
31. Pikor, N.B.; Astarita, J.L.; Summers-Deluca, L.; Galicia, G.; Qu, J.; Ward, L.A.; Armstrong, S.; Dominguez, C.X.; Malhotra, D.; Heiden, B.; et al. Integration of Th17- and Lymphotoxin-Derived Signals Initiates Meningeal-Resident Stromal Cell Remodeling to Propagate Neuroinflammation. *Immunity* **2015**, *43*, 1160–1173. [CrossRef] [PubMed]
32. Reali, C.; Magliozzi, R.; Roncaroli, F.; Nicholas, R.; Howell, O.W.; Reynolds, R. B cell rich meningeal inflammation associates with increased spinal cord pathology in multiple sclerosis. *Brain Pathol.* **2020**, *30*, 779–793. [CrossRef] [PubMed]
33. Bevan, R.J.; Evans, R.; Griffiths, L.; Watkins, L.M.; Rees, M.I.; Magliozzi, R.; Allen, I.; McDonnell, G.; Kee, R.; Naughton, M.; et al. Meningeal inflammation and cortical demyelination in acute multiple sclerosis. *Ann. Neurol.* **2018**, *84*, 829–842. [CrossRef] [PubMed]
34. Cañete, J.D.; Celis, R.; Moll, C.; Izquierdo, E.; Marsal, S.; Sanmartí, R.; Palacín, A.; Lora, D.; De La Cruz, J.; Pablos, J.L. Clinical significance of synovial lymphoid neogenesis and its reversal after anti-tumour necrosis factor α therapy in rheumatoid arthritis. *Ann. Rheum. Dis.* **2009**, *68*, 751–756. [CrossRef] [PubMed]
35. Klaasen, R.; Thurlings, R.M.; Wijbrandts, C.A.; Van Kuijk, A.W.; Baeten, D.; Gerlag, D.M.; Tak, P.P. The relationship between synovial lymphocyte aggregates and the clinical response to infliximab in rheumatoid arthritis: A prospective study. *Arthritis Rheum.* **2009**, *60*, 3217–3224. [CrossRef] [PubMed]
36. Serafini, B.; Rosicarelli, B.; Franciotta, D.; Magliozzi, R.; Reynolds, R.; Cinque, P.; Andreoni, L.; Trivedi, P.; Salvetti, M.; Faggioni, A.; et al. Dysregulated Epstein-Barr virus infection in the multiple sclerosis brain. *J. Exp. Med.* **2007**, *204*, 2899–2912. [CrossRef]
37. Kooi, E.J.; Geurts, J.J.G.; Van Horssen, J.; Bø, L.; Van Der Valk, P. Meningeal inflammation is not associated with cortical demyelination in chronic multiple sclerosis. *J. Neuropathol. Exp. Neurol.* **2009**, *68*, 1021–1028. [CrossRef]

38. Willis, S.N.; Stadelmann, C.; Rodig, S.J.; Caron, T.; Gattenloehner, S.; Mallozzi, S.S.; Roughan, J.E.; Almendinger, S.E.; Blewett, M.M.; Brück, W.; et al. Epstein–Barr virus infection is not a characteristic feature of multiple sclerosis brain. *Brain* **2009**, *132*, 3318–3328. [CrossRef]
39. Frischer, J.M.; Bramow, S.; Dal-Bianco, A.; Lucchinetti, C.F.; Rauschka, H.; Schmidbauer, M.; Laursen, H.; Sorensen, P.S.; Lassmann, H. The relation between inflammation and neurodegeneration in multiple sclerosis brains. *Brain* **2009**, *132*, 1175–1189. [CrossRef]
40. Peferoen, L.A.N.N.; Lamers, F.; Lodder, L.N.R.R.; Gerritsen, W.H.; Huitinga, I.; Melief, J.; Giovannoni, G.; Meier, U.; Hintzen, R.Q.; Verjans, G.M.G.M.G.M.; et al. Epstein Barr virus is not a characteristic feature in the central nervous system in established multiple sclerosis. *Brain* **2010**, *133*, e137. [CrossRef]
41. Torkildsen, O.; Stansberg, C.; Angelskar, S.M.; Kooi, E.-J.; Geurts, J.J.G.; van der Valk, P.; Myhr, K.-M.; Steen, V.M.; Bo, L. Upregulation of immunoglobulin-related genes in cortical sections from multiple sclerosis patients. *Brain Pathol.* **2010**, *20*, 720–729. [CrossRef] [PubMed]
42. Serafini, B.; Severa, M.; Columba-Cabezas, S.; Rosicarelli, B.; Veroni, C.; Chiappetta, G.; Magliozzi, R.; Reynolds, R.; Coccia, E.M.; Aloisi, F.; et al. Epstein-barr virus latent infection and baff expression in B cells in the multiple sclerosis brain: Implications for viral persistence and intrathecal B-cell activation. *J. Neuropathol. Exp. Neurol.* **2010**, *69*, 677–693. [CrossRef] [PubMed]
43. Lucchinetti, C.F.; Popescu, B.F.G.G.; Bunyan, R.F.; Moll, N.M.; Roemer, S.F.; Lassmann, H.; Brück, W.; Parisi, J.E.; Scheithauer, B.W.; Giannini, C.; et al. Inflammatory cortical demyelination in early multiple sclerosis. *N. Engl. J. Med.* **2011**, *365*, 2188–2197. [CrossRef]
44. Lovato, L.; Willis, S.N.; Rodig, S.J.; Caron, T.; Almendinger, S.E.; Howell, O.W.; Reynolds, R.; O'Connor, K.C.; Hafler, D.A.; Connor, K.C.O.; et al. Related B cell clones populate the meninges and parenchyma of patients with multiple sclerosis. *Brain* **2011**, *134*, 534–541. [CrossRef] [PubMed]
45. Magliozzi, R.; Serafini, B.; Rosicarelli, B.; Chiappetta, G.; Veroni, C.; Reynolds, R.; Aloisi, F. B-cell enrichment and Epstein-Barr virus infection in inflammatory cortical lesions in secondary progressive multiple sclerosis. *J. Neuropathol. Exp. Neurol.* **2013**, *72*, 29–41. [CrossRef]
46. Howell, O.W.; Schulz-Trieglaff, E.K.; Carassiti, D.; Gentleman, S.M.; Nicholas, R.; Roncaroli, F.; Reynolds, R. RR Extensive grey matter pathology in the cerebellum in multiple sclerosis is linked to inflammation in the subarachnoid space. *Neuropathol. Appl. Neurobiol.* **2015**, *41*, 798–813. [CrossRef]
47. Serafini, B.; Rosicarelli, B.; Veroni, C.; Zhou, L.; Reali, C.; Aloisi, F. RORgammat Expression and Lymphoid Neogenesis in the Brain of Patients with Secondary Progressive Multiple Sclerosis. *J. Neuropathol. Exp. Neurol.* **2016**, *75*, 877–888. [CrossRef]
48. Hassani, A.; Corboy, J.R.; Al-Salam, S.; Khan, G. Epstein-Barr virus is present in the brain of most cases of multiple sclerosis and may engage more than just B cells. *PLoS ONE* **2018**, *13*, e0192109. [CrossRef]
49. Bell, L.; Lenhart, A.; Rosenwald, A.; Monoranu, C.M.; Berberich-Siebelt, F. Lymphoid Aggregates in the CNS of Progressive Multiple Sclerosis Patients Lack Regulatory T Cells. *Front. Immunol.* **2019**, *10*, 3090. [CrossRef]
50. Engelhardt, B.; Sorokin, L. The blood–brain and the blood–cerebrospinal fluid barriers: Function and dysfunction. *Semin. Immunopathol.* **2009**, *31*, 497–511. [CrossRef]
51. Korin, B.; Ben-Shaanan, T.L.; Schiller, M.; Dubovik, T.; Azulay-Debby, H.; Boshnak, N.T.; Koren, T.; Rolls, A. High dimensional, single-cell characterization of the brain's immune compartment. *Nat. Neurosci.* **2017**, *20*, 1300–1309. [CrossRef] [PubMed]
52. Filiano, A.J.; Gadani, S.P.; Kipnis, J. How and why do T cells and their derived cytokines affect the injured and healthy brain? *Nat. Rev. Neurosci.* **2017**, *18*, 375–384. [CrossRef] [PubMed]
53. Mrdjen, D.; Pavlovic, A.; Hartmann, F.J.; Schreiner, B.; Utz, S.G.; Leung, B.P.; Lelios, I.; Heppner, F.L.; Kipnis, J.; Merkler, D.; et al. High-Dimensional Single-Cell Mapping of Central Nervous System Immune Cells Reveals Distinct Myeloid Subsets in Health, Aging, and Disease. *Immunity* **2018**, *48*, 380–395.e6. [CrossRef] [PubMed]
54. Derk, J.; Jones, H.E.; Como, C.; Pawlikowski, B.; Siegenthaler, J.A. Living on the Edge of the CNS: Meninges Cell Diversity in Health and Disease. *Front. Cell. Neurosci.* **2021**, *15*, 703944. [CrossRef]
55. Rua, R.; McGavern, D.B. Advances in Meningeal Immunity. *Trends Mol. Med.* **2018**, *24*, 542–559. [CrossRef] [PubMed]
56. Mascagni, P.; Sanctius, C. *Vasorum Lymphaticorum Corporis Humani Historia et Ichnographia*; Ex typographia Pazzini Carli: Siena, Italy, 1787.
57. Aspelund, A.; Antila, S.; Proulx, S.T.; Karlsen, T.V.; Karaman, S.; Detmar, M.; Wiig, H.; Alitalo, K. A dural lymphatic vascular system that drains brain interstitial fluid and macromolecules. *J. Exp. Med.* **2015**, *212*, 991–999. [CrossRef]
58. Louveau, A.; Smirnov, I.; Keyes, T.J.; Eccles, J.D.; Rouhani, S.J.; Peske, J.D.; Derecki, N.C.; Castle, D.; Mandell, J.W.; Lee, K.S.; et al. Structural and functional features of central nervous system lymphatic vessels. *Nature* **2015**, *523*, 337–341. [CrossRef] [PubMed]
59. Louveau, A.; Herz, J.; Alme, M.N.; Salvador, A.F.; Dong, M.Q.; Viar, K.E.; Herod, S.G.; Knopp, J.; Setliff, J.C.; Lupi, A.L.; et al. CNS lymphatic drainage and neuroinflammation are regulated by meningeal lymphatic vasculature. *Nat. Neurosci.* **2018**, *21*, 1380–1391. [CrossRef] [PubMed]
60. Rustenhoven, J.; Drieu, A.; Mamuladze, T.; de Lima, K.A.; Dykstra, T.; Wall, M.; Papadopoulos, Z.; Kanamori, M.; Salvador, A.F.; Baker, W.; et al. Functional characterization of the dural sinuses as a neuroimmune interface. *Cell* **2021**, *184*, 1000–1016.e27. [CrossRef] [PubMed]
61. Da Mesquita, S.; Louveau, A.; Vaccari, A.; Smirnov, I.; Cornelison, R.C.; Kingsmore, K.M.; Contarino, C.; Onengut-Gumuscu, S.; Farber, E.; Raper, D.; et al. Functional aspects of meningeal lymphatics in ageing and Alzheimer's disease. *Nature* **2018**, *560*, 185–191. [CrossRef] [PubMed]

62. Van Zwam, M.; Huizinga, R.; Heijmans, N.; van Meurs, M.; Wierenga-Wolf, A.F.; Melief, M.-J.; Hintzen, R.Q.; 't Hart, B.A.; Amor, S.; Boven, L.A.; et al. Surgical excision of CNS-draining lymph nodes reduces relapse severity in chronic-relapsing experimental autoimmune encephalomyelitis. *J. Pathol.* **2009**, *217*, 543–551. [CrossRef] [PubMed]
63. Herisson, F.; Frodermann, V.; Courties, G.; Rohde, D.; Sun, Y.; Vandoorne, K.; Wojtkiewicz, G.R.; Masson, G.S.; Vinegoni, C.; Kim, J.; et al. Direct vascular channels connect skull bone marrow and the brain surface enabling myeloid cell migration. *Nat. Neurosci.* **2018**, *21*, 1209–1217. [CrossRef]
64. Brioschi, S.; Wang, W.-L.; Peng, V.; Wang, M.; Shchukina, I.; Greenberg, Z.J.; Bando, J.K.; Jaeger, N.; Czepielewski, R.S.; Swain, A.; et al. Heterogeneity of meningeal B cells reveals a lymphopoietic niche at the CNS borders. *Science* **2021**, *373*, eabf9277. [CrossRef] [PubMed]
65. Aloisi, F.; Pujol-Borrell, R. Lymphoid neogenesis in chronic inflammatory diseases. *Nat. Rev. Immunol.* **2006**, *6*, 205–217. [CrossRef]
66. Corsiero, E.; Nerviani, A.; Bombardieri, M. PC Ectopic Lymphoid Structures: Powerhouse of Autoimmunity. *Front. Immunol.* **2016**, *7*, 430. [CrossRef] [PubMed]
67. Jones, G.W.; Hill, D.G.; Jones, S.A. Understanding immune cells in tertiary lymphoid organ development: It is all starting to come together. *Front. Immunol.* **2016**, *7*, 401. [CrossRef] [PubMed]
68. J Gunderson, A.; Rajamanickam, V.; Bui, C.; Bernard, B.; Pucilowska, J.; Ballesteros-Merino, C.; Schmidt, M.; McCarty, K.; Philips, M.; Piening, B.; et al. Germinal center reactions in tertiary lymphoid structures associate with neoantigen burden, humoral immunity and long-term survivorship in pancreatic cancer. *Oncoimmunology* **2021**, *10*, 1900635. [CrossRef] [PubMed]
69. Endres, R.; Alimzhanov, M.B.; Plitz, T.; Fütterer, A.; Kosco-Vilbois, M.H.; Nedospasov, S.A.; Rajewsky, K.; Pfeffer, K. Mature Follicular Dendritic Cell Networks Depend on Expression of Lymphotoxin β Receptor by Radioresistant Stromal Cells and of Lymphotoxin β and Tumor Necrosis Factor by B Cells. *J. Exp. Med.* **1999**, *189*, 159–168. [CrossRef]
70. Ansel, K.M.; Ngo, V.N.; Hyman, P.L.; Luther, S.A.; Förster, R.; Sedgwlck, J.D.; Browning, J.L.; Upp, M.; Cyster, J.G. A chemokine-driven positive feedback loop organizes lymphoid follicles. *Nature* **2000**, *406*, 309–314. [CrossRef] [PubMed]
71. Cyster, J.G.; Ansel, K.M.; Reif, K.; Ekland, E.H.; Hyman, P.L.; Tang, H.L.; Luther, S.A.; Ngo, V.N. Follicular stromal cells and lymphocyte homing to follicles. *Immunol. Rev.* **2000**, *176*, 181–193. [CrossRef] [PubMed]
72. Schneider, P.; MacKay, F.; Steiner, V.; Hofmann, K.; Bodmer, J.L.; Holler, N.; Ambrose, C.; Lawton, P.; Bixler, S.; Acha-Orbea, H.; et al. BAFF, a novel ligand of the tumor necrosis factor family, stimulates B cell growth. *J. Exp. Med.* **1999**, *189*, 1747–1756. [CrossRef]
73. Mackay, F.; Tangye, S.G. The role of the BAFF/APRIL system in B cell homeostasis and lymphoid cancers. *Curr. Opin. Pharmacol.* **2004**, *4*, 347–354. [CrossRef]
74. Thangarajh, M.; Gomes, A.; Masterman, T.; Hillert, J.; Hjelmström, P. Expression of B-cell-activating factor of the TNF family (BAFF) and its receptors in multiple sclerosis. *J. Neuroimmunol.* **2004**, *152*, 183–190. [CrossRef] [PubMed]
75. Krumbholz, M.; Theil, D.; Derfuss, T.; Rosenwald, A.; Schrader, F.; Monoranu, C.-M.; Kalled, S.L.; Hess, D.M.; Serafini, B.; Aloisi, F.; et al. BAFF is produced by astrocytes and up-regulated in multiple sclerosis lesions and primary central nervous system lymphoma. *J. Exp. Med.* **2005**, *201*, 195–200. [CrossRef] [PubMed]
76. Hjelmström, P.; Hjelmstrom, P. Lymphoid neogenesis: De novo formation of lymphoid tissue in chronic inflammation through expression of homing chemokines. *J. Leukoc. Biol.* **2001**, *69*, 331–339. [CrossRef] [PubMed]
77. Armengol, M.P.; Juan, M.; Lucas-Martin, A.; Fernandez-Figueras, M.T.; Jaraquemada, D.; Gallart, T.; Pujol-Borrell, R. Thyroid autoimmune disease: Demonstration of thyroid antigen-specific B cells and recombination-activating gene expression in chemokine-containing active intrathyroidal germinal centers. *Am. J. Pathol.* **2001**, *159*, 861–873. [CrossRef]
78. Ansel, K.M.; Cyster, J.G. Chemokines in lymphopoiesis and lymphoid organ development. *Curr. Opin. Immunol.* **2001**, *13*, 172–179. [CrossRef]
79. Mebius, R.E. Organogenesis of lymphoid tissues. *Nat. Rev. Immunol.* **2003**, *3*, 292–303. [CrossRef]
80. Cupedo, T.; Mebius, R.E. Role of chemokines in the development of secondary and tertiary lymphoid tissues. *Semin. Immunol.* **2003**, *15*, 243–248. [CrossRef]
81. Drayton, D.L.; Ying, X.; Lee, J.; Lesslauer, W.; Ruddle, N.H. Ectopic LTαβ directs lymphoid organ neogenesis with concomitant expression of peripheral node addressin and a HEV-restricted sulfotransferase. *J. Exp. Med.* **2003**, *197*, 1153–1163. [CrossRef] [PubMed]
82. Schropp, V.; Rohde, J.; Rovituso, D.M.; Jabari, S.; Bharti, R.; Kuerten, S. Contribution of LTi and TH17 cells to B cell aggregate formation in the central nervous system in a mouse model of multiple sclerosis. *J. Neuroinflamm.* **2019**, *16*, 111. [CrossRef] [PubMed]
83. Spits, H.; Artis, D.; Colonna, M.; Diefenbach, A.; Di Santo, J.P.; Eberl, G.; Koyasu, S.; Locksley, R.M.; McKenzie, A.N.J.; Mebius, R.E.; et al. Innate lymphoid cells–a proposal for uniform nomenclature. *Nat. Rev. Immunol.* **2013**, *13*, 145–149. [CrossRef]
84. Grogan, J.L.; Ouyang, W. A role for Th17 cells in the regulation of tertiary lymphoid follicles. *Eur. J. Immunol.* **2012**, *42*, 2255–2262. [CrossRef] [PubMed]
85. Stumhofer, J.S.; Laurence, A.; Wilson, E.H.; Huang, E.; Tato, C.M.; Johnson, L.M.; Villarino, A.V.; Huang, Q.; Yoshimura, A.; Sehy, D.; et al. Interleukin 27 negatively regulates the development of interleukin 17-producing T helper cells during chronic inflammation of the central nervous system. *Nat. Immunol.* **2006**, *7*, 937–945. [CrossRef]

86. Batten, M.; Li, J.; Yi, S.; Kljavin, N.M.; Danilenko, D.M.; Lucas, S.; Lee, J.; de Sauvage, F.J.; Ghilardi, N. Interleukin 27 limits autoimmune encephalomyelitis by suppressing the development of interleukin 17-producing T cells. *Nat. Immunol.* **2006**, *7*, 929–936. [CrossRef]
87. Fitzgerald, D.C.; Zhang, G.-X.; El-Behi, M.; Fonseca-Kelly, Z.; Li, H.; Yu, S.; Saris, C.J.M.; Gran, B.; Ciric, B.; Rostami, A. Suppression of autoimmune inflammation of the central nervous system by interleukin 10 secreted by interleukin 27-stimulated T cells. *Nat. Immunol.* **2007**, *8*, 1372–1379. [CrossRef]
88. Fitzgerald, D.C.; Ciric, B.; Touil, T.; Harle, H.; Grammatikopolou, J.; Das Sarma, J.; Gran, B.; Zhang, G.-X.; Rostami, A. Suppressive effect of IL-27 on encephalitogenic Th17 cells and the effector phase of experimental autoimmune encephalomyelitis. *J. Immunol.* **2007**, *179*, 3268–3275. [CrossRef]
89. Jones, G.W.; Bombardieri, M.; Greenhill, C.J.; McLeod, L.; Nerviani, A.; Rocher-Ros, V.; Cardus, A.; Williams, A.S.; Pitzalis, C.; Jenkins, B.J.; et al. Interleukin-27 inhibits ectopic lymphoid-like structure development in early inflammatory arthritis. *J. Exp. Med.* **2015**, *212*, 1793–1802. [CrossRef]
90. Babcock, G.J.; Decker, L.L.; Volk, M.; Thorley-Lawson, D.A. EBV persistence in memory B cells in vivo. *Immunity* **1998**, *9*, 395–404. [CrossRef]
91. Souza, T.A.; Stollar, B.D.; Sullivan, J.L.; Luzuriaga, K.; Thorley-Lawson, D.A. Peripheral B cells latently infected with Epstein–Barr virus display molecular hallmarks of classical antigen-selected memory B cells. *Proc. Natl. Acad. Sci. USA* **2005**, *102*, 18093–18098. [CrossRef]
92. Bjornevik, K.; Cortese, M.; Healy, B.C.; Kuhle, J.; Mina, M.J.; Leng, Y.; Elledge, S.J.; Niebuhr, D.W.; Scher, A.I.; Munger, K.L.; et al. Longitudinal analysis reveals high prevalence of Epstein-Barr virus associated with multiple sclerosis. *Science* **2022**, *375*, 296–301. [CrossRef] [PubMed]
93. Chu, A.B.; Sever, J.L.; Madden, D.L.; Iivanainen, M.; Leon, M.; Wallen, W.; Brooks, B.R.; Lee, Y.J.; Houff, S. Oligoclonal IgG bands in cerebrospinal fluid in various neurological diseases. *Ann. Neurol.* **1983**, *13*, 434–439. [CrossRef]
94. Thompson, A.J.; Banwell, B.L.; Barkhof, F.; Carroll, W.M.; Coetzee, T.; Comi, G.; Correale, J.; Fazekas, F.; Filippi, M.; Freedman, M.S.; et al. Diagnosis of multiple sclerosis: 2017 revisions of the McDonald criteria. *Lancet. Neurol.* **2018**, *17*, 162–173. [CrossRef]
95. Qin, Y.; Duquette, P.; Zhang, Y.; Talbot, P.; Poole, R.; Antel, J. Clonal expansion and somatic hypermutation of V(H) genes of B cells from cerebrospinal fluid in multiple sclerosis. *J. Clin. Investig.* **1998**, *102*, 1045–1050. [CrossRef]
96. Baranzini, S.E.; Jeong, M.C.; Butunoi, C.; Murray, R.S.; Bernard, C.C.; Oksenberg, J.R. B cell repertoire diversity and clonal expansion in multiple sclerosis brain lesions. *J. Immunol.* **1999**, *163*, 5133–5144. [PubMed]
97. Colombo, M.; Dono, M.; Gazzola, P.; Roncella, S.; Valetto, A.; Chiorazzi, N.; Mancardi, G.L.; Ferrarini, M. Accumulation of clonally related B lymphocytes in the cerebrospinal fluid of multiple sclerosis patients. *J. Immunol.* **2000**, *164*, 2782–2789. [CrossRef]
98. Palanichamy, A.; Apeltsin, L.; Kuo, T.C.; Sirota, M.; Wang, S.; Pitts, S.J.; Sundar, P.D.; Telman, D.; Zhao, L.Z.; Derstine, M.; et al. Immunoglobulin class-switched B cells form an active immune axis between CNS and periphery in multiple sclerosis. *Sci. Transl. Med.* **2014**, *6*, 248ra106. [CrossRef]
99. Uccelli, A.; Aloisi, F.; Pistoia, V. Unveiling the enigma of the CNS as a B-cell fostering environment. *Trends Immunol.* **2005**, *26*, 254–259. [CrossRef]
100. MacLennan, I.C. Germinal centers. *Annu. Rev. Immunol.* **1994**, *12*, 117–139. [CrossRef]
101. Liu, Y.J.; Arpin, C. Germinal center development. *Immunol. Rev.* **1997**, *156*, 111–126. [CrossRef]
102. Hamel, K.M.; Liarski, V.M.; Clark, M.R. Germinal center B-cells. *Autoimmunity* **2012**, *45*, 333–347. [CrossRef] [PubMed]
103. Salomonsson, S.; Jonsson, M.V.; Skarstein, K.; Brokstad, K.A.; Hjelmstrom, P.; Wahren-Herlenius, M.; Jonsson, R. Cellular basis of ectopic germinal center formation and autoantibody production in the target organ of patients with Sjogren's syndrome. *Arthritis Rheum.* **2003**, *48*, 3187–3201. [CrossRef] [PubMed]
104. Stott, D.I.; Hiepe, F.; Hummel, M.; Steinhauser, G.; Berek, C. Antigen-driven clonal proliferation of B cells within the target tissue of an autoimmune disease. The salivary glands of patients with Sjögren's syndrome. *J. Clin. Investig.* **1998**, *102*, 938–946. [CrossRef] [PubMed]
105. Humby, F.; Bombardieri, M.; Manzo, A.; Kelly, S.; Blades, M.C.; Kirkham, B.; Spencer, J.; Pitzalis, C. Ectopic lymphoid structures support ongoing production of class-switched autoantibodies in rheumatoid synovium. *PLoS Med.* **2009**, *6*, e1. [CrossRef]
106. Corcione, A.; Casazza, S.; Ferretti, E.; Giunti, D.; Zappia, E.; Pistorio, A.; Gambini, C.; Mancardi, G.L.; Uccelli, A.; Pistoia, V. Recapitulation of B cell differentiation in the central nervous system of patients with multiple sclerosis. *Proc. Natl. Acad. Sci. USA* **2004**, *101*, 11064–11069. [CrossRef]
107. James Bates, R.E.; Browne, E.; Schalks, R.; Jacobs, H.; Tan, L.; Parekh, P.; Magliozzi, R.; Calabrese, M.; Mazarakis, N.D.; Reynolds, R. Lymphotoxin-alpha expression in the meninges causes lymphoid tissue formation and neurodegeneration. *Brain* **2022**, awac232. [CrossRef]
108. Lassmann, H.; van Horssen, J.; Mahad, D. Progressive multiple sclerosis: Pathology and pathogenesis. *Nat. Rev. Neurol.* **2012**, *8*, 647–656. [CrossRef]
109. Gardner, C.; Magliozzi, R.; Durrenberger, P.F.; Howell, O.W.; Rundle, J.; Reynolds, R. Cortical grey matter demyelination can be induced by elevated pro-inflammatory cytokines in the subarachnoid space of MOG-immunized rats. *Brain* **2013**, *136*, 3596–3608. [CrossRef]

110. Magliozzi, R.; Howell, O.W.; Durrenberger, P.; Aricò, E.; James, R.; Cruciani, C.; Reeves, C.; Roncaroli, F.; Nicholas, R.; Reynolds, R. Meningeal inflammation changes the balance of TNF signalling in cortical grey matter in multiple sclerosis. *J. Neuroinflamm.* **2019**, *16*, 259. [CrossRef]
111. Picon, C.; Jayaraman, A.; James, R.; Beck, C.; Gallego, P.; Witte, M.E.; van Horssen, J.; Mazarakis, N.D.; Reynolds, R. Neuron-specific activation of necroptosis signaling in multiple sclerosis cortical grey matter. *Acta Neuropathol.* **2021**, *141*, 585–604. [CrossRef]
112. James, R.E.; Schalks, R.; Browne, E.; Eleftheriadou, I.; Munoz, C.P.; Mazarakis, N.D.; Reynolds, R. Persistent elevation of intrathecal pro-inflammatory cytokines leads to multiple sclerosis-like cortical demyelination and neurodegeneration. *Acta Neuropathol. Commun.* **2020**, *8*, 66. [CrossRef] [PubMed]
113. Komori, M.; Blake, A.; Greenwood, M.; Lin, Y.C.; Kosa, P.; Ghazali, D.; Winokur, P.; Natrajan, M.; Wuest, S.C.; Romm, E.; et al. Cerebrospinal fluid markers reveal intrathecal inflammation in progressive multiple sclerosis. *Ann. Neurol.* **2015**, *78*, 3–20. [CrossRef] [PubMed]
114. Magliozzi, R.; Howell, O.W.; Nicholas, R.; Cruciani, C.; Castellaro, M.; Romualdi, C.; Rossi, S.; Pitteri, M.; Benedetti, M.D.; Gajofatto, A.; et al. Inflammatory intrathecal profiles and cortical damage in multiple sclerosis. *Ann. Neurol.* **2018**, *83*, 739–755. [CrossRef]
115. Magliozzi, R.; Scalfari, A.; Pisani, A.I.; Ziccardi, S.; Marastoni, D.; Pizzini, F.B.; Bajrami, A.; Tamanti, A.; Guandalini, M.; Bonomi, S.; et al. The CSF Profile Linked to Cortical Damage Predicts Multiple Sclerosis Activity. *Ann. Neurol.* **2020**, *88*, 562–573. [CrossRef] [PubMed]
116. Kaunzner, U.W.; Gauthier, S.A. MRI in the assessment and monitoring of multiple sclerosis: An update on best practice. *Ther. Adv. Neurol. Disord.* **2017**, *10*, 247–261. [CrossRef]
117. Mainero, C.; Benner, T.; Radding, A.; van der Kouwe, A.; Jensen, R.; Rosen, B.R.; Kinkel, R.P. In vivo imaging of cortical pathology in multiple sclerosis using ultra-high field MRI. *Neurology* **2009**, *73*, 941–948. [CrossRef]
118. Metcalf, M.; Xu, D.; Okuda, D.T.; Carvajal, L.; Srinivasan, R.; Kelley, D.A.C.; Mukherjee, P.; Nelson, S.J.; Vigneron, D.B.; Pelletier, D. High-resolution phased-array MRI of the human brain at 7 tesla: Initial experience in multiple sclerosis patients. *J. Neuroimaging Off. J. Am. Soc. Neuroimaging* **2010**, *20*, 141–147. [CrossRef]
119. Kollia, K.; Maderwald, S.; Putzki, N.; Schlamann, M.; Theysohn, J.M.; Kraff, O.; Ladd, M.E.; Forsting, M.; Wanke, I. First clinical study on ultra-high-field MR imaging in patients with multiple sclerosis: Comparison of 1.5T and 7T. *AJNR. Am. J. Neuroradiol.* **2009**, *30*, 699–702. [CrossRef]
120. Simon, B.; Schmidt, S.; Lukas, C.; Gieseke, J.; Träber, F.; Knol, D.L.; Willinek, W.A.; Geurts, J.J.G.; Schild, H.H.; Barkhof, F.; et al. Improved in vivo detection of cortical lesions in multiple sclerosis using double inversion recovery MR imaging at 3 Tesla. *Eur. Radiol.* **2010**, *20*, 1675–1683. [CrossRef]
121. Geurts, J.J.G.; Pouwels, P.J.W.; Uitdehaag, B.M.J.; Polman, C.H.; Barkhof, F.; Castelijns, J.A. Intracortical lesions in multiple sclerosis: Improved detection with 3D double inversion-recovery MR imaging. *Radiology* **2005**, *236*, 254–260. [CrossRef]
122. Kilsdonk, I.D.; Jonkman, L.E.; Klaver, R.; van Veluw, S.J.; Zwanenburg, J.J.M.; Kuijer, J.P.A.; Pouwels, P.J.W.; Twisk, J.W.R.; Wattjes, M.P.; Luijten, P.R.; et al. Increased cortical grey matter lesion detection in multiple sclerosis with 7 T MRI: A post-mortem verification study. *Brain* **2016**, *139*, 1472–1481. [CrossRef] [PubMed]
123. Absinta, M.; Vuolo, L.; Rao, A.; Nair, G.; Sati, P.; Cortese, I.C.M.; Ohayon, J.; Fenton, K.; Reyes-Mantilla, M.I.; Maric, D.; et al. Gadolinium-based MRI characterization of leptomeningeal inflammation in multiple sclerosis. *Neurology* **2015**, *85*, 18–28. [CrossRef] [PubMed]
124. Harrison, D.M.; Wang, K.Y.; Fiol, J.; Naunton, K.; Royal, W., 3rd; Hua, J.; Izbudak, I. Leptomeningeal Enhancement at 7T in Multiple Sclerosis: Frequency, Morphology, and Relationship to Cortical Volume. *J. Neuroimaging Off. J. Am. Soc. Neuroimaging* **2017**, *27*, 461–468. [CrossRef] [PubMed]
125. Makshakov, G.; Magonov, E.; Totolyan, N.; Nazarov, V.; Lapin, S.; Mazing, A.; Verbitskaya, E.; Trofimova, T.; Krasnov, V.; Shumilina, M.; et al. Leptomeningeal Contrast Enhancement Is Associated with Disability Progression and Grey Matter Atrophy in Multiple Sclerosis. *Neurol. Res. Int.* **2017**, *2017*, 8652463. [CrossRef]
126. Zivadinov, R.; Ramasamy, D.P.; Vaneckova, M.; Gandhi, S.; Chandra, A.; Hagemeier, J.; Bergsland, N.; Polak, P.; Benedict, R.H.; Hojnacki, D.; et al. Leptomeningeal contrast enhancement is associated with progression of cortical atrophy in MS: A retrospective, pilot, observational longitudinal study. *Mult. Scler.* **2017**, *23*, 1336–1345. [CrossRef]
127. Jonas, S.N.; Izbudak, I.; Frazier, A.A.; Harrison, D.M. Longitudinal Persistence of Meningeal Enhancement on Postcontrast 7T 3D-FLAIR MRI in Multiple Sclerosis. *AJNR Am. J. Neuroradiol.* **2018**, *39*, 1799–1805. [CrossRef]
128. Hildesheim, F.E.; Ramasamy, D.P.; Bergsland, N.; Jakimovski, D.; Dwyer, M.G.; Hojnacki, D.; Lizarraga, A.A.; Kolb, C.; Eckert, S.; Weinstock-Guttman, B.; et al. Leptomeningeal, dura mater and meningeal vessel wall enhancements in multiple sclerosis. *Mult. Scler. Relat. Disord.* **2021**, *47*, 102653. [CrossRef]
129. Zivadinov, R.; Bergsland, N.; Carl, E.; Ramasamy, D.P.; Hagemeier, J.; Dwyer, M.G.; Lizarraga, A.A.; Kolb, C.; Hojnacki, D.; Weinstock-Guttman, B. Effect of Teriflunomide and Dimethyl Fumarate on Cortical Atrophy and Leptomeningeal Inflammation in Multiple Sclerosis: A Retrospective, Observational, Case-Control Pilot Study. *J. Clin. Med.* **2019**, *8*, 344. [CrossRef]
130. Bhargava, P.; Wicken, C.; Smith, M.D.; Strowd, R.E.; Cortese, I.; Reich, D.S.; Calabresi, P.A.; Mowry, E.M. Trial of intrathecal rituximab in progressive multiple sclerosis patients with evidence of leptomeningeal contrast enhancement. *Mult. Scler. Relat. Disord.* **2019**, *30*, 136–140. [CrossRef]

131. Zivadinov, R.; Jakimovski, D.; Ramanathan, M.; Benedict, R.H.; Bergsland, N.; Dwyer, M.G.; Weinstock-Guttman, B. Effect of ocrelizumab on leptomeningeal inflammation and humoral response to Epstein-Barr virus in multiple sclerosis. A pilot study. *Mult. Scler. Relat. Disord.* **2022**, *67*, 104094. [CrossRef]
132. Montalban, X.; Hauser, S.L.; Kappos, L.; Arnold, D.L.; Bar-Or, A.; Comi, G.; de Seze, J.; Giovannoni, G.; Hartung, H.-P.; Hemmer, B.; et al. Ocrelizumab versus Placebo in Primary Progressive Multiple Sclerosis. *N. Engl. J. Med.* **2017**, *376*, 209–220. [CrossRef] [PubMed]
133. Hauser, S.L.; Bar-Or, A.; Comi, G.; Giovannoni, G.; Hartung, H.-P.; Hemmer, B.; Lublin, F.; Montalban, X.; Rammohan, K.W.; Selmaj, K.; et al. Ocrelizumab versus Interferon Beta-1a in Relapsing Multiple Sclerosis. *N. Engl. J. Med.* **2017**, *376*, 221–234. [CrossRef]
134. Hauser, S.L.; Bar-Or, A.; Cohen, J.A.; Comi, G.; Correale, J.; Coyle, P.K.; Cross, A.H.; de Seze, J.; Leppert, D.; Montalban, X.; et al. Ofatumumab versus Teriflunomide in Multiple Sclerosis. *N. Engl. J. Med.* **2020**, *383*, 546–557. [CrossRef] [PubMed]
135. Naegelin, Y.; Naegelin, P.; von Felten, S.; Lorscheider, J.; Sonder, J.; Uitdehaag, B.M.J.; Scotti, B.; Zecca, C.; Gobbi, C.; Kappos, L.; et al. Association of Rituximab Treatment With Disability Progression Among Patients With Secondary Progressive Multiple Sclerosis. *JAMA Neurol.* **2019**, *76*, 274–281. [CrossRef]
136. Brand, R.M.; Friedrich, V.; Diddens, J.; Pfaller, M.; Romana de Franchis, F.; Radbruch, H.; Hemmer, B.; Steiger, K.; Lehmann-Horn, K. Anti-CD20 Depletes Meningeal B Cells but Does Not Halt the Formation of Meningeal Ectopic Lymphoid Tissue. *Neurol.-Neuroimmunol. Neuroinflamm.* **2021**, *8*, e1012. [CrossRef] [PubMed]
137. Mitsdoerffer, M.; Di Liberto, G.; Dötsch, S.; Sie, C.; Wagner, I.; Pfaller, M.; Kreutzfeldt, M.; Fräßle, S.; Aly, L.; Knier, B.; et al. Formation and immunomodulatory function of meningeal B cell aggregates in progressive CNS autoimmunity. *Brain* **2021**, *144*, 1697–1710. [CrossRef] [PubMed]
138. Brand, R.M.; Diddens, J.; Friedrich, V.; Pfaller, M.; Radbruch, H.; Hemmer, B.; Steiger, K.; Lehmann-Horn, K. Siponimod Inhibits the Formation of Meningeal Ectopic Lymphoid Tissue in Experimental Autoimmune Encephalomyelitis. *Neurol.-Neuroimmunol. Neuroinflamm.* **2022**, *9*, e1117. [CrossRef] [PubMed]
139. Gentile, A.; Musella, A.; Bullitta, S.; Fresegna, D.; De Vito, F.; Fantozzi, R.; Piras, E.; Gargano, F.; Borsellino, G.; Battistini, L.; et al. Siponimod (BAF312) prevents synaptic neurodegeneration in experimental multiple sclerosis. *J. Neuroinflamm.* **2016**, *13*, 207. [CrossRef] [PubMed]
140. Liang, C.; Tian, D.; Ren, X.; Ding, S.; Jia, M.; Xin, M.; Thareja, S. The development of Bruton's tyrosine kinase (BTK) inhibitors from 2012 to 2017: A mini-review. *Eur. J. Med. Chem.* **2018**, *151*, 315–326. [CrossRef] [PubMed]
141. Estupiñán, H.Y.; Berglöf, A.; Zain, R.; Smith, C.I.E. Comparative Analysis of BTK Inhibitors and Mechanisms Underlying Adverse Effects. *Front. Cell Dev. Biol.* **2021**, *9*, 630942. [CrossRef] [PubMed]
142. Bhargava, P.; Kim, S.; Reyes, A.A.; Grenningloh, R.; Boschert, U.; Absinta, M.; Pardo, C.; Van Zijl, P.; Zhang, J.; Calabresi, P.A. Imaging meningeal inflammation in CNS autoimmunity identifies a therapeutic role for BTK inhibition. *Brain* **2021**, *144*, 1396–1408. [CrossRef] [PubMed]
143. Montalban, X.; Arnold, D.L.; Weber, M.S.; Staikov, I.; Piasecka-Stryczynska, K.; Willmer, J.; Martin, E.C.; Dangond, F.; Syed, S.; Wolinsky, J.S. Placebo-Controlled Trial of an Oral BTK Inhibitor in Multiple Sclerosis. *N. Engl. J. Med.* **2019**, *380*, 2406–2417. [CrossRef] [PubMed]

biomedicines

MDPI

Communication

Genetic Markers for Thrombophilia and Cardiovascular Disease Associated with Multiple Sclerosis

Maria S. Hadjiagapiou [1], George Krashias [2], Elie Deeba [2], George Kallis [3], Andri Papaloizou [3], Paul Costeas [3], Christina Christodoulou [2], Marios Pantzaris [1] and Anastasia Lambrianides [1,*]

1 Department of Neuroimmunology, The Cyprus Institute of Neurology and Genetics, P.O. Box 23462, 1683 Nicosia, Cyprus
2 Department of Molecular Virology, The Cyprus Institute of Neurology and Genetics, P.O. Box 23462, 1683 Nicosia, Cyprus
3 Karaiskakio Foundation, P.O. Box 22680, 1523 Nicosia, Cyprus
* Correspondence: nancyl@cing.ac.cy; Tel.: +357-22-392885; Fax: +357-22-392738

Abstract: Multiple sclerosis (MS) is an autoimmune inflammatory disease of the central nervous system (CNS) with an unknown etiology, although genetic, epigenetic, and environmental factors are thought to play a role. Recently, coagulation components have been shown to provide immunomodulatory and pro-inflammatory effects in the CNS, leading to neuroinflammation and neurodegeneration. The current study aimed to determine whether patients with MS exhibited an overrepresentation of polymorphisms implicated in the coagulation and whether such polymorphisms are associated with advanced disability and disease progression. The cardiovascular disease (CVD) strip assay was applied to 48 MS patients and 25 controls to analyze 11 genetic polymorphisms associated with thrombosis and CVD. According to our results, FXIIIVal34Leu heterozygosity was less frequent (OR: 0.35 (95% CI: 0.12–0.99); $p = 0.04$), whereas PAI-1 5G/5G homozygosity was more frequent in MS (OR: 6.33 (95% CI: 1.32–30.24); $p = 0.016$). In addition, carriers of the HPA-1a/1b were likely to have advanced disability (OR: 1.47 (95% CI: 1.03–2.18); $p = 0.03$) and disease worsening (OR: 1.42 (95% CI: 1.05–2.01); $p = 0.02$). The results of a sex-based analysis revealed that male HPA-1a/1b carriers were associated with advanced disability (OR: 3.04 (95% CI: 1.22–19.54); $p = 0.01$), whereas female carriers had an increased likelihood of disease worsening (OR: 1.56 (95% CI: 1.04–2.61); $p = 0.03$). Our findings suggest that MS may be linked to thrombophilia-related polymorphisms, which warrants further investigation.

Keywords: multiple sclerosis; inflammation; thrombophilia; cardiovascular disease (CVD); expanded disability status scale (EDSS); multiple sclerosis severity score (MSSS)

1. Introduction

Multiple sclerosis (MS) is a chronic, autoimmune inflammatory disease of the central nervous system (CNS), characterized by demyelination and neurodegeneration; however, a growing body of evidence indicates the association of chronic, autoimmune disorders with the onset of cardiovascular disease (CVD), development of deep vein thrombosis (DVT), and pulmonary embolism (PE) [1,2]. In fact, a high risk of ischemic stroke, coronary artery disease, and venous thromboembolism (VTE) has been reported in patients with MS compared with the general population, especially during the early onset of the disease [3–5].

Recently, it has been discovered that VTE and CVD are caused by the interplay of environmental and genetic influences, identifying genetic polymorphisms that predispose for cardiovascular perturbation and prolonged thrombin formation [6].

One of the factors associated with VTE is a point mutation in the gene encoding the factor V (FV) that substitutes guanine for adenine (G>A) at nucleotide 1691, resulting in a missense mutation, also known as FV Leiden R506Q [7]. FV is the cofactor of activated FXa for the generation of thrombin and is negatively regulated by activated protein C (APC). The substituted 506 amino acid region constitutes one of the sites on the FVa molecule that the APC recognizes and binds to cleave the FVa protease. Thus, the presence of the mutation FV Leiden (R506Q) renders FVa resistant by up to 90%, suppressing the anticoagulant function of APC and promoting FXa–FVa complex formation and increased thrombin generation [7]. Interestingly, compound heterozygosity of FV Leiden and prothrombin mutation (G20210A) has also been reported as a critical thrombotic risk mediator with more than 40-fold increased risk for VTE [7]. The prothrombin G20210A variant has been found to increase both mRNA accumulation and protein synthesis, whereas its presence enhances approximately threefold the relative risk for thrombosis [8].

Another thrombosis-related mutation has been identified at nucleotide 4070 in the FV gene (FV R2, FV H1299R), and even though this variant does not have a significant impact on the clinical outcome, it can increase resistance to APC either in homozygous status or compound heterozygosity with FV Leiden [9].

The interaction between coagulation and inflammation has been reported in inflammatory and neurodegenerative diseases of the CNS, in which thrombin and fibrin(ogen) play a crucial role in triggering demyelination and neuroinflammation. Mutations in the fibrinogen gene, particularly the transition from guanine to adenine at nucleotide 455 of the beta-fibrinogen promoter, lead to elevated fibrinogen levels. Furthermore, the −455 G>A variant has been identified as a risk factor for fibrin clot formation in PE cases [10] and predisposes to coronary artery disease, as well as cerebral infarction [11, 12]. So far, in MS animal models, thrombin and fibrin(ogen) have been detected in predemyelinated CNS areas, attracting resident and infiltrating immune cells from the periphery, contributing further in abnormal BBB permeability, and stimulating the inflammatory process [13]. Consequently, analysis of the beta-fibrinogen −455 G>A should be considered with respect to the fibrinogen accumulation, since −455 G>A mutation could be associated with the abnormal deposition of elevated fibrinogen into the CNS, initiating inflammatory responses.

Genetic alterations have also been detected in the gene encoding the plasminogen activator inhibitor-1 (PAI-1), an essential inhibitor of the tissue plasminogen activator (tPA), leading to the suppression of plasminogen conversion to plasmin, interfering with fibrin lysis [14]. PAI-1 4G/5G polymorphism constitutes the most significant variant identified in the promoter region at nucleotide position 675 of the PAI-1 gene, and it is a guanine insertion or deletion (4G/5G) correlated with alterations in the transcription rate of the PAI-1 molecule [15]. While both 4G and 5G alleles have a transcriptional activator binding site, 5G has a transcriptional repressor binding site, resulting in a decreased transcription rate [14,15]. On the other hand, individuals homozygous for the 4G allele have an increased transcription rate and thus higher plasma levels of PAI-1 than the general population [16]. PAI-1 has been implicated in the inhibition of extracellular proteolysis and the suppression of fibrinolysis, promoting further the generation of fibrin clots, leading to thrombosis [15].

Fibrin clots are stabilized by the FXIII, a known zymogen that is activated by thrombin-mediated cleavage at amino acid residue 37 and cross-links fibrin [17]. In exon 2 of FXIII, the FXIII Val34Leu variant appears to provide increased activation but does not increase the plasma concentration levels of FXIII [17,18]. Paradoxically, the expression of this particular variant confers significant protection against CVD and VTE while affecting fibrin clot stabilization. In fact, the fibrin that cross-links with FXIII Val34Leu has smaller pores, thinner fibers, and altered findings of permeation [18,19].

Patients with MS have also shown lower folic acid levels and higher homocysteine concentration in plasma and cerebrovascular fluid (CSF) compared with healthy individuals [20]. A growing body of evidence supports the fact that increased homocysteine levels cause neurotoxic effects as a result of oxidized sulfhydryl groups and the release of reactive oxygen species following the overstimulation of excitatory N-methyl-D-aspartate receptors (NMDARs) in the membranes of neuronal cells [21,22]. The NMDAR triggers the activation of the ERK/MAPK pathway and phosphorylates the ERK1/2 kinases in the presence of calcium ions. When ERK1/2 phosphorylation is inhibited, homocysteine-induced neuronal death is reduced, clearly demonstrating the interplay between homocysteine, NMDAR, and MAPK signaling pathways [21]. Neurotoxicity triggers neuronal susceptibility to DNA damage and cellular apoptosis and affects the structural stability of myelin, promoting the degradation of the myelin sheath [23]. Since homocysteine is metabolized to methionine by the donation of methyl groups, low levels of methionine result in abnormally elevated homocysteine levels, which, in turn, reduce methyl groups donation and suppress methionine remethylation [23]. The influence of the methionine on the myelin basic protein (MBP) is significant as it makes the myelin sheath more stable by MBP methylation and retains hydrophobic properties [23]. Therefore, deficiency or suppression of methionine is associated with unstable myelin structure and myelin sheath rupture [23]. Methylenetetrahydrofolate reductase (MTHFR), which regulates both folate and homocysteine levels, plays a crucial role in the methionine synthesis pathway and ultimately is essential for the donation of methyl groups during the remethylation of methionine [20,24]. Mutations in the MTHFR gene impair the activity of the enzyme and, therefore, disrupt the regulation of plasma folate and homocysteine concentration [25]. Noteworthy, individuals homozygous for the MTHFR 677 C>T showed decreased activity of the enzyme at a rate between 35% and 70%, whereas the heterozygosity of the compound MTHFR 677 C>T and MTHFR 1298 A>C leads to a decreased activity rate from 50% to 60% [24,26]. Overall, elevated homocysteine levels have been linked to neuronal toxicity, stroke, coronary artery disease, and thrombophilia in either mutation [25,27].

Furthermore, predisposition to stroke, myocardial infarction (MI), or coronary artery disease was correlated with human platelet antigen (HPA-1) 1a/b polymorphisms [28,29], whereas MI was further associated with mutations linked to the gene that codes the angiotensin-converting enzyme (ACE) [29].

Given the significance of variants in genes encoding molecules involved in the coagulation cascade and the importance of coagulation–inflammation interplay in neuroinflammatory and neurodegenerative diseases, the purpose of our research was intended to examine such variants in MS. Specifically, we aimed to examine whether patients with MS displayed overrepresentations in the following genetic markers: FV Leiden polymorphism, FV R2, Prothrombin 20210 G>A, FXIII Val34Leu, beta-fibrinogen −455 G>A, HPA1a/1b, MTHFR 677 C>T, MTHFR 1298 A>T, PAI-1 4G/5G, ACE I/D, and Apo B R3500Q compared with healthy individuals. Moreover, we investigated whether such polymorphisms can serve as predictors of advanced disability and progression of the disease.

2. Materials and Methods

2.1. Study Participants

Forty-eight patients with MS were recruited into the study from the Department of Neuroimmunology at the Cyprus Institute of Neurology and Genetics between June 2021 and September 2021. The participants met all McDonald's revised criteria for inclusion [30] and strictly adhered to the following guidelines: age above 18 years old; patients with clearly identified classification (Relapsing–Remitting MS (RRMS), Secondary Progressive (SPMS), Primary Progressive MS (PPMS)); and sufficient demographic and clinical data (age of onset, expanded-disability status scale (EDSS), medication, other autoimmune and non-autoimmune disorders). The exclusion criteria were as follows: whether the patient is pregnant or has a history of drug and alcohol abuse.

The study also included 25 healthy controls (HCs) matched for sex with the patients selected. Table 1 demonstrates the demographic, clinical, and laboratory characteristics of the participants. All the participants were thoroughly informed about the objectives of the current study and signed written consent form, approved by the Cyprus National Bioethics Committee (EEBK/EΠ/2016/51).

Table 1. Demographic, clinical, and laboratory features of MS patients and healthy controls.

Features	MS Patients (n = 48)	HCs (n = 25)
Sex		
Women/Men	28/20	16/9
Age in years		
Mean ± S.D.	49.5 ± 13.8	40.7 ± 10.0
Min–max	23–80	21–55
Disease course (RRMS/SPMS/PPMS)	39/8/1	N/A
Disease duration		
Mean ± S.D.	15.52 ± 8.5	N/A
Median (interquartile range)	16 (10–21)	
EDSS		
Median (interquartile range, IQR)	3.25 (2.5–5.5)	
Mild: 0–3.0 [n (%)]	24 (50.0)	N/A
Moderate: 3.5–5.5 [n (%)]	17 (35.4)	
Severe: 6.0–9.5 [n (%)]	7 (14.6)	
Women/Men (median, IQR)	3.0 (2.5–4.75)/4.0 (2.5–6.0)	
MSSS		
Median (interquartile range)	3.65 (2.64–5.41)	
Benign MS: 0.01–1.99 [n (%)]	7 (14.6)	N/A
Moderate MS: 2.00–6.99 [n (%)]	36 (75.0)	
Severe MS: 7–10 [n (%)]	4 (8.3)	
N/A	1 (2.1)	
Women/Men (median, IQR)	3.14 (2.35–5.48)/4.20 (2.82–5.41)	
Laboratory findings		
Anti-FVIIa [n (%)]	11 (22.9)	
Anti-thrombin [n (%)]	6 (12.5)	
Anti-prothrombin [n (%)]	7 (14.6)	
Anti-FXa [n (%)]	11 (22.9)	N/A
Anti-FXII [n (%)]	9 (18.7)	
Anti-plasmin [n (%)]	15 (31.2)	
Anti-protein C [n (%)]	6 (12.5)	

MS: multiple sclerosis; HC: healthy controls; S.D.: standard deviation; RRMS: relapsing–remitting multiple sclerosis; SPMS: secondary progressive multiple sclerosis; PPMS: primary progressive multiple sclerosis; EDSS: expanded disability status scale; MSSS: multiple sclerosis severity score; N/A: not applicable.

2.2. Genetic Analysis for Thrombophilia and Cardiovascular Risk Factors in MS Patients

Fresh blood samples were collected in vacutainers containing ethylenediaminetetraacetic acid (EDTA) following the extraction of genetic material using a QIAamp DNA blood mini kit (Qiagen, Venlo, The Netherlands).

CVD Strip Assay (ViennaLab, Wien, Austria) was applied for the detection of genetic variants associated with thrombophilia and CVD, following the manufacturer's specifications [6]. The analyzed markers are presented in Table 2.

Table 2. Selected risk factors determined by sequence-specific oligonucleotides.

Protein	Gene	Mutation and Polymorphism	Ref SNP
Blood coagulation factor V	F5	1691 G>A (Leiden)	rs6025
		His1299Arg (HR2 haplotype)	rs1800595
Prothrombin (Blood coagulation factor II)	F2	20210 G>A	rs1799963
Blood coagulation factor XIII	F13A1	Val34Leu	rs5985
ß-Fibrinogen	FGB	−445 G>A	rs1800790
Human platelet antigen 1 (HPA1)	ITGB3	1a/1b (Leu33Pro)	rs5918
5,10-Methylenetetrahydrofolate reductase	MTHFR	677 C>T	rs1801133
		1298 A>C	rs1801131
Plasminogen activator inhibitor 1 (PAI-1)	Serpine1	4G/5G	rs1799762
Angiotensin-converting enzyme (ACE)	ACE	I/D (Insertion or Deletion)	rs1799752
Apolipoprotein B (Apo B)	ApoB	Arg3500Gln	rs5742904

SNP: single nucleotide polymorphism; His: histidine; Arg: arginine; Val: valine; Leu: leucine; Pro: proline; Gln: glutamine; Cys: cysteine.

All gene sequences were concurrently amplified by polymerase chain reaction (PCR) and labeled by biotin as follows. The initial denaturation step was conducted at 94 °C for 2 min, followed by 35 cycles of 94 °C for 15 s, 58 °C for 30 s, 72 °C for 30 s, and 72 °C for 3 min for the final extension step. PCR products were then hybridized to a test strip containing sequence-specific oligonucleotide probes for the wild-type and mutant sequences. The bound biotin-labeled sequences were detected by a streptavidin-alkaline phosphatase substrate.

2.3. Statistical Analysis

Fisher's exact test was used to assess sex matching between study groups, and the Hardy–Weinberg equilibrium test was used to examine whether frequencies in the control group matched the expected frequencies over time. The chi-square test, and, when necessary, Fisher's exact tests were used to determine genotype and allele frequency distributions, whereas logistic regression analysis was applied to evaluate possible associations between different variables. Significant results were determined when the p-value was less than 0.05.

3. Results

3.1. Demographic and Clinical Data of Study Participants

Forty-eight patients with MS who provided data on both clinical and nonclinical features were recruited in the current research. According to the data indicated in Table 1, the average duration of the disease was 15.52 ± 8.5 years, whereas 50% of the MS participants had mild disability status (EDSS: 0–3.0), 35.4% had moderate (EDSS: 3.5–5.5), and 14.6% showed severe disability (EDSS: 6.0–9.5). Additionally, 8.3% of individuals were experiencing an aggressive disease progression (MSSS: 7–10).

The results of a sex-specific analysis of the disability status and MS severity score revealed an increase in EDSS and MSSS in men compared with women. In particular, male patients showed an EDSS median of 4.00 (interquartile range, IQR: 2.5–6.0) and MSSS median of 4.20 (IQR: 2.82–5.41), whereas female patients had an EDSS median of 3.0 (IQR: 2.5–4.75) and MSSS of 3.14 (IQR: 2.35–5.48). The patients were selected on the basis that they tested positive for at least one IgG antibody against coagulation components in our previous research work [31]. Table 1 shows the IgG antibodies that were analyzed, whereas detailed laboratory findings for each patient are provided in Supplementary Tables S1–S5.

Twenty-five HCs were also recruited for the current study, matching their sex with the selected MS patients (p = 0.8).

3.2. Analysis of Genotype and Allele Distributions of Thrombophilia and Cardiovascular Polymorphisms in MS Patients and Healthy Controls

The distribution of genotype and allele frequencies of polymorphisms related to thrombophilia and CVD are presented in Tables 3–6. Genotypic frequencies for all loci tested in the control group satisfied the Hardy–Weinberg equilibrium.

Table 3. Genotype frequencies distributions of thrombophilia factors performed by sequence-specific oligonucleotide probing in MS patients and healthy controls.

Risk Factors	Genotype	MS (n (%))	HC (n (%))	* *p* Value	Hardy–Weinberg Equilibrium (Only for HCs)Chi-Square (χ^2)	Odds Ratio (95% CI)
Factor V Leiden	G/G	39 (81.25)	22 (88.0)			Ref
	G/A	9 (18.75)	3 (12.0)	0.53	0.10	1.69 (0.41–6.91)
	A/A	0	0	-		-
	G/A + A/A	9 (18.75)	3 (12.0)	0.53		1.69 (0.41–6.91)
Factor V R2	A/A	40 (83.33)	21 (84.0)			Ref
	A/G	8 (16.67)	4 (16.0)	1.00	0.19	1.05 (0.28–3.90)
	G/G	0	0	-		-
	A/G + G/G	8 (16.67)	4 (16.0)	1.00		1.05 (0.28–3.90)
Factor II	G/G	47 (97.92)	25 (100)			Ref
	G/A	1 (2.08)	0	1.00	-	1.61 (0.06–41.01)
	A/A	0	0	-		-
	G/A + A/A	1 (2.08)	0	1.00		1.61 (0.06–41.01)
Factor FXIII Val34Leu	G/G	34 (70.83)	12 (48.0)	-		Ref
	G/T	12 (25.0)	12 (48.0)	0.04 *	0.91	0.35 (0.12–0.99)
	T/T	2 (4.17)	1 (4.0)	1.00		0.70 (0.05–8.51)
	G/T + T/T	14 (29.17)	13 (52.0)	0.055		0.38 (0.14–1.03)
β-Fibrinogen	G/G	23 (47.92)	16 (64.0)	-		Ref
	G/A	21 (43.75)	9 (36.0)	0.34	1.20	1.62 (0.59–4.45)
	A/A	4 (8.33)	0	0.27		6.32 (0.32–125.6)
	G/A + A/A	25 (52.08)	9 (36.0)	0.19		1.93 (0.71–5.22)
HPA-1	1a/1a	34 (70.83)	17 (68.0)	-		Ref
	1a/1b	14 (29.17)	7 (28.0)	1.00	0.06	1.00 (0.34–2.94)
	1b/1b	0	1 (4.0)	0.34		0.17 (0.0–4.37)

* Chi-square test and, when necessary, Fisher's exact tests were used to determine genotype and allele frequency distributions, whereas logistic regression analysis was applied to evaluate possible associations. MS: multiple sclerosis; HC: healthy controls; HPA-1: human platelet antigen 1. Statistically significant values $p < 0.05$ (*).

Table 4. Genotype frequencies distributions of cardiovascular risk factors performed by sequence-specific oligonucleotide probing in MS patients and healthy controls.

Risk Factors	Genotype	MS (n (%))	HC (n (%))	* *p* Value	Hardy–Weinberg Equilibrium (Only for HCs) Chi-Square (χ^2)	Odds Ratio (95% CI)
PAI-1	4G/4G	8 (16.67)	8 (32.0)	-		Ref
	4G/5G	21 (43.75)	14 (56.0)	0.50	0.69	1.50 (0.46–4.93)
	5G/5G	19 (39.58)	3 (12.0)	0.02 *		6.33 (1.32–30.24)
	4G/4G + 4G/5G	29 (60.42)	22 (88.0)	-		Ref
	5G/5G	19 (39.58)	3 (12.0)	0.016 *		4.80 (1.26–18.31)
MTHFR (C677T)	C/C	18 (37.5)	12 (48.0)	-		Ref
	C/T	25 (52.08)	9 (36.0)	0.25	0.98	1.85 (0.64–5.32)
	T/T	5 (10.42)	4 (16.0)	1.00		0.83 (0.18–3.75)
	C/T + T/T	30 (62.50)	13 (52.0)	0.38		1.54 (0.57–4.09)
MTHFR (A1298C)	A/A	21 (43.75)	10 (40.0)	-		Ref
	A/C	23 (47.92)	12 (48.0)	0.86	0.04	0.91 (0.32–2.55)
	C/C	4 (8.33)	3 (12.0)	0.67		0.63 (0.12–3.39)
	A/C + C/C	27 (56.25)	15 (60.0)	0.76		0.85 (0.32–2.29)
ACE	I/I	3 (6.25)	4 (16.0)	-		Ref
	I/D	26 (54.17)	9 (36.0)	0.17	0.98	3.85 (0.72–20.63)
	D/D	19 (39.58)	12 (48.0)	0.42		2.11 (0.40–11.13)
Apo B	G/G	48(100)	25 (100)			
	G/A	0	0	-	-	-
	A/A	0	0			

* Chi-square test and, when necessary, Fisher's exact tests were used to determine genotype and allele frequency distributions, whereas logistic regression analysis was applied to evaluate possible associations. MS: multiple sclerosis; HC: healthy controls; PAI-1: plasminogen activator inhibitor-1; MTHFR: methylenetetrahydrofolate reductase; ACE: angiotensin-converting enzyme; Apo: apolipoprotein. Statistically significant value $p < 0.05$ (*).

Table 5. Allele frequencies distributions of thrombophilia factors performed by sequence-specific oligonucleotide probing in MS patients and healthy controls.

Risk Factors	Allele	MS (%)	HC (%)	* *p* Value	Odds Ratio (95% CI)
Factor V Leiden	G A	87 (90.62) 9 (9.38)	47 (94.0) 3 (6.0)	0.75	Ref 1.62 (0.42–6.28)
Factor V R2	A G	88 (91.67) 8 (8.33)	46 (92.0) 4 (8.0)	1.00	Ref 1.04 (0.30–3.66)
Factor II	G A	95 (98.96) 1 (1.04)	50 (100) 0	1.00	Ref 1.59 (0.06–39.69)
Factor FXIII Val34Leu	G T	80 (83.33) 16 (16.67)	36 (72.0) 14 (28.0)	0.10	Ref 0.51 (0.22–1.17)
beta-Fibrinogen	G A	67 (69.80) 29 (30.20)	41 (82.0) 9 (18.0)	0.11	Ref 1.97 (0.85–4.58)
HPA-1	1a 1b	82 (85.42) 14 (14.58)	41 (82.0) 9 (18.0)	0.59	Ref 0.77 (0.31–1.95)

* Chi-square test and, when necessary, Fisher's exact tests were used to determine genotype and allele frequency distributions, whereas logistic regression analysis was applied to evaluate possible associations. MS: multiple sclerosis; HC: healthy controls; HPA-1: human platelet antigen 1.

Table 6. Allele frequencies distributions of cardiovascular risk factors performed by sequence-specific oligonucleotide probing in MS patients and healthy controls.

Risk Factors	Allele	MS (%)	HC (%)	* *p* Value	Odds Ratio (95% CI)
PAI-1	4G 5G	37 (38.54) 59 (61.46)	30 (60.0) 20 (40.0)	0.013 *	Ref 2.39 (1.19–4.81)
MTHFR (C677T)	C T	61 (63.54) 35 (36.46)	33 (66.0) 17 (34.0)	0.77	Ref 1.11 (0.54–2.28)
MTHFR (A1298C)	A C	65 (67.71) 31 (32.29)	32 (64.0) 18 (36.0)	0.65	Ref 0.85 (0.41–1.74)
ACE	I D	32 (33.33) 64 (66.67)	17 (34.0) 33 (66.0)	0.93	Ref 1.03 (0.50–2.12)
Apo B	G A	96 (100) 0	50 (100) 0	-	-

* Chi-square test and, when necessary, Fisher's exact tests were used to determine genotype and allele frequency distributions, whereas logistic regression analysis was applied to evaluate possible associations. MS: multiple sclerosis; HC: healthy controls; PAI-1: plasminogen activator inhibitor-1; MTHFR: methylenetetrahydrofolate reductase; ACE: angiotensin-converting enzyme; Apo: apolipoprotein. Statistically significant value $p < 0.05$ (*).

Individuals homozygous for the FV Leiden, FV R2, and prothrombin G20210A polymorphisms were identified neither in the disease group nor the controls, and the same observation was found when analyzing the Apo B R3500Q variant.

Although there was no significant difference between MS patients and HCs for most of the tested mutations, a statistically significant difference was revealed in the genotype frequencies between MS patients and HCs for the FXIIIVal34Leu and PAI-1 4G/5G polymorphisms, as indicated in Tables 3 and 4, respectively. More specifically, the genotype frequency of heterozygous FXIII V34L was significantly lower in MS patients compared with that in HCs ($p < 0.05$), and simultaneously, it was less associated with the disease occurrence according to the odds ratio (OR: 0.35 (0.12–0.99); $p < 0.05$). Moreover, the frequencies of PAI-1 polymorphisms were 16% for 4G/4G, 46% for 4G/5G, and 38% for 5G/5G in the patient group, whereas the corresponding frequencies in the healthy participants were 32%, 56%, and 12%, respectively. Following a comparison between 4G/4G and 5G/5G homozygous variants, the presence of 5G/5G appears to predominate in the MS group compared with controls ($p = 0.02$), and in regard to the 4G/4G genotype, the presence of the 5G/5G genotype was more likely to be associated with the disease

(OR: 6.33 (95% CI: 1.32–30.24)) (Table 4). This finding was supported further by the analysis of the 5G/5G genotype against the 4G/4G + 4G/5G compound genotypes in both study groups, demonstrating a significant difference ($p = 0.016$) in terms of genotypic frequency, revealing once again that the homozygous 5G/5G genotype was correlated with the disease onset as opposed to the 4G/4G or compound 4G/4G + 4G/5G polymorphisms (OR: 4.80 (1.26–18.31); $p < 0.05$). Similarly, assessing the allele frequency, we observed that the 5G allele distribution was significantly frequent and more likely to be associated with the disease group compared with HCs (OR: 2.39 (1.19–4.81); $p = 0.013$) (Table 6).

3.3. Mutant Allele Presence and Disability Progression in MS

The results of the analysis of MS disability and progression revealed significant findings in terms of genetic variants related to thrombophilia and CVD (Tables 7 and 8). Namely, the presence of the FV Leiden GA genotype was 47% less likely to be associated with advanced disability (OR: 0.53 (0.25–0.90); $p < 0.05$), and this was extended to the FV R2 AG, which had a 54% decrease in the likelihood of increased EDSS (OR: 0.46 (95% CI: 0.19–0.84); $p < 0.001$) and a 40% decrease in MSSS (OR: 0.60 (95% CI: 0.30–0.97)) (Table 7). Furthermore, the results of the analysis of the EDSS and MSSS median indices in regard to the FV polymorphisms demonstrated a lower median index being associated with the mutant genotype compared with the wild type (Table 7).

Table 7. Association of thrombophilia factor genotype with EDSS and MSSS scores.

Risk Factors	Genotype	EDSS			MSSS		
		Median (IQR)	Odds Ratio (95% CI)	*p* Value for OR	Median (IQR)	Odds Ratio (95% CI)	*p* Value for OR
Factor V Leiden	G/G	3.25 (2.50–5.50)	Ref		3.65 (2.64–5.41)	Ref	
	G/A	3.00 (1.75–3.50)	0.53 (0.25–0.90)	0.016 (*)	2.73 (1.90–3.93)	0.70 (0.44–1.06)	0.10
Factor V R2	A/A	3.25 (2.50–5.50)	Ref		3.65 (2.64–5.41)	Ref	
	A/G	1.75 (1.00–4.75)	0.46 (0.19–0.84)	0.008 (**)	2.10 (1.45–4.49)	0.60 (0.30–0.97)	0.038 (*)
Factor FXIII Val34Leu	G/G	3.50 (2.50–5.50)	Ref		3.65 (2.64–5.60)	Ref	
	G/T, T/T	3.00 (2.50–5.75)	1.02 (0.71–1.44)	0.90	4.16 (2.55–6.28)	1.16 (0.87–1.57)	0.31
beta-Fibrinogen −455 G>A	G/G	3.50 (2.50–5.50)	Ref		3.65 (2.50–5.41)	Ref	
	G/A, A/A	3.50 (2.50–5.50)	0.99 (0.72–1.37)	0.99	4.21 (3.02–5.26)	1.06 (0.81–1.40)	0.66
HPA-1	1a/1a	3.25 (2.50–5.50)	Ref		3.65 (2.64–5.41)	Ref	
	1a/1b	4.50 (2.87–6.12)	1.47 (1.03–2.18)	0.03 (*)	4.54 (3.08–6.47)	1.42 (1.05–2.01)	0.02 (*)

EDSS: expanded disability status scale; MSSS: multiple sclerosis severity score; IQR: interquartile range; HPA-1: human platelet antigen 1. Statistically significant values $p < 0.05$ (*), $p < 0.01$ (**).

Interestingly, another significant correlation was observed when assessing the HPA-1a/1b genotype regarding the EDSS ($p < 0.05$) and MSSS ($p < 0.05$). Patients with HPA-1a/1b had a 47% possibility of having an increased disability score (OR: 1.47 (95% CI: 1.03–2.18); $p < 0.05$), whereas the results of the analysis of disease progression, according to the MSSS score, also showed a correlation with the presence of such genotype (OR: 1.42 (95% CI: 1.05–2.01); $p < 0.05$). In parallel, the median index of EDSS was higher in the presence of HPA-1a/1b (median index: 4.5 (IQR: 2.87–6.12)) compared with the HPA-1a/1a genotype (median index: 3.25 (IQR: 2.50–5.50)), which also holds true for MSSS (Table 7).

Table 8. Association of cardiovascular risk factor genotype with EDSS and MSSS scores.

Risk Factors	Genotype	EDSS			MSSS		
		Median (IQR)	**Odds Ratio (95% CI)**	***p* Value for OR**	**Median (IQR)**	**Odds Ratio (95% CI)**	***p* Value for OR**
PAI-1	4G/4G	4.00 (2.75–5.50)	Ref		3.65 (2.40–5.63)	Ref	
	4G/5G, 5G/5G	3.00 (2.50–5.12)	0.79 (0.52–1.20)	0.27	3.50 (2.64–5.03)	0.88 (0.62–1.25)	0.46
MTHFR (C677T)	CC	3.50 (2.50–5.50)	Ref		3.69 (2.64–5.50)	Ref	
	CT, TT	3.50 (2.50–5.50)	1.05 (0.75–1.47)	0.78	3.57 (2.30–5.12)	0.92 (0.70–1.23)	0.60
MTHFR (A1298C)	AA	3.50 (2.50–5.50)	Ref		3.65 (2.64–5.03)	Ref	
	AC, CC	3.00 (2.50–5.50)	1.09 (0.79–1.52)	0.60	4.25 (2.77–6.45)	1.33 (0.99–1.87)	0.055
ACE	I/I	3.00 (2.50–5.50)	Ref		3.50 (2.57–4.64)	Ref	
	I/D, D/D	3.50 (2.50–5.50)	0.81 (0.43–1.58)	0.52	3.57 (2.53–4.98)	0.69 (0.39–1.16)	0.16

EDSS: expanded disability status scale; MSSS: multiple sclerosis severity score; IQR: interquartile range; PAI-1: plasminogen activator inhibitor-1; MTHFR: methylenetetrahydrofolate reductase; ACE: angiotensin-converting enzyme; Apo: apolipoprotein.

The results of a detailed analysis of HPA-1a/1b genotype frequencies indicated that there was a significant difference between male and female patients with MS. As shown in Table 9, male HPA-1a/1b carriers were significantly more likely to have a high EDSS score (OR: 3.04 (1.22–19.54); $p < 0.05$), whereas female carriers showed no significant association. On the other hand, female MS patients carrying the HPA-1a/1b genotype had an increased likelihood to be correlated with an increased MSSS score (OR: 1.56 (1.04–2.61), $p < 0.05$); however, such a correlation was not observed in the group of male patients.

Table 9. Sex-based association of genetic polymorphisms that were correlated with increased EDSS and MSSS scores.

Risk Factors	Genotype	EDSS			MSSS		
		Median (IQR)	**Odds Ratio (95% CI)**	***p* Value for OR**	**Median (IQR)**	**Odds Ratio (95% CI)**	***p* Value for OR**
HPA-1 (Women)	1a/1a	3.00 (2.50–4.00)	Ref		2.64 (1.60–4.25)	Ref	
	1a/1b	4.00 (2.50–5.50)	1.54 (0.90–2.99)	0.11	4.49 (3.01–6.24)	1.56 (1.04–2.61)	0.03 (*)
HPA-1 (Men)	1a/1a	3.50 (2.25–5.50)	Ref		3.69 (2.68–4.98)	Ref	
	1a/1b	6.50 (6.00–8.00)	3.04 (1.22–19.54)	0.01 (*)	6.43 (4.5408.47)	1.63 (0.93–3.35)	0.08
MTHFR (A1298C) (Women)	AA	3.50 (3.00–4.00)	Ref		2.97 (2.30–3.79)	Ref	
	AC, CC	3.00 (2.50–5.25)	0.97 (0.57–1.70)	0.93	4.21 (2.47–6.01)	1.23 (0.84–1.92)	0.29
MTHFR (A1298C) (Men)	AA	3.25 (2.37–5.62)	Ref		3.62 (2.42–4.87)	Ref	
	AC, CC	4.00 (2.62–7.12)	1.21 (0.80–1.91)	0.37	4.38 (3.35–8.35)	1.66 (1.02–3.43)	0.04 (*)

EDSS: expanded disability status scale; MSSS: multiple sclerosis severity score; IQR: interquartile range; HPA-1: human platelet antigen 1; MTHFR: methylenetetrahydrofolate reductase. Statistically significant values $p < 0.05$ (*).

Another important observation was revealed when analyzing the MTHFR A1298C polymorphism. Although there was no association between heterozygous or homozygous genotypes for the MTHFR A1298C polymorphism and the clinical outcomes of the disease, the results of a further analysis in male patients carrying the mutant C allele demonstrated an increased likelihood of having worse MS progression (OR: 1.66 (1.02–3.43), $p < 0.05$), a finding that was not observed in female patients (Table 9).

4. Discussion

MS is a chronic complex disease in which underlying mechanisms influenced by genetic, epigenetic, and environmental factors play a crucial role in disease onset. Although the etiology of MS is still under investigation, changes in the genetic makeup can affect the signaling pathways involved in the onset of MS. Previous studies have highlighted the importance of the interaction between coagulation components and inflammation [5,13,31,32], and, therefore, mutations in genes encoding procoagulant serine proteases or regulators of the coagulation cascade could be essential risk factors for MS.

In this case-control study, we analyzed different mutations identified in related genes to thrombophilia and CVD, and we examined their frequency and impact in patients with MS. In detail, we investigated the FV Leiden polymorphism, FV R2, prothrombin 20210 G>A, FXIII Val34Leu, beta-fibrinogen −455 G>A, HPA1a/1b, MTHFR 677 C>T, MTHFR 1298 A>T, PAI-1 4G/5G, ACE I/D, and Apo B R3500Q, and, to the best of our knowledge, this is the first study assessing such polymorphisms that may increase the predisposition of thrombotic episodes or cardiovascular events in MS, known pathological conditions in early disease occurrence [33,34].

The studied mutations in the FV gene, namely FV Leiden (FV R506Q) and FV R2 (FV H1299R), affect the sensitivity of the FV molecule to APC and disrupt the APC-mediated anticoagulant mechanism. These mutations prevent the binding of the APC to the FVa cleavage site, increasing the resistance to the APC and disrupting the anticoagulant mechanism [35]. In addition, the FV R2 mutation (FV H1299R) promotes the expression of the FV in plasma, which results in increased thrombin generation [36]. FV Leiden is a major risk factor for inherited thrombophilia and is identified in 20–50% of individuals with VTE, whereas the FV R2 mutation increases the risk of VTE and CVD in the presence of FV Leiden. Researchers found that Greek Cypriots from the general population showed heterozygosity of FV Leiden and FV R2 at frequencies of 7% and 10%, respectively [6]. For both mutations, no homozygous cases were identified. In other studies, assessing different ethnic groups, the frequency of heterozygous FV Leiden genotype ranged between 2% and 4% in healthy individuals [29,37], whereas in patients with coronary artery disease, it was 3.7% [29]. Furthermore, a frequency of 9.5% to 16.5% for FV R2 heterozygosity was shown in patients with VTE, in contrast to 5.8% to 10.4% in the general population, having a fluctuation in the proportion due to different ethnicities and sample sizes [38–40]. Our findings were in accordance with previous studies, showing that no homozygous individuals were identified in either the disease group or the control group, revealing similar heterozygous genotype frequencies as well as allele distribution in both study groups. Based on a comprehensive analysis of our findings regarding disability status and disease worsening, it was found that MS patients carrying heterozygous FV Leiden and FV R2 mutations had a reduced risk of developing advanced disability and were less likely to progress to advanced stages of the disease. As far as we know, this is the first study that aimed to correlate the FV Leiden and FV R2 vascular risk factors with clinical outcomes in MS and to deal with their potentially harmful effects on disease progression.

Importantly, FV Leiden carriers are four times more likely to experience recurrent thrombosis, and this finding is further extended to those individuals carrying the compound FV Leiden and prothrombin G20210A mutations, as they are 40% more prone to recurrence of thrombosis and having the first episode under the age of 45 years [7,41]. The prothrombin G20210A variant is correlated with elevated prothrombin levels in plasma, leading to an increased rate of thrombin generation and activation [42]. Studies in patients with coronary artery disease found a low frequency (3.3%) of the prothrombin G20210A heterozygous genotype, whereas the homozygous genotype was not identified [29]. Similarly, patients who developed thromboembolic episodes showed low frequency for the G20210A heterozygous genotype, and no homozygous individual was identified [7]. The findings of our study were consistent with other studies as we detected only one heterozygous case for the prothrombin G20210A variant in the entire cohort of MS participants. In addition, we found no healthy individuals being heterozygous or homozygous for such mutation, further confirming studies from European and non-European countries, in which the G20210A polymorphism is rarely detected in the general population [6].

Interestingly, when analyzing the genotype distribution of FXIII Val34Leu mutation between patients and healthy controls, we found a significant linkage between wild-type FXIII and the disease. Conversely, the heterozygous model of such polymorphism was associated with the control individuals rather than the disease group. It has previously been suggested that FXIII Val34Leu provides a protective effect against thrombosis as it affects the cross-linked structure of fibrin clots and suppresses the mass of thrombi [19,43]. Other researchers reported a high allele frequency, ranging between 21% and 28% for the Val34Leu variant in patients with VTE. Furthermore, they speculated that the Val34Leu variant in the presence of mutations known to promote VTE development, such as FV Leiden and prothrombin G20210A, might disrupt the mechanisms underlying VTE development [6,44]. Our results are consistent with such observations from previous research, highlighting the importance of FXIII in the study of neuroinflammatory diseases like MS.

The results of the analysis of the HPA-1 polymorphism showed differences when assessing disability and disease progression. Based on logistic regression analysis, the HPA-1a/1b genotype was more likely to be associated with increased EDSS and MSSS scores, whereas the HPA-1a/1a genotype was less likely to be associated.

Recent studies highlighted the fact that male MS patients annually experienced a greater deterioration in disability status compared with female patients, and, at the same time, male patients also exhibited disease worsening, including atrophy of the gray matter [45,46]. With regard to the HPA-1 polymorphism, our study showed significant findings due to the sex differences in MS. In comparison with male MS patients with the HPA-1a/1a genotype, male MS patients with the HPA-1a/1b genotype showed a significant association with advanced disability status; however, such an association was not demonstrated for female MS patients harboring the 1b allele. Furthermore, the results of our analysis indicated that in female patients carrying the HPA-1a/1b genotype, there was an increased likelihood of disease progression; however, this was not true for male patients carrying the 1b allele. In view of these findings, it is increasingly clear that sex plays a role in MS severity, even in genetic predispositions that show significant sex differences.

Substitution of proline for leucine at position 33 of the extracellular beta-3 domain of aIIb3 platelet integrin results in a change from HPA-1a to HPA-1b and disrupts the balance of local structure, thereby enhancing the adhesion of platelets to fibrinogen, increasing the flexibility of integrin, and the risk of thrombosis [47]. Our findings support the notion of the HPA-1b contribution to the cross-talk between thrombosis and inflammation, and further studies are required to investigate its role in neuroinflammatory diseases. In addition, the results of the analysis of the HPA-1 polymorphisms in the groups studied showed that only HPA-1a/1a and HPA-1a/1b genotypes were detected, whereas nonhomozygous individuals for the 1b allele were identified. Earlier studies in patients with coronary artery disease reported the presence of HPA-1a/1a and HPA-1a/1b genotypes in the study participants, whereas only HPA-1a/1a was identified in the control group [29]. In contrast, screening Greek Cypriots from the general population showed the presence of the HPA-1b/1b variant at a frequency of 4%, and this supports the notion of further analysis of such polymorphisms to better validate the results [6]. Interestingly, the 1b allele has been associated with the early onset of MI and ischemic stroke, and this has been demonstrated by a large case-control study including 1211 patients from Germany and 510 patients from the U.S.A. with coronary artery disease in which participants carrying the 1b allele had an increased risk of early onset of MI [29].

Moreover, our results showed no significant difference when assessing the frequency distribution of the beta-fibrinogen (−455 G>A) genotype in the studied groups or the association between beta-fibrinogen (−455 G>A) and disability or disease progression.

Consistent with our findings, a large investigation involving 426 patients who had suffered an ischemic stroke and 234 healthy volunteers showed no difference in the frequency of the beta-fibrinogen 455 G>A mutation between the study groups [29]. In addition, a study on MS found a weak association between the −455 G>A mutation and disease, further supporting a weak contribution to disease susceptibility [48]. Nonetheless, homozygosity for −455 G>A represents an increased risk factor for VTE and ischemic stroke, which are pathological conditions that occur at the early stages of MS [11,43]. Since fibrinogen deposition in the CNS of MS animal models has been shown to affect microglial activity, cause abnormal BBB permeability that contributes to T lymphocyte infiltration, and enhance the interplay between coagulation and inflammation in pre-demyelinated regions [49], the beta-fibrinogen 455 G>A mutation should be further investigated with respect to the content of fibrinogen accumulation, since 455 G>A mutation associated with elevated plasma fibrinogen levels.

Importantly, the underlying mechanisms that are involved in the VTE and CVD onset have also been linked to the presence of the PAI-1 4G/5G polymorphism [16,43]. Although PAI-1 plays an essential role in the fibrinolytic system by inhibiting tPA, hence suppressing plasmin formation, only a few studies have examined the impact of the PAI-1 4G/5G polymorphism on the coagulation–neuroinflammation circuit [50]. Research on CVD, especially on MI, has demonstrated that the 4G allele is a high-risk factor for disease onset [6], whereas in patients with coronary artery disease, the 4G allele was detected more frequently than the 5G allele [51,52]. On the contrary, the 4G allele seems to have a neuroprotective effect against cerebral ischemia, whereas the 5G allele and 5G/5G genotype have been correlated with hemorrhage in post-lysis stroke patients [53]. In the current study, we achieved to show that the 5G allele and 5G/5G genotype were associated with MS susceptibility, demonstrating an increased prevalence compared with healthy participants, which can serve as a predictor risk factor for the occurrence of the disease. Similarly, a previous study on MS found that 5G/5G was associated with harmful effects on MS susceptibility, and the genotype PAI-1 5G/5G by itself or together with the tPA I allele could be crucial risk factors for MS onset [16].

No significant difference in the genotype distribution was observed between MS patients and controls when analyzing MTHFR 677 C>T and 1298 A>C polymorphisms. According to the results of the odds analysis, there was no significant probability of correlating the genotypes with the onset of MS. Previous research on MS showed that the MTHFR 1298 A>C variant was more likely to be associated with disease onset than the MTHFR 6777 C>T variant [54]. Nonetheless, other studies have not found any correlation between mutations and MS, but this may be due to a small study population and different ethnicity, which could account for a different genetic makeup between the study groups [55,56]. In a comprehensive analysis regarding sex, we discovered that men who carried the mutant allele had a greater likelihood of experiencing worse MS progression, but female carriers were not affected. In addition to confirming that disease progression is more severe in male MS patients than in female patients, our results indicate that genetic markers not only may serve as potential biomarkers for the disease but also could be predictive of disease worsening or advanced disability in male patients [45,46].

ACE I/D and Apo B R3500Q polymorphisms have also been associated with thrombosis and CVD since they increase the risk of MI and thrombotic episodes, whereas the ACE D/D variant has also been linked to elevated plasma levels of ACE and suppression of fibrinolysis [57,58]. In the current study, we observed similar frequencies of the ACE I/D and Apo B R3500Q variants between MS patients and healthy controls, and our findings were in agreement with previous studies in the coronary artery that did not demonstrate any correlation between disease occurrence and such mutations [29].

The current research project has some limitations that warrant discussion. Considering the small sample size of participants and the fact that they represent only one population, the statistical power may be diminished, affecting the validity of substantial conclusions. Moreover, the study was limited to patients who tested positive for IgG antibodies against seven coagulant serine proteases, i.e., FVIIa, thrombin, prothrombin, FXa, FXII, plasmin, and protein C. Therefore, further studies are needed to validate our results, recruiting large case-control groups from a wide range of ethnicities to shed more light on the context of gene–gene interactions, combined mutations, and molecular mechanisms that play a crucial role in the coagulation–inflammation interplay. In addition, a comparison of patients who tested positive for antibodies against serine proteases of the coagulation cascade and those who were negative will provide further data on neuroinflammation and neurodegeneration regarding the genetic polymorphisms related to coagulation or thrombosis. Furthermore, the present study focused on identifying high-risk polymorphisms in MS patients. To characterize the role of such polymorphisms and gain a better understanding of the mechanisms that underlie MS pathology, preclinical studies should also be considered. Genetic polymorphisms related to thrombosis could serve as biomarkers for disease prognosis and monitoring and could also be a potential target in therapeutic strategies.

5. Conclusions

In conclusion, compelling evidence was revealed when assessing MS occurrence with genetic markers related to thrombophilia and CVD. Among the eleven polymorphisms studied, the homozygous PAI-1 5G/5G genotype and PAI-1 5G allele were found to play a role in MS, whereas the FXIII Val34Leu polymorphism demonstrated a protective role. According to the best of our knowledge, this is the first study to examine such polymorphisms and disease outcomes, finding a positive association between HPA-1a/1b and advanced disability as well as disease severity. The results of an in-depth analysis further revealed the differences regarding sex, demonstrating that disability was associated with male patients carrying the HPA-1b allele, whereas female carriers of HPA-1b were more likely to be correlated with an increase in MS severity. The severity of MS was also significantly increased in male patients carrying the mutant allele of MTHFR 1298 A>C but not in female carriers. Consequently, our findings emphasize the importance of genetics in the MS population and the impact that different genotypes may have on patients' clinical outcomes.

Supplementary Materials: The following supporting information can be downloaded at: https://www.mdpi.com/article/10.3390/biomedicines10102665/s1, Table S1: Demographic and laboratory findings of healthy controls (HC) for thrombophilia risk factors; Table S2: Demographic and laboratory findings of healthy controls (HC) for cardiovascular risk factors; Table S3: Demographic, clinical, and laboratory findings of patients with multiple sclerosis (MS); Table S4: Laboratory findings of patients with multiple sclerosis (MS) for thrombophilia risk factors; Table S5: Laboratory findings of patients with multiple sclerosis (MS) for cardiovascular risk factors.

Author Contributions: A.L. conceived and designed the study. M.P. and E.D. recruited the patients. M.S.H., G.K. (George Kallis) and A.P. performed the main experiment work and analyzed and interpreted the data. M.S.H., A.L., G.K. (George Krashias), C.C., P.C. and M.P. drafted the manuscript. M.S.H. prepared the tables. All authors revised the manuscript. All authors provided substantial input throughout the process. All authors have read and agreed to the published version of the manuscript.

Funding: This work was funded by the Cyprus Institute of Neurology and Genetics.

Institutional Review Board Statement: The study was conducted in accordance with the Declaration of Helsinki, and approved by the Institutional Review Board (or Ethics Committee) of the Cyprus National Bioethics Committee (EEBK/EΠ/2016/51 obtained in 2016).

Informed Consent Statement: All procedures were carried out according to the ethical standards of the Cyprus National Bioethics Committee. Informed consent was obtained from all subjects involved in the study (EEBK/EΠ/2016/51).

Data Availability Statement: The data that support the findings of this study are available from the corresponding author upon reasonable request.

Acknowledgments: We would like to thank all patients and healthy participants at the Cyprus Institute of Neurology and Genetics for donating blood for this research. We would like to express our deepest gratitude to Kyriaki Michailidou for guidance on statistical analysis. Special thanks are given to Efthychia Gagglia, Irene Smoleski, and Andria Xyrichi for their assistance in blood sample collection.

Conflicts of Interest: All authors have no potential conflict of interest to report.

References

1. Lennon, R.P.; Claussen, K.A.; Kuersteiner, K.A. State of the Heart: An Overview of the Disease Burden of Cardiovascular Disease from an Epidemiologic Perspective. *Prim. Care-Clin. Off. Pract.* **2018**, *45*, 1–15. [CrossRef] [PubMed]
2. Jadidi, E.; Mohammadi, M.; Moradi, T. High Risk of Cardiovascular Diseases after Diagnosis of Multiple Sclerosis. *Mult. Scler. J.* **2013**, *19*, 1336–1340. [CrossRef] [PubMed]
3. Tseng, C.H.; Huang, W.S.; Lin, C.L.; Chang, Y.J. Increased Risk of Ischaemic Stroke among Patients with Multiple Sclerosis. *Eur. J. Neurol.* **2015**, *22*, 500–506. [CrossRef] [PubMed]
4. Palladino, R.; Marrie, R.A.; Majeed, A.; Chataway, J. Evaluating the Risk of Macrovascular Events and Mortality among People with Multiple Sclerosis in England. *JAMA Neurol.* **2020**, *77*, 820–828. [CrossRef]
5. Koudriavtseva, T. Thrombotic Processes in Multiple Sclerosis as Manifestation of Innate Immune Activation. *Front. Neurol.* **2014**, *5*, 119. [CrossRef] [PubMed]
6. Koumas, L.; Costeas, P.A.; Papaloizou, A.; Giantsiou-Kyriakou, A. Genetic Assessment of Cardiovascular Risk Factors in the Greek Cypriot Population. *Thromb. Res.* **2003**, *112*, 143–146. [CrossRef]
7. Friedline, J.A.; Ahmad, E.; Garcia, D.; Blue, D.; Ceniza, N.; Mattson, J.C.; Crisan, D. Combined Factor V Leiden and Prothrombin Genotyping in Patients Presenting with Thromboembolic Episodes. *Arch. Pathol. Lab. Med.* **2001**, *125*, 105–111. [CrossRef] [PubMed]
8. Gehring, N.H.; Frede, U.; Neu-Yilik, G.; Hundsdoerfer, P.; Vetter, B.; Hentze, M.W.; Kulozik, A.E. Increased Efficiency of MRNA 3′ End Formation: A New Genetic Mechanism Contributing to Hereditary Thrombophilia. *Nat. Genet.* **2001**, *28*, 389–392. [CrossRef]
9. Spiroski, I. Factor V Leiden (G1691A), Factor V R2 (A4070G), and Prothrombin (G20210A) Genetic Polymorphisms in Macedonian Patients with Occlusive Artery Disease and Deep Vein Thrombosis. *South East Eur. J. Cardiol.* **2015**, 2015. [CrossRef]
10. Klajmon, A.; Chmiel, J.; Ząbczyk, M.; Pociask, E.; Wypasek, E.; Malinowski, K.P.; Undas, A.; Natorska, J. Fibrinogen β Chain and FXIII Polymorphisms Affect Fibrin Clot Properties in Acute Pulmonary Embolism. *Eur. J. Clin. Investig.* **2022**, *52*, e13718. [CrossRef]
11. Hu, X.; Wang, J.; Li, Y.; Wu, J.; Qiao, S.; Xu, S.; Huang, J.; Chen, L. The β-Fibrinogen Gene 455G/A Polymorphism Associated with Cardioembolic Stroke in Atrial Fibrillation with Low CHA2DS2-VaSc Score. *Sci. Rep.* **2017**, *7*, 17517. [CrossRef] [PubMed]
12. Martiskainen, M.; Oksala, N.; Pohjasvaara, T.; Kaste, M.; Oksala, A.; Karhunen, P.J.; Erkinjuntti, T. Beta-Fibrinogen Gene Promoter A -455 Allele Associated with Poor Longterm Survival among 55 71 Years Old Caucasian Women in Finnish Stroke Cohort. *BMC Neurol.* **2014**, *14*, 137. [CrossRef] [PubMed]
13. Davalos, D.; Baeten, K.M.; Whitney, M.A.; Mullins, E.S.; Friedman, B.; Olson, E.S.; Ryu, J.K.; Smirnoff, D.S.; Petersen, M.A.; Bedard, C.; et al. Early Detection of Thrombin Activity in Neuroinflammatory Disease. *Ann. Neurol.* **2014**, *75*, 303–308. [CrossRef] [PubMed]
14. Shammaa, D.M.R.; Sabbagh, A.S.; Taher, A.T.; Zaatari, G.S.; Mahfouz, R.A.R. Plasminogen Activator Inhibitor-1 (PAI-1) Gene 4G/5G Alleles Frequency Distribution in the Lebanese Population. *Mol. Biol. Rep.* **2008**, *35*, 453–457. [CrossRef]
15. Zhang, T.; Pang, C.; Li, N.; Zhou, E.; Zhao, K. Plasminogen Activator Inhibitor-1 4G/5G Polymorphism and Retinopathy Risk in Type 2 Diabetes: A Meta-Analysis. *BMC Med.* **2013**, *11*, 1–9. [CrossRef] [PubMed]
16. Živković, M.; Starčević Čizmarević, N.; Lovrečić, L.; Klupka-Sarić, I.; Stanković, A.; Gašparović, I.; Lavtar, P.; Dinčić, E.; Stojković, L.; Rudolf, G.; et al. The Role of TPA I/D and PAI-1 4G/5G Polymorphisms in Multiple Sclerosis. *Dis. Mark.* **2014**, *2014*, 362708. [CrossRef] [PubMed]
17. Duval, C.; Ali, M.; Chaudhry, W.W.; Ridger, V.C.; Ariëns, R.A.S.; Philippou, H. Factor XIII A-Subunit V34L Variant Affects Thrombus Cross-Linking in a Murine Model of Thrombosis. *Arterioscler. Thromb. Vasc. Biol.* **2016**, *36*, 308–316. [CrossRef]
18. Wells, P.S.; Anderson, J.L.; Scarvelis, D.K.; Doucette, S.P.; Gagnon, F. Factor XIII Val34Leu Variant Is Protective against Venous Thromboembolism: A HuGE Review and Meta-Analysis. *Am. J. Epidemiol.* **2006**, *164*, 101–109. [CrossRef] [PubMed]
19. Kattula, S.; Bagoly, Z.; Tóth, N.K.; Muszbek, L.; Wolberg, A.S. The Factor XIII-A Val34Leu Polymorphism Decreases Whole Blood Clot Mass at High Fibrinogen Concentrations. *J. Thromb. Haemost.* **2020**, *18*, 885–894. [CrossRef]
20. Naghibalhossaini, F.; Ehyakonandeh, H.; Nikseresht, A.; Kamali, E. Association Between MTHFR Genetic Variants and Multiple Sclerosis in a Southern Iranian Population. *Int. J. Mol. Cell. Med.* **2015**, *4*, 82.
21. Poddar, R.; Paul, S. Homocysteine-NMDA Receptor-Mediated Activation of Extracellular Signal-Regulated Kinase Leads to Neuronal Cell Death. *J. Neurochem.* **2009**, *110*, 1095–1106. [CrossRef] [PubMed]
22. Deep, S.N.; Mitra, S.; Rajagopal, S.; Paul, S.; Poddar, R. GluN2A-NMDA Receptor-Mediated Sustained Ca2+ Influx Leads to Homocysteine-Induced Neuronal Cell Death. *J. Biol. Chem.* **2019**, *294*, 11154–11165. [CrossRef] [PubMed]

23. Ramsaransing, G.S.M.; Fokkema, M.R.; Teelken, A.; Arutjunyan, A.V.; Koch, M.; De Keyser, J. Plasma Homocysteine Levels in Multiple Sclerosis. *J. Neurol. Neurosurg. Psychiatry* **2006**, *77*, 189–192. [CrossRef] [PubMed]
24. Li, Y.; Qiu, S.; Shi, J.; Guo, Y.; Li, Z.; Cheng, Y.; Liu, Y. Association between MTHFR C677T/A1298C and Susceptibility to Autism Spectrum Disorders: A Meta-Analysis. *BMC Pediatr.* **2020**, *20*, 449. [CrossRef] [PubMed]
25. Brown, N.M.; Pratt, V.M.; Buller, A.; Pike-Buchanan, L.; Redman, J.B.; Sun, W.; Chen, R.; Crossley, B.; McGinniss, M.J.; Quan, F.; et al. Detection of 677CT/1298AC "Double Variant" Chromosomes: Implications for Interpretation of MTHFR Genotyping Results. *Genet. Med.* **2005**, *7*, 278–282. [CrossRef] [PubMed]
26. Bouzidi, N.; Hassine, M.; Fodha, H.; Ben Messaoud, M.; Maatouk, F.; Gamra, H.; Ferchichi, S. Association of the Methylene-Tetrahydrofolate Reductase Gene Rs1801133 C677T Variant with Serum Homocysteine Levels, and the Severity of Coronary Artery Disease. *Sci. Rep.* **2020**, *10*, 10064. [CrossRef] [PubMed]
27. Ghazouani, L.; Abboud, N.; Mtiraoui, N.; Zammiti, W.; Addad, F.; Amin, H.; Almawi, W.Y.; Mahjoub, T. Homocysteine and Methylenetetrahydrofolate Reductase C677T and A1298C Polymorphisms in Tunisian Patients with Severe Coronary Artery Disease. *J. Thromb. Thrombolysis* **2009**, *27*, 191–197. [CrossRef] [PubMed]
28. Saidi, S.; Mahjoub, T.; Slamia, L.B.; Ammou, S.B.; Al-Subaie, A.M.; Almawi, W.Y. Polymorphisms of the Human Platelet Alloantigens HPA-1, HPA-2, HPA-3, and HPA-4 in Ischemic Stroke. *Am. J. Hematol.* **2008**, *83*, 570–573. [CrossRef] [PubMed]
29. Gulsah, D.; Nevin, K.; Serkan, Y.; Nurten, K. Analysis of Twelve Cardiovascular Disease Related Gene Mutations among Turkish Patients with Coronary Artery Disease. *Int. J. Blood Res. Disord.* **2020**, *7*, 074. [CrossRef]
30. Polman, C.H.; Reingold, S.C.; Banwell, B.; Clanet, M.; Cohen, J.A.; Filippi, M.; Fujihara, K.; Havrdova, E.; Hutchinson, M.; Kappos, L.; et al. Diagnostic Criteria for Multiple Sclerosis: 2010 Revisions to the McDonald Criteria. *Ann. Neurol.* **2011**, *69*, 292–302. [CrossRef] [PubMed]
31. Hadjiagapiou, M.S.; Krashias, G.; Deeba, E.; Christodoulou, C.; Pantzaris, M.; Lambrianides, A. Antibodies to Blood Coagulation Components Are Implicated in Patients with Multiple Sclerosis. *Mult. Scler. Relat. Disord.* **2022**, *62*, 103775. [CrossRef]
32. Göbel, K.; Kraft, P.; Pankratz, S.; Gross, C.C.; Korsukewitz, C.; Kwiecien, R.; Mesters, R.; Kehrel, B.E.; Wiendl, H.; Kleinschnitz, C.; et al. Prothrombin and Factor X Are Elevated in Multiple Sclerosis Patients. *Ann. Neurol.* **2016**, *80*, 946–951. [CrossRef] [PubMed]
33. Ahmed, O.; Geraldes, R.; DeLuca, G.C.; Palace, J. Multiple Sclerosis and the Risk of Systemic Venous Thrombosis: A Systematic Review. *Mult. Scler. Relat. Disord.* **2019**, *27*, 424–430. [CrossRef] [PubMed]
34. Christiansen, C.F. Risk of Vascular Disease in Patients with Multiple Sclerosis: A Review. *Neurol. Res.* **2012**, *34*, 746–753. [CrossRef] [PubMed]
35. Castoldi, E. FV and APC Resistance: The Plot Thickens. *Blood* **2014**, *123*, 2288–2289. [CrossRef]
36. Castoldi, E.; Simioni, P.; Kalafatis, M.; Lunghi, B.; Tormene, D.; Girelli, D.; Girolami, A.; Bernardi, F. Combinations of 4 Mutations (FV R506Q, FV H1299R, FV Y1702C, PT 20210G/A) Affecting the Prothrombinase Complex in a Thrombophilic Family. *Blood* **2000**, *96*, 1443–1448. [CrossRef]
37. Slowik, A.; Dziedzic, T.; Turaj, W.; Pera, J.; Glodzik-Sobanska, L.; Szermer, P.; Malecki, M.T.; Figlewicz, D.A.; Szczudlik, A. A2 Alelle of GpIIIa Gene Is a Risk Factor for Stroke Caused by Large-Vessel Disease in Males. *Stroke* **2004**, *35*, 1589–1593. [CrossRef] [PubMed]
38. Faioni, E.M.; Castaman, G.; Asti, D.; Lussana, F.; Rodeghiero, F. Association of Factor V Deficiency with Factor V HR2. *Haematologica* **2004**, *89*, 195–200. [PubMed]
39. Margaglione, M.; Bossone, A.; Coalizzo, D.; D'Andrea, G.; Brancaccio, V.; Ciampa, A.; Grandone, E.; Di Minno, G. FV HR2 Haplotype as Additional Inherited Risk Factor for Deep Vein Thrombosis in Individuals with a High-Risk Profile. *Thromb. Haemost.* **2002**, *87*, 32–36. [CrossRef]
40. Pecheniuk, N.M.; Morris, C.P.; Walsh, T.P.; Marsh, N.A. The Factor V HR2 Haplotype: Prevalence and Association of the A4070G and A6755G Polymorphisms. *Blood Coagul. Fibrinolysis* **2001**, *12*, 201–206. [CrossRef] [PubMed]
41. Federici, E.H.; Al-Mondhiry, H. High Risk of Thrombosis Recurrence in Patients with Homozygous and Compound Heterozygous Factor V R506Q (Factor V Leiden) and Prothrombin G20210A. *Thromb. Res.* **2019**, *182*, 75–78. [CrossRef]
42. Demirci, F.Y.K.; Dressen, A.S.; Kammerer, C.M.; Barmada, M.M.; Kao, A.H.; Ramsey-Goldman, R.; Manzi, S.; Kamboh, M.I. Functional Polymorphisms of the Coagulation Factor II Gene (F2) and Susceptibility to Systemic Lupus Erythematosus. *J. Rheumatol.* **2011**, *38*, 652–657. [CrossRef] [PubMed]
43. Hoteit, R.; Abbas, F.; Antar, A.; Abdel Khalek, R.; Shammaa, D.; Mahfouz, R. Significance of the Use of the ViennaLab "Cardiovascular Disease Panel" (CVD) Assay as a Reflex Test for the "Factor V/II/MTHFR Assay.". *Meta Gene* **2013**, *1*, 76–81. [CrossRef]
44. Renner, W.; Köppel, H.; Hoffmann, C.; Schallmoser, K.; Stanger, O.; Toplak, H.; Wascher, T.C.; Pilger, E. Prothrombin G20210A, Factor V Leiden, and Factor XIII Val34Leu: Common Mutations of Blood Coagulation Factors and Deep Vein Thrombosis in Austria. *Thromb. Res.* **2000**, *99*, 35–39. [CrossRef]
45. Voskuhl, R.R.; Patel, K.; Paul, F.; Gold, S.M.; Scheel, M.; Kuchling, J.; Cooper, G.; Asseyer, S.; Chien, C.; Brandt, A.U.; et al. Sex Differences in Brain Atrophy in Multiple Sclerosis. *Biol. Sex Differ.* **2020**, *11*, 49. [CrossRef] [PubMed]
46. Coyle, P.K. What Can We Learn from Sex Differences in MS? *J. Pers. Med.* **2021**, *11*, 1006. [CrossRef] [PubMed]
47. Jallu, V.; Poulain, P.; Fuchs, P.F.J.; Kaplan, C.; de Brevern, A.G. Modeling and Molecular Dynamics of HPA-1a and -1b Polymorphisms: Effects on the Structure of the B3 Subunit of the AIIbβ3 Integrin. *PLoS ONE* **2012**, *7*, e47304. [CrossRef] [PubMed]

48. Abbadessa, G.; Miele, G.; Di Pietro, A.; Sparaco, M.; Palladino, R.; Armetta, I.; D'Elia, G.; Trojsi, F.; Signoriello, E.; Giacomo Lus, G.; et al. Multiple Sclerosis and Genetic Polymorphisms in Fbrinogen-mediated Hemostatic Pathways: A Case–Control Study. *Neurol. Sci.* **2022**, *43*, 2601–2609. [CrossRef] [PubMed]
49. Davalos, D.; Akassoglou, K. Fibrinogen as a Key Regulator of Inflammation in Disease. *Semin. Immunopathol.* **2012**, *34*, 43–62. [CrossRef]
50. Sillen, M.; Declerck, P.J. Targeting PAI-1 in Cardiovascular Disease: Structural Insights Into PAI-1 Functionality and Inhibition. *Front. Cardiovasc. Med.* **2020**, *7*, 364. [CrossRef]
51. Abboud, N.; Ghazouani, L.; Saidi, S.; Ben-Hadj-Khalifa, S.; Addad, F.; Almawi, W.Y.; Mahjoub, T. Association of PAI-1 4G/5G and -844G/A Gene Polymorphisms and Changes in PAI-1/Tissue Plasminogen Activator Levels in Myocardial Infarction: A Case-Control Study. *Genet. Test. Mol. Biomark.* **2010**, *14*, 23–27. [CrossRef] [PubMed]
52. Isordia-Salas, I.; Leaños-Miranda, A.; Sainz, I.M.; Reyes-Maldonado, E.; Borrayo-Sánchez, G. Association of the Plasminogen Activator Inhibitor-1 Gene 4G/5G Polymorphism With ST Elevation Acute Myocardial Infarction in Young Patients. *Rev. Esp. Cardiol. (Engl. Ed.)* **2009**, *62*, 365–372. [CrossRef]
53. Szegedi, I.; Nagy, A.; Székely, E.G.; Czuriga-Kovács, K.R.; Sarkady, F.; Lánczi, L.I.; Berényi, E.; Csiba, L.; Bagoly, Z. PAI-1 5G/5G Genotype Is an Independent Risk of Intracranial Hemorrhage in Post-Lysis Stroke Patients. *Ann. Clin. Transl. Neurol.* **2019**, *6*, 2240–2250. [CrossRef] [PubMed]
54. Ineichen, B.V.; Keskitalo, S.; Farkas, M.; Bain, N.; Kallweit, U.; Weller, M.; Klotz, L.; Linnebank, M. Genetic Variants of Homocysteine Metabolism and Multiple Sclerosis: A Case-Control Study. *Neurosci. Lett.* **2014**, *562*, 75–78. [CrossRef] [PubMed]
55. Szvetko, A.L.; Fowdar, J.; Nelson, J.; Colson, N.; Tajouri, L.; Csurhes, P.A.; Pender, M.P.; Griffiths, L.R. No Association between MTHFR A1298C and MTRR A66G Polymorphisms, and MS in an Australian Cohort. *J. Neurol. Sci.* **2007**, *252*, 49–52. [CrossRef]
56. Tajouri, L.; Martin, V.; Gasparini, C.; Ovcaric, M.; Curtain, R.; Lea, R.A.; Haupt, L.M.; Csurhes, P.; Pender, M.P.; Griffiths, L.R. Genetic Investigation of Methylenetetrahydrofolate Reductase (MTHFR) and Catechol-O-Methyl Transferase (COMT) in Multiple Sclerosis. *Brain Res. Bull.* **2006**, *69*, 327–331. [CrossRef] [PubMed]
57. Fawzy, M.S.; Toraih, E.A.; Aly, N.M.; Fakhr-Eldeen, A.; Badran, D.I.; Hussein, M.H. Atherosclerotic and Thrombotic Genetic and Environmental Determinants in Egyptian Coronary Artery Disease Patients: A Pilot Study. *BMC Cardiovasc. Disord.* **2017**, *17*, 26. [CrossRef]
58. Ohira, N.; Matsumoto, T.; Tamaki, S.; Takashima, H.; Tarutani, Y.; Yamane, T.; Yasuda, Y.; Horie, M. Angiotensin-Converting Enzyme Insertion/Deletion Polymorphism Modulates Coronary Release of Tissue Plasminogen Activator in Response to Bradykinin. *Hypertens. Res.* **2004**, *27*, 39–45. [CrossRef]

biomedicines

MDPI

Article

Countermovement Jumps Detect Subtle Motor Deficits in People with Multiple Sclerosis below the Clinical Threshold

Anne Geßner †, Heidi Stölzer-Hutsch †, Katrin Trentzsch, Dirk Schriefer and Tjalf Ziemssen *

Center of Clinical Neuroscience, Neurological Clinic, University Hospital Carl Gustav Carus, TU Dresden, Fetscherstr. 74, 01307 Dresden, Germany

* Correspondence: tjalf.ziemssen@uniklinikum-dresden.de; Tel.: +49-351-458-4465; Fax: +49-351-458-5717

† These authors contributed equally to this work.

Abstract: In the early stages of multiple sclerosis (MS), there are currently no sensitive assessments to evaluate complex motor functions. The countermovement jump (CMJ), a high-challenge task in form of a maximal vertical bipedal jump, has already been investigated as a reliable assessment in healthy subjects for lower extremity motor function. The aim was to investigate whether it is possible to use CMJ to identify subthreshold motor deficits in people with multiple sclerosis (pwMS). All participants (99 pwMS and 33 healthy controls) performed three maximal CMJs on a force plate. PwMS with full motor function and healthy controls (HC) did not differ significantly in age, disease duration, Body Mass Index and the Expanded Disability Scale Score. In comparison to HC, pwMS with full motor function demonstrated a significantly decreased CMJ performance in almost all observed kinetic, temporal and performance parameters ($p < 0.05$). With increasing disability in pwMS, it was also observed that jump performance decreased significantly. This study showed that the CMJ, as a high challenge task, could detect motor deficits in pwMS below the clinical threshold of careful neurological examination. Longitudinal studies are pending to evaluate whether the CMJ can be used as a standardized measure of disease progression.

Keywords: multiple sclerosis; motor deficits; assessment; jump analysis; countermovement jump

1. Introduction

Multiple sclerosis (MS) is an inflammatory chronic disease of the central nervous system, which damages the myelin layer of the nerve fibers [1]. Therefore, early initiation of therapy is critical for a more favourable progression of disease [2]. MS often results in decreased motor functions, which may rely upon integrated involvement of neuromuscular, neurosensory, musculoskeletal, and cardiopulmonary systems [3]. Equally as complex as the motor system is the identification of subtle motor deficits in people with multiple sclerosis (pwMS).

In the early stage of disease in MS, when pwMS have no or minimal disability, there are currently no sensitive objective assessments to identify subtle motor deficits in the lower extremities as well as to identify and quantify early deficits in complex movements. However, the ability to identify, specify and monitor subtle motor impairments is critical to the management of optimal disease-modifying and symptomatic treatment [4]. In the early stages of MS, neurological reserve can functionally compensate for neuronal damage caused by the demyelinating lesions through various mechanisms involving, for example, cerebral reorganization [5,6]. Currently, the assessment of MS patients occurs as a neurological examination and on rare occasions by a standardized functional test.

Neurological examination is standardized using the Expanded Disability Status Scale (EDSS) [7]

Krieger et al. [8] reported in their study, that traditional clinical measures (i.e., EDSS) did not distinguish neurologically "normal" pwMS (i.e., EDSS 0) from healthy controls

(HC). High-challenge tasks were more sensitive to subtle deficits than traditional clinical measures in pwMS with an EDSS 0 and could detect subthreshold impairments and identify underlying disease burden [8]. Assessments such as the EDSS are quite subjective in evaluating the different functional systems separately [9]. In contrast, high-challenge tasks represent a complex integration of different functional systems (e.g., motor, cerebellar, sensory) requiring great physical effort.

The countermovement jump (CMJ) exemplifies a high-challenge task, challenging the neuromuscular system by combining strength, balance, coordination and muscle timing in one assessment. As a type of vertical jump, the CMJ works on the principle of the stretch-shortening cycle (SSC). The SSC is defined as a high-intensity eccentric contraction immediately before a rapid concentric contraction and occurs in natural movements such as walking and running [10].

The CMJ is commonly used in professional sports to assess lower-body ballistic performance and monitor the effectiveness of training programs [11–13]. Many research studies confirm the high validity and reliability of the CMJ on force plates to assess motor function of the lower extremity in a variety of clinical settings [12,14–20].

To our knowledge, there are no studies that investigate CMJ performance in MS. Two pilot studies from Kirkland et al. [21,22] provide the first evidence that jump tasks can detect differences between pwMS with mild disability and healthy controls and that they are a potentially useful measurement of lower limb function in pwMS. However, in contrast to our study, Kirkland et al. assessed the use of horizontal jumps on an instrumental walkway system with small sample size. The combination of multiple domains in one test enables the identification of deficits and facilitates adequate rehabilitation [4].

In this study, we created a MS group equal to HC according to the degree of disability, motor function assessed with EDSS and physical activity. We aimed first (i) to investigate the CMJ performance between pwMS groups and HC and second (ii) to evaluate the suitability of the CMJ for detecting motor deficits in pwMS below the clinical threshold of the pyramidal FSS. The clinical threshold is defined by clinical signs of an underlying burden of disease. Below the clinical threshold, clinical signs may not be apparent on routine clinical examination, and when lesions cross the clinical threshold, clinical symptoms occur [8]. The third aim (iii) was to assess the CMJ performance complementary to subthreshold EDSS measures in sensory and cerebellar FSS.

2. Materials and Methods

2.1. Participants

We conducted a cross-sectional study in the MS Center at the Center of Clinical Neuroscience of the Department of Neurology, University Hospital Carl Gustav Carus, Dresden, Germany. HC without neurological disease and pwMS were invited to participate. We recruited 189 subjects between April 2021 and September 2021. All participants provided written informed consent for the study. The study was approved by the local ethics committee (BO-EK-320062021).

Inclusion criteria were as follows: (a) presence of confirmed MS diagnosis according to McDonald's criteria, (b) relapse-free status in the past 3 months, (c) EDSS Score between 0 and 5.0, (d) age between 18 and 65 years, (e) ability to walk without aid and rest for $\geq$500 m and (f) to perform heel rise, stand on heels and perform squats. Prior to jump testing, physical activity was assessed by patients using Godin Leisure Time Exercise Questionnaire (GLTEQ). Exclusion criteria were with the presence of orthopedic and surgical disorders that affect jumping, history of falls in the past month, fear of falling while jumping and current pregnancy. In all study participants, first the EDSS was recorded, followed by the GLTEQ and finally the CMJs.

To standardize physical performance, a GLTEQ-Score $\geq$ 24 provided the basis of participants included in the analysis. Further, for comparability in terms of motor skills between pwMS and HC, two groups were divided retrospectively in pwMS with normal (full) motor function (pwMS $_{\text{motor normal}}$) and pwMS with impaired motor function (pwMS $_{motor\ impaired}$). PwMS $_{motor\ normal}$ were defined as having an EDSS score $\leq$ 1.5, with no motor abnormalities and disability appearing below this clinical threshold. As per the EDSS classification, an EDSS Score $\leq$ 1.5 resulted in pyramidal FSS of 0–1, normal muscle strength and unimpaired monopedal hopping. In all these items, the pwMS $_{motor\ normal}$ were equal to the HC. The pwMS $_{motor\ impaired}$ showed an EDSS score $\geq$ 2 and therefore a pyramidal FSS of 2–4, reduced muscle strength and impaired monopedal hopping. Hence, this group was above the clinical threshold. In a final step, to test the suitability of the CMJ, only pwMS $_{unimpaired}$ and HC were compared. Notably, both groups showed normal results in the cerebellar and sensory functional systems which affect the neuromuscular control and motor function.

2.2. Assessments

2.2.1. Expanded Disability Status Scale (EDSS)

To examine the clinical status, the EDSS was assessed by certified raters in pwMS including MS-specific pyramidal, cerebellar and sensory FSS [9]. The EDSS is the most used disability scale in MS and is well established among neurologists [23]. In this study, HC were also examined with the complete EDSS. Participants were classified according to Kurtzke [9] as follows:

(a) No disability in pyramidal FSS: pyramidal $\leq$ 1.
(b) Normal sensory and cerebellar function: sensory FSS = 0 and cerebellar FSS = 0.

As part of the EDSS in the pyramidal FSS, the British Medical Research Council Rating Scale (BMRC) was assessed for lower extremity muscles [24]. Participants were classified according to BMRC as follows:

(a) Participants with normal muscle strength: full strength in all assessed muscle groups of the lower extremity.
(b) Participants with reduced muscle strength: not full strength in one or more muscle groups of the lower extremity.

Monopedal hopping was also performed as a part of the pyramidal FSS in the EDSS. Participants were classified according to monopedal hopping as follows:

(a) Participants with monopedal hopping unimpaired: normal, 10 jumps performed on one leg right and left.
(b) Participants with monopedal hopping impaired: less than 10 jumps on one or both legs.

2.2.2. Godin Leisure Time Exercise Questionnaire (GLTEQ)

The GLTEQ is a validated patient-reported outcome (PRO) for measuring simple and effective physical activity in pwMS [25]. It is a three-item questionnaire to record the frequency at which the subjects performed physically strenuous, moderate, and mild exercise per week in the past month. A GLTEQ score of less than 14 units indicates insufficient activity, 14 to 23 indicated moderate activity and 24 units or more indicated high activity [25].

2.2.3. Countermovement Jump (CMJ)

All participants performed three maximal CMJs without arm swing on a single force plate. Before the jumps, a physiotherapist verbally explained and demonstrated the jumping technique to each subject. The participants were instructed to jump as high as possible with their hands on their hips and to keep their legs extended during the flight phase of the jump (Figure 1). A 5 s rest was performed between the jumps, as described in previous studies [26–28]. Any CMJs that were inadvertently performed with the inclusion of arm swing or tucking of the legs during the flight phase of the jumps were excluded. All of the participants completed a practice jump before data collection. The jumping trials were performed wearing socks and everyday clothes.

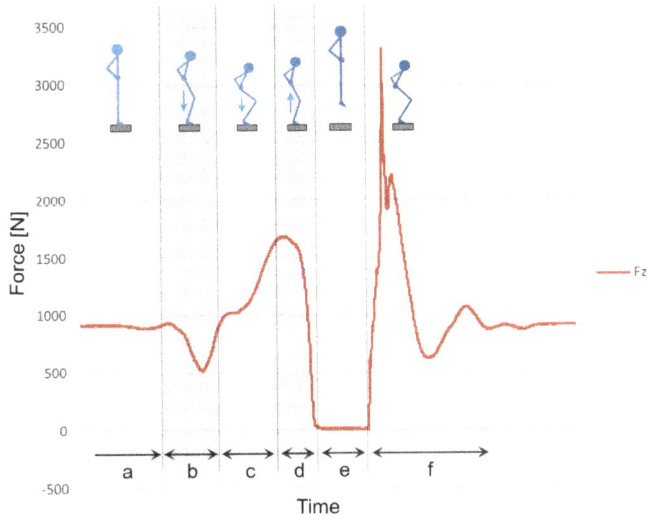

Figure 1. Countermovement jump phases in ground reaction curve. a = weight phase, b = unweight phase, c = eccentric phase, d = concentric phase, e = flight phase, f = landing phase; Fz = resultant force.

The CMJ can be divided into 6 phases (Figure 1.) First (a), the patient stands still on the force plate and the body weight is measured. In the second phase (b), the patient begins a short countermovement with flexion of the hips and knees in which the body weight is reduced below a threshold value of 5%. The phase ends when the body weight in the force–time curve is reached again. Third is the braking or eccentric phase (c), characterized by flexion of the hip, knee, and ankle until the center of mass (COM) is lowest and velocity is zero. During the braking phase, the following leg muscles work eccentrically: M. gluteus maximus, M. iliopsoas, M. quadriceps femoris, and M. triceps surae. Next is the propulsion or concentric phase (d). It begins with a forceful extension of the hips, knees, and ankles to move COM upwards and push off the force plate. The muscles which previously, in the braking phase, worked eccentrically now work concentrically. The time after take-off from the force plate to the highest point of the COM is described as the flight phase (e). The CMJ ends with the landing phase (f) when both feet touch the force plate and the initial position is reached again [29].

2.3. Data Collection

Ground reaction forces and moments of force were recorded using a portable single force plate from AMTI (Advanced Mechanical Technology Inc., Watertown, MA, USA, AccuPower-O) and sampled at 1000 Hz. Force plates are the gold standard and a valid method of measuring vertical jump performance [30,31]. The reliability of the AMTI force plate is good to excellent and shows a low error rate of 2.5% [32].

A dedicated biomechanical analysis software (AccuPower Solutions, Version 1.5.4.2082, Watertown, MA, USA) was used to record the parameters during the different jump phases. The most common and reliable jump parameters in sports medicine depending on the different CMJ phases were selected [33]. An important consideration in the extraction of the jump parameter was to analyse not only force parameters, but also time-based parameters, as these are more indicative of neuromuscular performance [14,34]. Table 1 shows a description of the recorded jump parameters.

Table 1. Measured jump parameters by force plate.

Jump Parameters	Description	Interpretation
Temporal parameters		
Flight time (s)	time in the air from jump take-off to landing	longer = better
Braking time (s)	duration of the eccentric phase	shorter = better
Propulsive time (s)	duration of the concentric phase	shorter = better
FTCTR	ratio of flight to contraction time	higher = better
Kinetic parameters		
FZV (N/kg)	maximum force during eccentric phase	higher = better
Peak force (N/kg)	maximum force during concentric phase	higher = better
ANP (W/kg)	average power during eccentric phase	higher = better
APP (W/kg)	average power during concentric phase	higher = better
BPIR	ratio of braking to propulsive impulse	lower = better
Performance parameter		
Jump height (cm)	jump height calculated by force impact	higher = better

Abbreviations: FTCTR = flight time to contraction time ratio; FZV = force at zero velocity; ANP = average negative power; APP = average positive power; BPIR = brake to propulsive impulse ratio.

2.4. Statistical Analysis

For all three jumps, the mean values of the individual parameters were used for the statistical analyses. Force values were converted to values relative to body mass. The distribution of all jump parameters was visually inspected and supplemented with the Shapiro–Wilk test for the assessment of normality.

In the evaluation of jump parameters, a descriptive specification of mean values and standard deviations occurred. Generalized linear mixed models (GLMM) were applied to determine the differences in jump parameters between the groups (HC, pwMS $_{\text{motor normal}}$ and pwMS $_{\text{motor impaired}}$) and subgroups according to normal cerebellar and sensory FSS (HC and pwMS $_{\text{unimpaired}}$) adjusted for age, gender and Body Mass Index (BMI). For normally distributed outcomes, the Gaussian distribution with identity link was used, while for right-skewed outcomes, the Gamma distribution with log link function was used. Statistical significance was fixed at $p < 0.05$. The significance level α was Bonferroni corrected for multiple testing. Effect sizes in between-group comparisons were quantified using Cohen's d, with effect sizes defined as small (d = 0.20–0.49), moderate (d = 0.50–0.79) or large (d > 0.80) [35]. Spearman rank correlations were calculated to study bivariate relations of jump parameters with EDSS and FSS. Statistical analyses were performed using IBM Statistical Package for the Social Sciences (SPSS) for Windows, Version 28 (IBM Corp, Armonk, NY, USA).

3. Results

3.1. Participants

A total of 189 study participants were examined in the study. After evaluation of the GLTEQ, $n = 132$ study participants emerged as physically active and were therefore included in the analysis (Figure 2). PwMS $_{\text{motor normal}}$ and HC are equal regarding to degree of disability, motor function according to EDSS and physical activity and did not differ based on age, BMI or gender (Table 2). The pwMS $_{\text{motor impaired}}$ had a significant higher age ($p < 0.05$), EDSS score ($p < 0.001$) as well as pyramidal FSS, sensory FSS and cerebellar FSS ($p < 0.001$), as expected. An overview of the participants' characteristics is shown in Table 2.

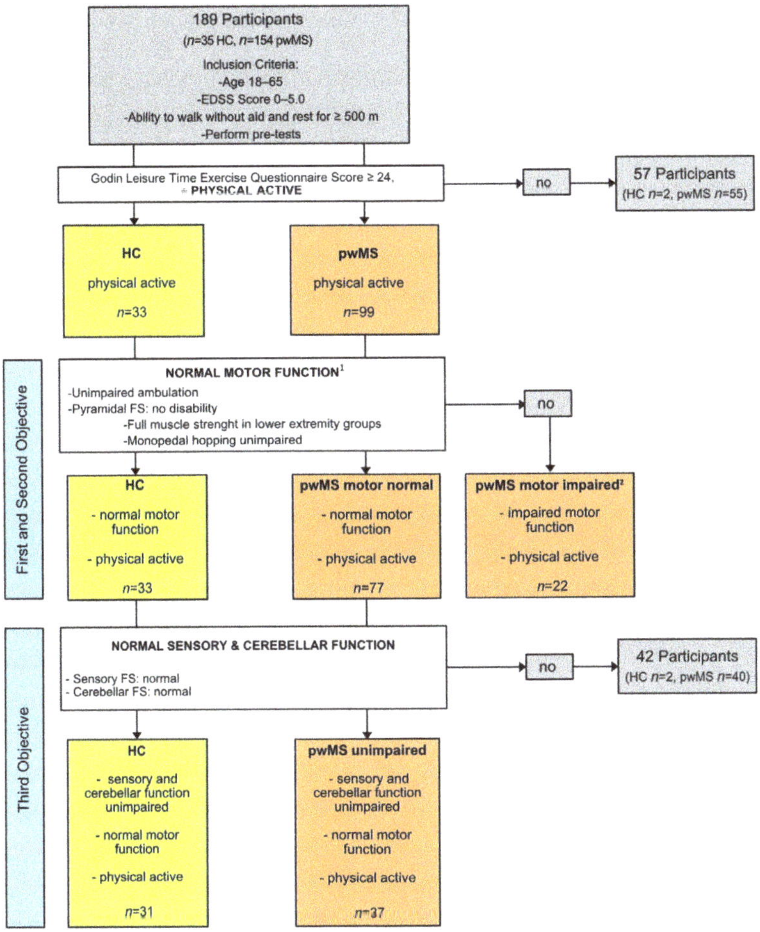

Figure 2. Flowchart of the study population. In order to create the best possible basis for comparability between groups, only participants with a GLTEQ $\geq$ 24, i.e., physically active, were included in the analysis. In a next adjustment step, the group of pwMS was divided according to the degree of disability and motor impairment assessed with EDSS. This resulted in a pwMS group with motor disability (pwMS $_{\text{motor impaired}}$) and a pwMS group without motor disability (pwMS $_{\text{motor normal}}$). PwMS $_{\text{motor normal}}$ thus corresponds to the HC group (all participants were examined with EDSS). In this study, the jumping performances between these three groups were analysed in two steps (first and second objective). Because sensory and cerebellar dysfunction can influence motor function, only participants without sensory and cerebellar dysfunction according to the EDSS were included in a finally analysis step (tertiary objective). [1] Normal motor function: EDSS score $\leq$ 1.5 with pyramidal FSS $\leq$ 1. [2] PwMS motor impaired: EDSS score $\geq$ 2 with pyramidal FSS of 2–4, reduced muscle strength and impaired monopedal hopping. Abbreviation: EDSS = Expanded Disability Status Scale; GLTEQ = Godin Leisure Time Exercise Questionnaire; FSS = functional system score; pwMS = people with multiple sclerosis; HC = healthy controls.

Table 2. Baseline characteristics of the study population. Data presented as mean (±standard deviation) unless specified otherwise.

	HC (n = 33)	pwMS Motor Normal (n = 77)	pwMS Motor Impaired (n = 22)
Age (years)	34.82 (±9.68) [a]	35.86 (±8.83) [a]	41.91 (±10.63)
Gender (female) n (%)	21 (63.6%)	54 (70.1%)	16 (72.7%)
Disease duration (years)	n.a	7.05 (±5.86)	9.27 (±6.63)
MS Subtype			
RRMS (%)	n.a	100%	100%
BMI	24.95 (±4.97)	24.58 (±4.26)	25.63 (±5.26)
EDSS (median, IQR)	1.0 (0–1.0) [a]	1.5 (1.0–1.5) [a]	3.0 (2.5–3.5)
Pyramidal FSS	1.0 (0–1.0) [a]	1.0 (1.0–1.0) [a]	2.0 (2.0–2.5)
Cerebellar FSS	0 (0–0) [a]	0 (0–1.0) [a]	1.0 (1.0–2.0)
Sensory FSS	0 (0–0) [a]	0 (0–1.0) [a]	1.5 (1.0–2.0)

Abbreviations: pwMS = people with multiple sclerosis; HC = healthy controls; RRMS = relapsing-remitting multiple sclerosis; BMI= Body Mass Index; EDSS = Expanded Disability Status Scale; FSS = functional system score; IQR = interquartile range. [a] significant difference from motor impaired pwMS ($p < 0.05$).

3.2. Group Comparison between MS Groups and HC in CMJ Performance

Significant differences between the three groups could be observed in almost all jump parameters, except jump height (Table 3). PwMS $_{\text{motor normal}}$ showed a better jump performance than pwMS $_{\text{motor impaired}}$ and HC better than pwMS $_{\text{motor normal}}$ (pwMS $_{\text{motor impaired}}$ < pwMS $_{\text{motor normal}}$ < HC). Significant differences were detected between the MS groups regarding to temporal parameters (except braking time), kinetic parameters (except peak force) and performance parameter. PwMS $_{\text{motor impaired}}$ differed significantly in all jump parameters from the HC. The comparison of examples of the CMJ force–time curves during the contraction time between pwMS $_{\text{motor normal}}$, pwMS $_{\text{motor impaired}}$ and HC is shown in Figure 3.

Table 3. Jump parameters in pwMS and HC.

Jump Parameters	HC (n = 33)	pwMS Motor Normal (n = 77)	pwMS Motor Impaired (n = 22)	F (2,126)	p-Value
Temporal parameters					
Flight time (s)	0.36 ± 0.06 [b,c]	0.32 ± 0.05 [a,c]	0.27 ± 0.06 [a,b]	22.24	<0.001 *
Braking time (s)	0.18 ± 0.05 [b,c]	0.25 ± 0.15 [a]	0.30 ± 0.19 [a]	9.49	<0.001 *
Propulsive time (s)	0.28 ± 0.06 [c]	0.30 ± 0.07 [c]	0.43 ± 0.19 [a,b]	10.57	<0.001 *
FTCTR	0.51 ± 0.12 [b,c]	0.45 ± 0.11 [a,c]	0.34 ± 0.12 [a,b]	11.86	<0.001 *
Kinetic parameters					
FZV (N/kg)	19.61 ± 3.0 [b,c]	17.52 ± 2.93 [a,c]	14.99 ± 3.63 [a,b]	11.43	<0.001 *
Peak force (N/kg)	20.57 ± 2.30 [b,c]	19.34 ± 2.18 [a]	17.92 ± 2.69 [a]	5.711	0.004 *
ANP (W/kg)	−4.53 ± 3.86 [b,c]	−3.41 ± 1.07 [a,c]	−2.29 ± 0.89 [a,b]	10.66	<0.001 *
APP (W/kg)	16.38 ± 3.86 [b,c]	15.08 ± 3.22 [a,c]	11.51 ± 3.76 [a,b]	25.56	<0.001 *
BPIR	1.92 ± 0.31 [b,c]	2.29 ± 1.14 [a,c]	2.29 ± 1.14 [a,b]	13.71	<0.001 *
Performance parameter					
Jump height (cm)	15.38 ± 4.78 [c]	13.73 ± 4.28	11.03 ± 5.22 [a]	3.07	0.050

Data presented as mean (± standard deviation) unless specified. Abbreviations: HC = healthy controls; pwMS = people with multiple sclerosis; FTCTR = flight time to contraction time ratio; FZV = force at zero velocity; ANP = average negative power; APP = average positive power; BPIR = brake to propulsive impulse ratio; * = significant ($p < 0.05$). [a] significant difference with healthy group ($p < 0.05$). [b] significant difference with MS motor normal ($p < 0.05$). [c] significant difference with MS motor impaired ($p < 0.05$).

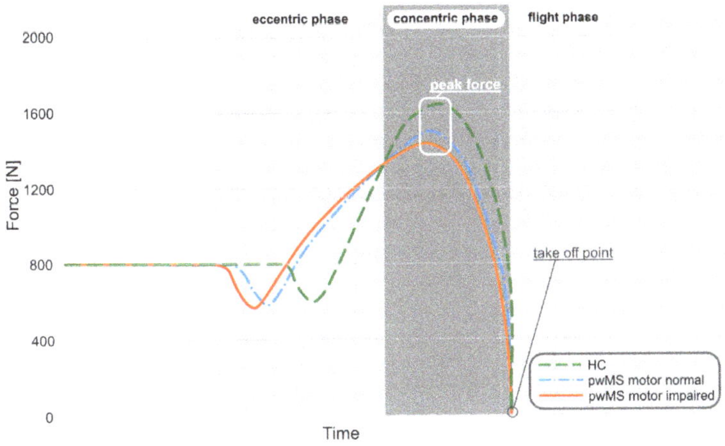

Figure 3. Examples of the countermovement jump force–time curves during the contraction time for pwMS $_{motor\ normal}$, pwMS $_{motor\ impaired}$, and HC. HC shows a rapid increase in force in the eccentric phase and a higher peak force than pwMS. Compared to HC and pwMS $_{motor\ normal}$, the pwMS $_{motor\ impaired}$ show the longest contraction phase (eccentric + concentric phase). Abbreviations: HC = healthy controls; pwMS = people with multiple sclerosis.

3.3. Group Comparision between pwMS with Normal Motor Function and HC

Significant differences between the HC and pwMS $_{motor\ normal}$ could be observed in all kinetic and temporal parameters (except propulsive time) (Table 3). PwMS $_{motor\ normal}$ showed a significantly decreased eccentric and concentric force, resulting in significantly shorter flight time. A significant imbalance in the ratio between flight time and contraction time as well as between braking impulse and propulsive impulse could be observed for pwMS $_{motor\ normal}$ in comparison to HC. Small effect sizes were detected for all jump parameters. The largest effect sizes were shown for flight time (d = 0.461), average negative power (d = 0.404) and braking time (d = 0.358).

3.4. Group Comparision between HC and pwMS with Full Motor, Sensory and Cerebellar Function

Significant group differences in jumping performance between pwMS $_{unimpaired}$ and HC, both with normal sensory and cerebellar function, were observed in the eccentric phase (braking time, force at zero velocity, average negative power), flight phase (flight time, jump height) and peak force of the CMJ (see Figure 4). The highest effect size, with small effects for sensory and cerebellar FSS of 0, was detected for the same parameters as in the group comparison between pwMS $_{motor\ normal}$ and HC.

3.5. Correlation of Jump Parameters According to EDSS

Overall, the bivariate comparison of the jump parameters and clinical outcome scores (EDSS) showed mild to moderate association (Table 4). The highest correlation coefficients were detected between kinetic parameters and EDSS with FSS. All jump parameters showed significant correlation with pyramidal FSS, but the highest correlation coefficients were obtained for the parameter average positive power and average negative power. The highest correlation was detected between cerebellar FSS and kinetic parameters from the eccentric phase of CMJ (force at zero velocity and average negative power). Similarly, the highest correlation for sensory FSS was also detected for average negative power.

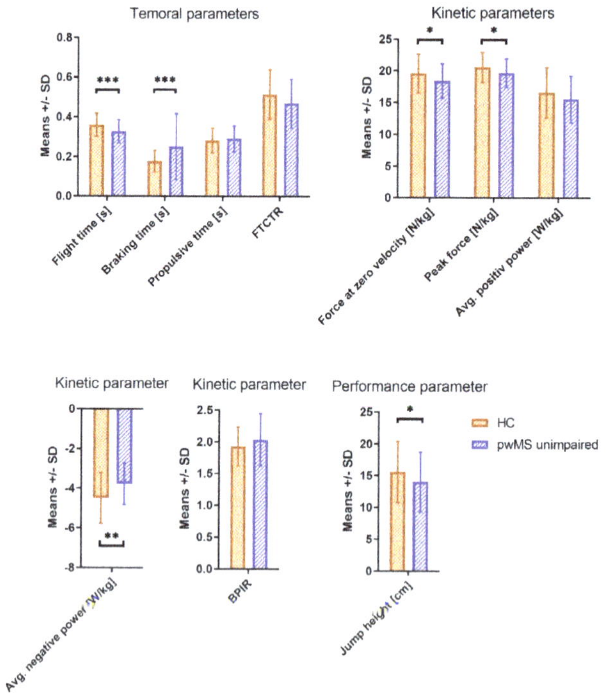

Figure 4. Group comparison between pwMS $_{unimpaired}$ and HC according to normal sensory and cerebellar FSS for temporal, kinetic and performance jump parameters. Data presented as mean with standard deviation and significance indicators (*** $p \leq 0.001$; ** $p < 0.01$; * $p < 0.05$). Abbreviations: HC = healthy controls; pwMS = people with multiple sclerosis; FTCTR = flight time to contraction time ratio; Avg. = average; BPIR= brake to propulsive impulse ratio.

Table 4. Correlation between jump parameters and EDSS including pyramidal, cerebellar and sensory FSS in pwMS (n = 99) according to Spearman.

Jump Parameters	EDSS	Pyramidal FSS	Cerebellar FSS	Sensory FSS
Temporal parameters				
Flight time (s)	−0.295 **	−0.382 **	−0.263 **	−0.248 **
Braking time (s)	0.125	0.290 **	0.149	−0.68
Propulsive time (s)	0.225 *	0.267 **	0.337 **	0.143
FTCTR	−0.338 **	−0.391 **	−0.405 **	−0.188
Kinetic parameters				
FZV (N/kg)	−0.299 **	−0.336 **	−0.417 **	−0.239 *
Peak force (N/kg)	−0.249 *	−0.305 **	−0.348 **	−0.163
ANP (W/kg)	0.385 **	0.421 **	0.408 **	0.354**
APP (W/kg)	−0.374 **	−0.440 **	−0.358 **	−0.203 *
BPIR	0.274	0.283 **	0.314 **	0.325 **
Performance parameter				
Jump height (cm)	−0.248 *	−0.275 **	−0.108	−0.166

Abbreviations: FSS = functional system score; FTCTR = flight time to contraction time ratio; FZV = force at zero velocity; ANP = average negative power; APP = average positive power; BPIR = brake to propulsive impulse ratio; EDSS = Expanded Disability Status Scale; ** = $p < 0.001$, * = $p < 0.05$.

4. Discussion

This study aimed to investigate the CMJ performance between pwMS groups and HC, as well as to evaluate the suitability of the CMJ on a force plate for detecting motor deficits in pwMS below different thresholds of neurological examination as part of EDSS. To our knowledge, this study is the first description of CMJ performance in pwMS.

First, we were able to create a MS group (pwMS $_{\text{motor normal}}$) equal to HC according to the degree of disability, motor function assessed with EDSS and physical activity. We determined that pwMS showed decreased CMJ performances in comparison to HC. In comparison of the motor normal group of pwMS, it was shown that CMJ performance decreased in all kinetic and temporal parameters (except propulsive time) compared to HC. With increasing disability in pwMS, it was also observed that jump performance decreased significantly. Furthermore, the CMJ could detect significant deficits in flight time, peak force and eccentric-based parameter (braking time, force at zero velocity and average negative power) for pwMS $_{\text{motor normal}}$ with additionally normal cerebellar and sensory function.

As we assumed, our results suggest that pwMS without obvious strength, coordination and sensory abnormalities of the legs require a more challenging task such as the CMJ to demonstrate motor deficits below the clinical threshold of the EDSS. These results confirm the findings of Krieger et al. [8] and suggest that pwMS, with full muscle strength, normal cerebellar and sensory function as assessed by EDSS, indeed demonstrate motor impairments. The correlation results suggest that jump parameters are appropriate outcome measures indicating disability deterioration in pwMS, especially disability in motor function. In addition, the jump parameters could supplement the EDSS with sensorimotor and neuromuscular outcomes as metric variables.

Our study findings are consistent with Kirkland et al. in showing that bipedal hopping can detect and monitor sensorimotor control in pwMS who do not currently experience clinical deficits [4]. Compared to Kirkland et al., we used the CMJ instead of horizontal jumps as it is already a reliable and valid measure of muscle strength and neuromuscular control in sports medicine [14,36]. Furthermore, vertical jumps require less space and, with appropriate upholstering, can be performed safely.

We determined that CMJ performances in pwMS are characterized by a significantly lower force at zero velocity in the eccentric phase, in which participants squat to the lowest COM. Overall, the braking phase was significantly longer in pwMS (pwMS $_{\text{motor normal}}$: +39%; pwMS $_{\text{motor impaired}}$: +67%) than in HC (see Figure 3). To achieve a rapid change between eccentric and concentric phases, a high eccentric force is necessary to develop an even higher concentric force [29]. The low eccentric force in pwMS is therefore followed by a significantly lower peak force compared to HC (see Figure 3). This suggests a reduction in the strength of the lower limbs in pwMS, even in those with normal muscle strength according to the BMRC scale. In the eccentric to concentric phase ratio, pwMS demonstrated an inefficient SSC, as indicated by an increased BPIR compared to HC.

These findings have clinical relevance in the care of pwMS. Identifying early sensorimotor deficits is important to initiate early rehabilitative intervention [4,37]. The CMJ in MS can be useful not only for early detection but also for determining the exact movement impairment. By measuring multiple domains (coordination, balance, proprioception and strength) of impairment in one test, complex movement functions can be assessed, specific deficits can be identified and finally appropriate rehabilitation can be performed. For clinical practice, besides the force plate as the gold standard, there are also other possibilities such as video analysis, IPhone apps ("My Jump") and optical-based systems to objectively assess CMJ performance [4,26].

Compared to the BMRC muscle strength assessment, which is part of the EDSS and tests only isolating concentric muscle strength, the CMJ measures the functional activity of the total muscle chain of the lower extremity. This functional assessment of muscle activity provides a better simulation of everyday movements as it is based on the principal of the slow stretch shortening cycle that occurs in natural movements such as walking and running [38].

Our study has the limitations of a cross-sectional study. Future studies with repeated measurements should be conducted to investigate whether the CMJ can be used as a standardized measure for the mid- and long-term assessment of disease progression and treatment response in MS. Furthermore, pwMS with a very low degree of disability, especially without limitation in the motor area according to EDSS, were examined; therefore, the EDSS total scores were very low, but not zero. To increase objectivity, isolated strength measurements should be included in future studies.

5. Conclusions

Our study is the first to provide evidence that the CMJ on a force plate, as a new assessment tool in MS, appears to be able to detect early motor and neuromuscular deficits in pwMS who have normal motor, cerebellar and sensory FSS according to the EDSS. Using the CMJ as a part of motor diagnosis, the deficits of eccentric and concentric muscle activity can be determined. These findings are useful in facilitating early and detailed rehabilitation approaches. The CMJ on a force plate as an objective and sensitive assessment could be a subthreshold test complementary to the neurological EDSS in the early stages of MS.

Author Contributions: Conceptualization A.G., H.S.-H., K.T., D.S. and T.Z.; methodology A.G., H.S.-H., K.T. and D.S.; software A.G. validation A.G. and H.S.-H.; formal analysis A.G., H.S.-H., K.T. and D.S.; investigation A.G.; data curation A.G.; writing—original draft preparation A.G., H.S.-H. and K.T.; writing—review and editing K.T., D.S. and T.Z.; visualization A.G, H.S.-H. and D.S.; supervision T.Z.; project administration A.G.; funding acquisition T.Z. All authors have read and agreed to the published version of the manuscript.

Funding: The Article Processing Charges (APC) were funded by the joint publication fund of the TU Dresden, the Medical Faculty Carl Gustav Carus, and the SLUB Dresden.

Institutional Review Board Statement: The study was conducted in accordance with the Declaration of Helsinki and approved by the local ethics committee (BO-EK-320062021).

Informed Consent Statement: Informed consent was obtained from all subjects involved in the study.

Data Availability Statement: All data produced in the present study are available upon reasonable request to the authors.

Acknowledgments: The authors acknowledge to all participants for their time and to Maximilian Hartmann for recruiting and testing participants.

Conflicts of Interest: The authors declare no conflict of interest.

References

1. Goldenberg, M.M. Multiple Sclerosis Review. *Pharm. Ther.* **2012**, *37*, 175–184.
2. Ziemssen, T.; Kern, R.; Thomas, K. Multiple sclerosis: Clinical profiling and data collection as prerequisite for personalized medicine approach. *BMC Neurol.* **2016**, *16*, 124. [CrossRef]
3. Reuben, D.B.; Magasi, S.; McCreath, H.E.; Bohannon, R.W.; Wang, Y.-C.; Bubela, D.J.; Rymer, W.Z.; Beaumont, J.; Rine, R.M.; Lai, J.-S.; et al. Motor assessment using the NIH Toolbox. *Neurology* **2013**, *80*, S65–S75. [CrossRef]
4. Kirkland, M.C.; Wadden, K.P.; Ploughman, M. Bipedal hopping as a new measure to detect subtle sensorimotor impairment in people with multiple sclerosis. *Disabil. Rehabil.* **2020**, *44*, 1544–1555. [CrossRef]
5. Ziemssen, T.; De Stefano, N.; Sormani, M.P.; Van Wijmeersch, B.; Wiendl, H.; Kieseier, B.C. Optimizing therapy early in multiple sclerosis: An evidence-based view. *Mult. Scler. Relat. Disord.* **2015**, *4*, 460–469. [CrossRef]
6. Ziemssen, T.; Derfuss, T.; de Stefano, N.; Giovannoni, G.; Palavra, F.; Tomic, D.; Vollmer, T.; Schippling, S. Optimizing treatment success in multiple sclerosis. *J. Neurol.* **2015**, *263*, 1053–1065. [CrossRef]
7. Francis, D.A.; Bain, P.; Swan, A.V.; Hughes, R.A.C. An Assessment of Disability Rating Scales Used in Multiple Sclerosis. *Arch. Neurol.* **1991**, *48*, 299–301. [CrossRef]
8. Krieger, S.C.; Antoine, A.; Sumowski, J.F. EDSS 0 is not normal: Multiple sclerosis disease burden below the clinical threshold. *Mult. Scler. J.* **2022**, *28*, 2299–2303. [CrossRef]
9. Kurtzke, J.F. Rating neurologic impairment in multiple sclerosis: An expanded disability status scale (EDSS). *Neurology* **1983**, *33*, 1444–1452. [CrossRef]

10. Van Hooren, B.; Zolotarjova, J. The Difference Between Countermovement and Squat Jump Performances: A Review of Underlying Mechanisms With Practical Applications. *J. Strength Cond. Res.* **2017**, *31*, 2011–2020. [CrossRef]
11. Quagliarella, L.; Sasanelli, N.; Belgiovine, G.; Accettura, D.; Notarnicola, A.; Moretti, B. Evaluation of counter movement jump parameters in young male soccer players. *J. Appl. Biomater. Funct. Mater.* **2011**, *9*, 40–46. [CrossRef]
12. Gannon, E.A.; Higham, D.G.; Gardner, B.W.; Nan, N.; Zhao, J.; Bisson, L.J. Changes in Neuromuscular Status Across a Season of Professional Men's Ice Hockey. *J. Strength Cond. Res.* **2021**, *35*, 1338–1344. [CrossRef]
13. Helland, C.; Midttun, M.; Saeland, F.; Haugvad, L.; Olstad, D.S.; Solberg, P.A.; Paulsen, G. A strength-oriented exercise session required more recovery time than a power-oriented exercise session with equal work. *PeerJ* **2020**, *8*, e10044. [CrossRef]
14. Lombard, W.; Reid, S.; Pearson, K.; Lambert, M. Reliability of metrics associated with a counter-movement jump performed on a force plate. *Meas. Phys. Educ. Exerc. Sci.* **2017**, *21*, 235–243. [CrossRef]
15. Aragón, L.F. Evaluation of Four Vertical Jump Tests: Methodology, Reliability, Validity, and Accuracy. *Meas. Phys. Educ. Exerc. Sci.* **2000**, *4*, 215–228. [CrossRef]
16. Slinde, F.; Suber, C.; Suber, L.; Edwén, C.E.; Svantesson, U. Test-Retest Reliability of Three Different Countermovement Jumping Tests. *J. Strength Cond. Res.* **2008**, *22*, 640–644. [CrossRef]
17. Hori, N.; Newton, R.U.; Kawamori, N.; McGuigan, M.R.; Kraemer, W.J.; Nosaka, K. Reliability of Performance Measurements Derived From Ground Reaction Force Data During Countermovement Jump and the Influence of Sampling Frequency. *J. Strength Cond. Res.* **2009**, *23*, 874–882. [CrossRef]
18. Meylan, C.; McMaster, T.; Cronin, J.; Mohammad, N.I.; Rogers, C.; Deklerk, M. Single-Leg Lateral, Horizontal, and Vertical Jump Assessment: Reliability, Interrelationships, and Ability to Predict Sprint and Change-of-Direction Performance. *J. Strength Cond. Res.* **2009**, *23*, 1140–1147. [CrossRef]
19. Rauch, R.; Veilleux, L.; Rauch, F.; Bock, D.; Welisch, E.; Filler, G.; Robinson, T.; Burrill, E.; Norozi, K.R. Muscle force and power in obese and overweight children. *J. Musculoskelet. Neuronal Interact.* **2012**, *12*, 80–83.
20. Singh, H.; Kim, D.; Kim, E.; Bemben, M.G.; Anderson, M.; Seo, D.-I.; Bemben, D.A. Jump Test Performance and Sarcopenia Status in Men and Women, 55 to 75 Years of Age. *J. Geriatr. Phys. Ther.* **2014**, *37*, 76–82. [CrossRef]
21. Kirkland, M.C.; Downer, M.B.; Holloway, B.J.; Wallack, E.M.; Lockyer, E.J.; Buckle, N.C.M.; Abbott, C.L.; Ploughman, M. Bipedal Hopping Reveals Evidence of Advanced Neuromuscular Aging Among People With Mild Multiple Sclerosis. *J. Mot. Behav.* **2016**, *49*, 505–513. [CrossRef] [PubMed]
22. Kirkland, M.C.; Chen, A.; Downer, M.B.; Holloway, B.J.; Wallack, E.M.; Lockyer, E.J.; Buckle, N.C.; Abbott, C.L.; Ploughman, M. Bipedal hopping timed to a metronome to detect impairments in anticipatory motor control in people with mild multiple sclerosis. *Clin. Biomech.* **2018**, *55*, 45–52. [CrossRef]
23. Van Munster, C.E.P.; Uitdehaag, B.M.J. Outcome Measures in Clinical Trials for Multiple Sclerosis. *CNS Drugs* **2017**, *31*, 217–236. [CrossRef] [PubMed]
24. Vanhoutte, E.K.; Faber, C.G.; Van Nes, S.I.; Jacobs, B.C.; Van Doorn, P.A.; Van Koningsveld, R.; Cornblath, D.R.; Van Der Kooi, A.J.; Cats, E.A.; Berg, L.H.V.D.; et al. Modifying the Medical Research Council grading system through Rasch analyses. *Brain* **2011**, *135*, 1639–1649. [CrossRef]
25. Godin, G. The Godin-Shephard Leisure-Time Physical Activity Questionnaire. *Health Fit. J. Can.* **2011**, *4*, 18–22. [CrossRef]
26. Yingling, V.R.; Castro, D.A.; Duong, J.T.; Malpartida, F.J.; Usher, J.R.; Jenny, O. The Reliability of Vertical Jump Tests between the Vertec and My Jump Phone Application. *PeerJ* **2018**, *6*, e4669. [CrossRef]
27. Kershner, A.L.; Fry, A.C.; Cabarkapa, D. Effect of Internal vs. External Focus of Attention Instructions on Countermovement Jump Variables in NCAA Division I Student-Athletes. *J. Strength Cond. Res.* **2019**, *33*, 1467–1473. [CrossRef] [PubMed]
28. Ruffieux, J.; Wälchli, M.; Kim, K.-M.; Taube, W. Countermovement Jump Training Is More Effective Than Drop Jump Training in Enhancing Jump Height in Non-professional Female Volleyball Players. *Front. Physiol.* **2020**, *11*, 231. [CrossRef]
29. McMahon, J.J.; Suchomel, T.J.; Lake, J.P.; Comfort, P. Understanding the Key Phases of the Countermovement Jump Force-Time Curve. *Strength Cond. J.* **2018**, *40*, 96–106. [CrossRef]
30. Buckthorpe, M.; Morris, J.; Folland, J.P. Validity of vertical jump measurement devices. *J. Sports Sci.* **2012**, *30*, 63–69. [CrossRef]
31. Cronin, J.B.; Hing, R.D.; McNair, P.J. Reliability and Validity of a Linear Position Transducer for Measuring Jump Performance. *J. Strength Cond. Res.* **2004**, *18*, 590–593. [CrossRef] [PubMed]
32. Koltermann, J.J.; Gerber, M.; Beck, H.; Beck, M. Validation of the HUMAC Balance System in Comparison with Conventional Force Plates. *Technologies* **2017**, *5*, 44. [CrossRef]
33. Eagles, A.N.; Sayers, M.G.L.; Bousson, M.; Lovell, D.I. Current Methodologies and Implications of Phase Identification of the Vertical Jump: A Systematic Review and Meta-analysis. *Sports Med.* **2015**, *45*, 1311–1323. [CrossRef]
34. Gathercole, R.; Sporer, B.; Stellingwerff, T.; Sleivert, G. Alternative Countermovement-Jump Analysis to Quantify Acute Neuromuscular Fatigue. *Int. J. Sports Physiol. Perform.* **2015**, *10*, 84–92. [CrossRef]
35. Cohen, J. A power primer. *Psychol. Bull.* **1992**, *112*, 155–159. [CrossRef] [PubMed]
36. Markovic, G.; Dizdar, D.; Jukic, I.; Cardinale, M. Reliability and Factorial Validity of Squat and Countermovement Jump Tests. *J. Strength Cond. Res.* **2004**, *18*, 551–555. [CrossRef] [PubMed]

37. Riemenschneider, M.; Hvid, L.G.; Stenager, E.; Dalgas, U. Is there an overlooked "window of opportunity" in MS exercise therapy? Perspectives for early MS rehabilitation. *Mult. Scler. J.* **2018**, *24*, 886–894. [CrossRef]
38. Aeles, J.; Vanwanseele, B. Do Stretch-Shortening Cycles Really Occur in the Medial Gastrocnemius? A Detailed Bilateral Analysis of the Muscle-Tendon Interaction During Jumping. *Front. Physiol.* **2019**, *10*, 1504. [CrossRef]

biomedicines

Review

Health Disparities in Multiple Sclerosis among Hispanic and Black Populations in the United States

Michael Z. Moore, Carlos A. Pérez, George J. Hutton, Hemali Patel and Fernando X. Cuascut *

Maxine Mesinger Multiple Sclerosis Center, Baylor College of Medicine, Houston, TX 77030, USA
* Correspondence: fernando.cuascut@bcm.edu

Abstract: Multiple sclerosis (MS) is an acquired demyelinating disease of the central nervous system (CNS). Historically, research on MS has focused on White persons with MS. This preponderance of representation has important possible implications for minority populations with MS, from developing effective therapeutic agents to understanding the role of unique constellations of social determinants of health. A growing body of literature involving persons of historically underrepresented races and ethnicities in the field of multiple sclerosis is assembling. Our purpose in this narrative review is to highlight two populations in the United States: Black and Hispanic persons with multiple sclerosis. We will review the current understanding about the patterns of disease presentation, genetic considerations, response to treatment, roles of social determinants of health, and healthcare utilization. In addition, we explore future directions of inquiry as well as practical methods of meeting these challenges.

Keywords: MS—multiple sclerosis; DMT—disease modifying therapies; pwMS—persons with multiple sclerosis; SDOH—social determinants of health; EDSS—Expanded Disability Severity Scale; SES—socioeconomic status; nSES—neighborhood socioeconomic status

1. Introduction

Multiple sclerosis (MS) is an acquired demyelinating disease of the central nervous system (CNS). A recent study estimates that in 2017, nearly 1 million adults had MS in the United States (US) [1]. The burden of this disease is well established, as it represents the most common progressive neurologic disorder in young adults worldwide [1]. The most recent estimated total economic burden in the United States (US) exceeded $85 billion [2]. However, there has been great pharmacologic advancement in the treatment of MS over the past few decades, and MS is now considered a less disabling condition with appropriate intervention [3].

Previous studies have shown that different genetic, environmental, and immunological risk factors play a role in the pathogenesis of the disease. Moreover, MS may be influenced by multiple social determinants of health, such as income, education, and cultural perceptions [4–7]. These have ranged from decreased access to healthcare, increased frequency of lower incomes correlating with increased disease severity, and decreased representation in clinical trials.

Increasing evidence suggests that racial disparities are important factors that may explain differences in the disease course, incidence, prevalence, and outcomes [8]. Still, Black and Hispanic populations in the United States remain largely underrepresented and understudied in clinical trials [9–12]. Recently, a cumulative number of studies have been focusing on improving our understanding of the disease course and disparities across underrepresented populations [13]. A more comprehensive understanding of the disparities can help improve disease management in patients of diverse backgrounds. This narrative review aims to explore these topics as it applies to historically understudied minority populations in the US, specifically Black and Hispanic persons with multiple sclerosis (pwMS).

2. Methods/Definitions

Utilizing the Texas Medical Center Library OneSearch and Pubmed, we performed a literature search for English language studies including the phrases "multiple sclerosis", "disparities", "social determinants of health", "African-American", "Black", "Hispanic", "Latino", "LatinX" from 2014 to the date of search in October 2022, and similar searches were carried out periodically in subsequent reviews of the text. Additional studies were reviewed guided by the reference lists of relevant studies and further elements of interest emerging from this literature review.

We will use Black, Hispanic, and White racial/ethnic designations for this paper. To ensure accuracy, the term Black is substituted to reference patients defined as "African-American" or "Non-Hispanic Black," White is substituted for "Non-Hispanic White," and Hispanic for those of Latin American descent. While the term also applies to persons from Spain, we will limit its use to the Latin American population in this article. If a population in a study does not meet one of these designations, or if the use of these general terms would impair the appropriate interpretation of the study in question, we will revert to the terminology used by the original authors. While a diverse array of populations of different races are affected by MS and important considerations likely exist in the management of MS, the focus in this review is largely limited to the three populations detailed above under their positions as those with the highest representation of MS disease burden in the United States.

3. Multiple Sclerosis & Its Course in Black Persons

Historically, the incidence of MS in the US was thought to be substantially higher in White persons of European background than in most minority groups, including Black individuals. More recent studies have challenged this position. A large cohort study from 1990 to 2007 within the United States military served by the Veterans Affairs system demonstrated an incidence rate of 12.1 per 100,000 among Black persons, compared to an incidence of 9.3 per 100,000 among White persons [14]. This is further corroborated by a retrospective cohort study in Southern California that reported an incidence of MS in Blacks that exceeds that of Whites (10.2 per 100,000 and 6.9 per 100,000, respectively) [15].

In addition to the increased incidence rate, Black pwMS may have a less favorable disease course and morbidity than their White counterparts. For example, a 2003 study among patients of the New York State Multiple Sclerosis Consortium (NYSMSC) demonstrated a younger age at diagnosis and greater disability with increased disease duration among Black pwMS [16]. Other studies have corroborated these data and have demonstrated faster progression to require ambulatory assistance [17,18]. Furthermore, other studies showed that Blacks consistently had higher disability than Whites when measuring cognitive, ambulatory, and manual dexterity functions [19].

Black pwMS have been noted to be more likely to have spinal cord lesions and multifocal clinical presentations [17]. They also were less likely to experience full recovery from relapses, had shorter times to a second relapse, and had more frequent relapses overall [16]. A faster transition from relapsing–remitting MS (RRMS) to secondary progressive MS (SPMS) was also observed in Black pwMS [20]. Moreover, a multicenter study across 3 academic hospitals revealed significantly lower visual acuity in Black patients in both high- and low-contrast visual acuity, as well as faster retinal nerve fiber layer (RNFL) thinning [21].

MRI volumetrics and lesion burden studies have also suggested less favorable outcomes for Black pwMS. One study demonstrated that Black pwMS had diffusely lower brain volumes, more brain lesions on MRI, lower gray matter volumes, and lower cortical and thalamic volumes [19]. An additional study comparing MRIs between Black and White pwMS demonstrated a higher burden of T2 hyperintense lesions and T1 hypointense lesions in the former group, which correlate with greater associated disability [22].

4. Multiple Sclerosis & Its Course in Hispanic Persons

Available literature on MS and its course in Hispanic pwMS is more limited than in White and Black pwMS in the US. Historically, data have largely been drawn from patient registries and retrospective cohort studies. As previously stated, there is an additional limitation in identifying consistent patient grouping due to variations in terminology (Hispanic, Latino, LatinX, etc.). With that qualification, available population studies seem to reflect a lower incidence and prevalence in Hispanic populations than in White and Black Americans [14,15,23–25]. Similarly, mortality associated with MS, as measured by death certificate analysis, appears lower in Hispanic pwMS compared to their Black and White counterparts [8].

Over the last few decades, cohort study observations regarding morbidity, disease course, and severity across racial groups have shown some inconsistencies. A study utilizing retrospective chart review and patient interviews in southern California demonstrated earlier age of disease onset and diagnosis and more frequent myelitis presentations among Hispanics. Hispanic and White pwMS appeared to have similar rates of ambulatory disability [26]. In contrast, a study comparing disability as measured by the Patient Derived Multiple Sclerosis Severity Score (PDMSS) demonstrated higher disability in Hispanic pwMS compared to White pwMS, following a trajectory similar to Black pwMS [27]. In a single institution cross-sectional study involving primarily Hispanic pwMS of Caribbean descent, an increase in ambulatory disability was reported in Hispanics compared to White pwMS [28]. A separate single academic center registry review found that, like Blacks, Hispanic pwMS were more likely to have a lower survival time ratio than Whites [29]. They were also more likely to present at a younger age and to have optic neuritis at presentation [29]. Additionally, Hispanic pwMS have been found to have significantly lower baseline thalamic volume measures correlating with a higher median baseline Expanded Disability Severity Scale (EDSS) [30]. Taken together, these studies suggest differences in the type and degree of morbidity associated with MS in Hispanic populations.

5. Genetics

While the immunopathophysiology and phenotypic expression of MS is complex, genetic factors play a substantial role. Variations in the human leukocyte antigen (HLA) complex genotypes have been shown to correlate with differences in the incidence of MS [31]. For example, HLA DRB1*15:01 is associated with an increased risk of disease development, while HLA-A*02 is associated with a decreased corresponding risk [5]. Extending beyond the HLA complex, single nucleotide polymorphisms (SNPs) in other exome regions have been associated with less significant effects on the risk of MS development [7].

It should be recognized that most of these studies have been carried out in persons of European ancestry, and it should not be taken for granted that these genetic risk factors are equally present in or have an equivalent effect on those of different races and ethnicities.

Recent studies have utilized genotyping within a broader range of races, whole exome sequencing, and tools such as admixture mapping to correlate disease incidence and expression with trends in ancestral haplotypes in key regions. In a study involving HLA genotyping and admixture mapping in Black and White pwMS, HLA DRB1*15 was appreciated in both groups. It was present at a higher frequency in pwMS compared to the unaffected controls [32]. In this study, admixture evidence of African origin at HLA DRB1*15 was associated with higher disability as measured by Multiple Sclerosis Severity Score (MSSS) after controlling for other factors. However, more recent studies using admixture mapping have demonstrated the opposite correlation with incidence. In an admixture mapping study involving Black, Hispanic, and Asian pwMS in the US, individuals with the European haplotype of HLA DRB1*15 experienced three times the disease risk compared to those with the African haplotype [33]. Similar literature on specific genetic variation in the Hispanic pwMS is somewhat more limited.

Outside the HLA complex, ancestral variation in other areas is also being studied. A whole exome scan of a sample of Black pwMS in the US indicates an increased risk for MS development in those who inherit European haplotypes in two loci on chromosome 1 [34]. Within a previously mentioned study, a genome-wide admixture search demonstrated a new region of interest on chromosome 8 with a significantly higher representation of European origin haplotypes in Hispanic pwMS than in controls [33]. A different study utilizing a custom SNP array to investigate a sample set of Black pwMS (2319 total, 803 with MS, 1516 without) found significant overlap in the variants associated with increased risk in SNPs previously identified in those of primarily European ancestry [35]. These findings were not corroborated by a more recent study in Black, Hispanic, and Asian pwMS and controls in the US, in which the majority of the 200 SNPs of interest identified in those of European ancestry were not significantly associated with MS [33].

Multiple considerations above invite further inquiry, including the prospect of genetic variations specific to minority populations and mixed evidence in admixture mapping and SNP data. Further progress in this area could have future implications in pharmacogenomics and personalized medicine in MS.

6. Response to Disease Modifying Therapies

Much of our understanding of MS clinical course in minority populations comes from limited studies. A systematic review of phase III disease-modifying treatment (DMT) clinical trials found that most trial subjects were White, raising questions about expectations of treatment tolerability and effectiveness across minorities [36]. These questions are rendered more compelling by evidence from post hoc drug trial analyses demonstrating increased rates of disease progression and lesion formation in Black pwMS treated with interferon β 1a [37,38]. While further investigations into other DMTs have commenced, they have generally consisted of post hoc analyses. These have demonstrated similar treatment benefits in the case of natalizumab and ocrelizumab in trials with Black participants, though with slightly more adverse events and hypersensitivity reactions in the case of ocrelizumab [38,39]. In the case of dimethyl fumarate, post hoc analyses of phase III clinical studies appeared to demonstrate similar clinical efficacy and tolerability among Black, Hispanic, and Asian pwMS subgroups as appreciated in the full study population [40]. Similarly, subgroup analyses of a multinational prospective cohort study on pwMS treated with dimethyl fumarate found similar relapse rate reductions and safety profiles in Hispanic and Black pwMS compared to non-Hispanic and non-Black pwMS. However, they demonstrated a less pronounced lymphocyte count decrease in Blacks [41,42].

It remains difficult to cite discrete mechanisms to account for differences in disease severity and response to DMTs among these populations and literature on this topic remains sparse. However, there is some evidence of factors that could underlie these disparities. For example, a cross-sectional study of White, Black, and Hispanic pwMS off DMT or on natalizumab compared to healthy controls of matched self-reported racial/ethnic background demonstrated a significant elevation in circulating plasmablasts among Black and Hispanic pwMS compared to White pwMS [11].

Observational studies not focused on a single DMT have also raised concerns about worsened outcomes. In a single academic center retrospective electronic medical record review (EMR) comparing sociodemographic characteristics, treatment response, and disability outcomes between 300 age and gender-matched cohorts, Hispanic and Black pwMS had a higher median EDSS score at baseline. This was despite similar patterns of DMTs used, average therapeutic lag, duration of individual therapies, and frequency of medication change [29]. Altogether, these studies underscore the importance of further research on the effectiveness and tolerability of existing DMTs in non-White populations and increased minority representation in future DMT trials [13].

7. Social Determinants of Health and Healthcare Utilization

There is increasing awareness about the impact of social determinants of health (SDOH), such as where a person is born, grows, works, lives, and ages, amidst the wider set of forces and systems shaping the conditions of daily life, on disease outcome and quality of life in MS [43,44]. Though the impact of these factors remains incompletely understood, available data suggest that significant differences in SDOH exist across racial groups [4]. Differential patterns and degree of healthcare utilization across minority populations have been described [45]. However, current data regarding these trends and their effects on minority populations among pwMS are limited.

Regarding general neurologic care, significant disparities in healthcare utilization between Whites and minority populations have been described. Data from the Medical Expenditure Panel Survey (MEPS) from 2006 to 2013 involving patients with neurologic conditions demonstrated that Blacks and Hispanics were approximately 30% and 40% less likely to see an outpatient neurologist compared to Whites, respectively [45]. This disparity has also been reported in pwMS, as demonstrated in a national cross-sectional study showing that the probability of seeing a neurologist was significantly lower among patients who did not have health insurance, were poor, lived in rural areas, and, notably, Black individuals [46]. Since adequate MS treatment requires a comprehensive and multidisciplinary approach, the presence of these risk factors can suggest a potential increased risk of disability and disease progression in minority populations. In a previous single-center retrospective study, after adjustment for race and age, MS patients who were evaluated by a neurologist at diagnosis were found to have 60% lower odds of attaining an EDSS > 4.5 at subsequent follow-up visits compared to patients evaluated by a non-neurologist [47].

Nevertheless, disparities in healthcare utilization appear to extend beyond direct access to care by a neurologist into other areas equally worth noting. In this regard, community-based services, in a study of Medicare/Medicaid eligible pwMS who were identified as Black or White (race limited to a dichotomous variable), Black pwMS utilized multiple services less frequently than their White counterparts, including case management (64% less likely), nursing services (48% less likely), and equipment, technology, and modification services (31% less likely) [48]. This trend mirrors previously reported trends toward greater disability among Black pwMS. In fact, in this study, Black pwMS utilizing Medicaid-funded services were more likely to have mobility impairment despite a younger average age than their White counterparts [48].

Important correlations have emerged regarding income and its effect on morbidity and management. White patients with lower socioeconomic status (SES) had a worse mean performance score on walking, manual dexterity, and cognitive processing tests [19]. One study of approximately 8500 individuals showed that Black pwMS were more likely to have Medicaid, be unemployed, and have higher rates of disability, both on self-reported and objective measures [19].

The area deprivation index (ADI) is a widely used and multidimensional tool comprised of seventeen variables to assess for socioeconomic disadvantage [49]. In White pwMS, higher ADI scores (indicating higher disadvantage) correlated with slower cognitive processing and manual dexterity speeds. A correlation was also noted between slower walking speeds and residence in low-income households. In Black participants, lower household income was associated with slower manual dexterity, but there was no clear association between ADI scores and other neurologic performance measures [19]. Similarly, correlations between income and mental health comorbidities in pwMS have been described. A study involving pwMS identified as Black, Hispanic, or White correlated neighborhood socioeconomic status (nSES) scores with results of screening tests for multiple mental health disorders, including anxiety, depression, and alcohol use disorder. This study found that patients in the lowest quartile of nSES (lower relative income) in all groups had lower screening test scores for mental health disorders overall [50]. In addition, Black and Hispanic pwMS more frequently occupied the lower quartile of nSES in this study population.

Of particular interest is the role of perception of healthcare and MS research participation among Black and Hispanic pwMS. Specifically, in a web-based survey among members of the MS Minority Research Engagement Partnership Network (MSREPN), important differences between Hispanic, Black, and White participants were described. Specifically,

Hispanic and Black participants more frequently reported concerns of "being taken advantage of or used by" the research team than White participants. Hispanic participants more frequently reported concern about research participation affecting their legal status [51].

Additional social determinants of health, including cultural dispositions towards illness and disease mitigation, health literacy, regional/geographical barriers to care, insurance coverage, and support community involvement have been identified [4]. Increased research into the type and degree of effect of these factors on disease management among historically underrepresented populations in MS care is necessary. Healthcare systems serving these populations should be structured to account for these differences.

8. Limitations

There are several limitations to this narrative review. First is the limitation of the focus to a particular region (i.e., United States) and the limited subset of races and ethnicities (i.e., White, Black, Hispanic). It is important to recognize that many races are not reviewed here, many of whom have a presence in the United States and have unique trends in disease incidence, phenotype, morbidity, genetic/epigenetic factors, and social determinants. Their omission from this review is due in part to a present paucity of data relative to the populations discussed herein, highlighting the importance of further and more inclusive studies in this field. Additionally, in the formation of this narrative review, there is the prospect of sampling bias of included articles.

Importantly, in a review of the literature on historically understudied racial groups, the use of inconsistent terminology used to describe different populations presents itself. Though race identification is a heavily personal decision, issues in the terms used can complicate the interpretation of results. Terminology referring to minority populations in the US has been inconsistent. Various terms are used to refer to different populations in the literature, including African-American, Afro-Caribbean, Black, White, Caucasian, Hispanic, Hispanic Black, Hispanic White, Hispanic non-White, Mestizo, Latino, LatinX, etc. We must practice caution when analyzing these terms as they are not synonymous. For example, as a matter of etymological integrity, the term Hispanic is not used to refer to people from Brazil, as the term carries a linguistic association with Spanish-speaking countries. The term African-American usually pertains to those with lineage tracing to Africa, but it might not apply to those whose known lineage traces no further than the country in which they live. Another important distinction is that some studies classify individuals by self-identified methodology, whereas in other studies authors assign these classifications. Even in the cases of self-identification, there exists a variance in the options provided and their range and clarity. This presents a difficulty in properly representing, comparing, and contrasting population trends between studies over different regions and periods. In attempting to identify trends and patterns, we risk false equivalencies as a function of unclear terminology about race and ethnicity.

9. Discussion and Future Directions

Emerging literature demonstrates important differences in incidence, prevalence, phenotypic features, and associated disability in Hispanic and Black pwMS as compared to White pwMS as well as unique elements in genetic predisposing features and risk factors across these populations. Moreover, an increasing number of community-based MS observational studies describe important racial and ethnic disparities in SDOH.

Considering these differences, we would like to identify future directions of research and practice strategies to better serve these populations (Figure 1). First, increased efforts are needed in education amongst healthcare professionals regarding the incidence and prevalence of MS in minority populations. This may decrease unconscious diagnostic biases regarding pretest probability delaying timely diagnosis [52]. This is particularly important among Black pwMS given estimates of incidence now exceeding those of their White counterparts. Additionally, healthcare providers' awareness of the variability in disease severity and expression among Black and Hispanic pwMS may improve proper comprehensive care and patient counseling.

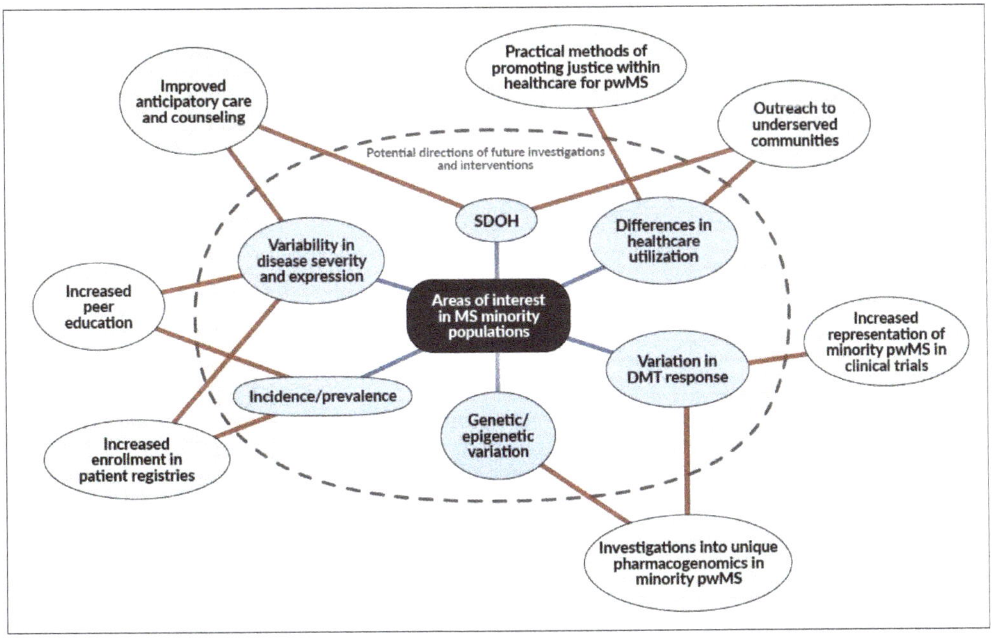

Figure 1. Areas of emphasis in care of minority populations with multiple sclerosis and future directions. The diagram illustrates points of emphasis emerging from a review of literature on multiple sclerosis (MS) in minority populations, specifically Hispanic and Black persons with multiple sclerosis (pwMS). Items beyond the dashed line indicate areas of future research and practice strategy changes.

Next, increased enrollment of minority pwMS in registries can assist in advancing research efforts among minority populations. The evidence of variation in response to some DMTs among minority groups underscores the importance of increased representation of non-White pwMS in clinical trials. There is evidence of recognition of this need and attempts to better meet it in the design of more recent drug trials, including those involving multiple sclerosis therapeutics [12]. To this end, investigators and participating clinical study sites should be conscious of differences in the perception of healthcare research by study participants. These can be addressed in several ways: increased representation of these populations amongst investigators and associated healthcare teams, outreach in minority communities and collaboration with community leaders, and increased availability of counseling and educational materials appropriate to the participant's native language and degree of health literacy. With these and other measures in place, increased minority representation in DMT clinical trials and future research in genetic/epigenetic variation across non-White pwMS can help advance pharmacogenomics among historically underserved populations.

Considering the differences in SDOH and healthcare utilization patterns in Black and Hispanic pwMS, many practical adjustments in care strategies may prove useful. A few publications have outlined some measures in improving care with a view to these needs, but this remains a poorly understood topic [4,13]. Reliable communication strategies should be established between healthcare providers and patients to promote comprehensive outpatient care and minimize unnecessary hospital visits and economic burden. Ideally, pwMS should have an associated healthcare provider such as a nurse navigator to decrease this reliance further. Likewise, there is evidence that co-locating allied care services (mental health, physical medicine and rehabilitation, etc.) may increase utilization among Black and Hispanic pwMS [50]. In a previously mentioned report on correlations of income and mental health comorbidities, Black and Hispanic pwMS were more likely to seek mental health care if it was co-located with sites at which their MS care was provided [50].

In addition to the elements described above, practical measures should be placed to best meet the needs of minority pwMS. Strategies to develop cultural competence among care teams should be employed to detect and correct possible deficiencies. Proactive outreach in communities with high minority representation by MS societies and centers of excellence may have many benefits, including increasing community awareness and fundraising efforts. Attention should also be paid to decreasing obstacles in access to care. Potential strategies include increased utilization of telemedicine, satellite clinic sites, and cultivating practical referral networks from primary care providers.

10. Conclusions

There is increasing recognition of significant differences in incidence patterns, prevalence, and outcomes in Black and Hispanic pwMS. However, the underpinnings of these differences remain an area that requires future study. The role of genetic and biological determinants of health has long been understudied and therefore underrecognized. Race and ethnicity are also associated with genetic ancestry and therefore indirectly related to genetic variants that may affect disease and health outcomes in MS. Discrepancies in socioeconomic constructs are becoming important interventional targets to help alleviate disease severity by race and ethnicity. While further research remains a high priority in this field, evidence now exists to guide improvements in the delivery of MS care to historically underserved minority populations.

Author Contributions: Conceptualization: F.X.C., G.J.H. and C.A.P.; Writing—Original Draft Preparation: M.Z.M. and H.P.; Writing—Review & Editing: M.Z.M., F.X.C., C.A.P. and G.J.H.; Figure conceptualization, creation: M.Z.M. and C.A.P.; Review, final editing: F.X.C., G.J.H. and C.A.P. All authors have read and agreed to the published version of the manuscript.

Funding: This research received no external funding.

Conflicts of Interest: The authors declare no conflict of interest.

References

1. Wallin, M.T.; Culpepper, W.J.; Campbell, J.D.; Nelson, L.M.; Langer-Gould, A.; Marrie, R.A.; Cutter, G.R.; Kaye, W.E.; Wagner, L.; Tremlett, H.; et al. The prevalence of MS in the United States: A population-based estimate using health claims data. *Neurology* **2019**, *92*, e1029–e1040. [CrossRef] [PubMed]
2. Bebo, B.; Cintina, I.; LaRocca, N.; Ritter, L.; Talente, B.; Hartung, D.; Ngorsuraches, S.; Wallin, M.; Yang, G. The Economic Burden of Multiple Sclerosis in the United States: Estimate of Direct and Indirect Costs. *Neurology* **2022**, *98*, e1810–e1817. [CrossRef]
3. Giovannoni, G. Disease-modifying treatments for early and advanced multiple sclerosis: A new treatment paradigm. *Curr. Opin. Neurol.* **2018**, *31*, 233–243. [CrossRef]
4. Amezcua, L.; Rivera, V.M.; Vazquez, T.C.; Baezconde-Garbanati, L.; Langer-Gould, A. Health Disparities, Inequities, and Social Determinants of Health in Multiple Sclerosis and Related Disorders in the US: A Review. *Arch. Neurol.* **2021**, *78*, 1515–1524. [CrossRef]
5. Olsson, T.; Barcellos, L.F.; Alfredsson, L. Interactions between genetic, lifestyle and environmental risk factors for multiple sclerosis. *Nat. Rev. Neurol.* **2017**, *13*, 25–36. [CrossRef]
6. Reich, D.S.; Lucchinetti, C.F.; Calabresi, P.A. Multiple Sclerosis. *N. Engl. J. Med.* **2018**, *378*, 169. [CrossRef] [PubMed]
7. Waubant, E.; Lucas, R.; Mowry, E.; Graves, J.; Olsson, T.; Alfredsson, L.; Langer-Gould, A. Environmental and genetic risk factors for MS: An integrated review. *Ann. Clin. Transl. Neurol.* **2019**, *6*, 1905–1922. [CrossRef]
8. Amezcua, L.; Rivas, E.; Joseph, S.; Zhang, J.; Liu, L. Multiple Sclerosis Mortality by Race/Ethnicity, Age, Sex, and Time Period in the United States, 1999–2015. *Neuroepidemiology* **2018**, *50*, 35–40. [CrossRef] [PubMed]
9. Diaz, V.M.D. Encouraging Participation of Minorities in Research Studies. *Ann. Fam. Med.* **2012**, *10*, 372–373. [CrossRef]
10. Avasarala, J. Inadequacy of Clinical Trial Designs and Data to Control for the Confounding Impact of Race/Ethnicity in Response to Treatment in Multiple Sclerosis. *JAMA Neurol.* **2014**, *71*, 943–944. [CrossRef]

11. Telesford, K.M.; Kaunzner, U.W.; Perumal, J.; Gauthier, S.A.; Wu, X.; Diaz, I.; Kruse-Hoyer, M.; Engel, C.; Marcille, M.; Vartanian, T. Black African and Latino/a identity correlates with increased plasmablasts in MS. *Neurol. Neuroimmunol. Neuroinflamm.* **2020**, *7*, e634. [CrossRef]
12. Mohan, S.V.; Freedman, J. A Review of the Evolving Landscape of Inclusive Research and Improved Clinical Trial Access. *Clin. Pharmacol. Ther.* **2023**, *113*, 518–527. [CrossRef] [PubMed]
13. Khan, O.; Williams, M.J.; Amezcua, L.; Javed, A.; Larsen, K.E.; Smrtka, J.M. Multiple sclerosis in US minority populations: Clinical practice insights. *Neurol. Clin. Pract.* **2015**, *5*, 132–142. [CrossRef] [PubMed]
14. Wallin, M.T.; Culpepper, W.J.; Coftman, P.; Pulaski, S.; Maloni, H.; Mahan, C.M.; Haselkorn, J.K.; Kurtzke, J.F. The Gulf War era multiple sclerosis cohort: Age and incidence rates by race, sex and service. *Brain* **2012**, *135*, 1778–1785. [CrossRef]
15. Langer-Gould, A.; Brara, S.M.; Beaber, B.E.; Zhang, J.L. Incidence of multiple sclerosis in multiple racial and ethnic groups. *Neurology* **2013**, *80*, 1734–1739. [CrossRef]
16. Weinstock-Guttman, B.; Jacobs, L.D.; Gottesman, M.H.; Herbert, J.; Holub, R.; Lava, N.S.; Lenihan, M.; Lusins, J.; Mihai, C.; Miller, A.E.; et al. Multiple sclerosis characteristics in African American patients in the New York State Multiple Sclerosis Consortium. *Mult. Scler.* **2003**, *9*, 293–298. [CrossRef] [PubMed]
17. Cree, B.A.C.; Khan, O.; Haines, J.L.; Pericak-Vance, M.; Deloa, C.; Oksenberg, J.R.; Hauser, S.L.; Bourdette, D.; Goodin, D.S.; Cohen, J.A.; et al. Clinical characteristics of African Americans vs Caucasian Americans with multiple sclerosis. *Neurology* **2004**, *63*, 2039–2045. [CrossRef]
18. Marrie, R.A.; Cutter, G.; Tyry, T.; Vollmer, T.; Campagnolo, D. Does multiple sclerosis-associated disability differ between races? *Neurology* **2006**, *66*, 1235–1240. [CrossRef]
19. Gray-Roncal, K.; Fitzgerald, K.C.; Ryerson, L.Z.; Charvet, L.; Cassard, S.D.; Naismith, R.; Ontaneda, D.; Mahajan, K.; Castro-Borrero, W.; Mowry, E.M. Association of Disease Severity and Socioeconomic Status in Black and White Americans with Multiple Sclerosis. *Neurology* **2021**, *97*, e881–e889. [CrossRef]
20. Amezcua, L.; McCauley, J.L. Race and ethnicity on MS presentation and disease course. *Mult. Scler.* **2020**, *26*, 561–567. [CrossRef]
21. Kimbrough, D.J.; Sotirchos, E.S.; Wilson, J.A.; Al-Louzi, O.; Conger, A.; Conger, D.; Frohman, T.C.; Saidha, S.; Green, A.J.; Frohman, E.M.; et al. Retinal damage and vision loss in African American multiple sclerosis patients. *Ann. Neurol.* **2015**, *77*, 228–236. [CrossRef]
22. Howard, J.; Battaglini, M.; Babb, J.S.; Arienzo, D.; Holst, B.; Omari, M.; De Stefano, N.; Herbert, J.; Inglese, M. MRI correlates of disability in African-Americans with multiple sclerosis. *PLoS ONE* **2012**, *7*, e43061. [CrossRef]
23. Abarca, E.; Davis, P.; Marrie, R.A.; Cutter, G.; Campagnolo, D.; Vollmer, T. NARCOMS Latino cohort. *Mult. Scler.* **2008**, *14*, S56.
24. Langer-Gould, A.M.; Gonzales, E.G.; Smith, J.B.; Li, B.H.; Nelson, L.M. Racial and Ethnic Disparities in Multiple Sclerosis Prevalence. *Neurology* **2022**, *98*, e1818–e1827. [CrossRef] [PubMed]
25. Romanelli, R.J.; Huang, Q.; Lacy, J.; Hashemi, L.; Wong, A.; Smith, A. Multiple sclerosis in a multi-ethnic population from Northern California: A retrospective analysis, 2010-2016. *BMC Neurol.* **2020**, *20*, 163. [CrossRef]
26. Amezcua, L.; Lund, B.T.; Weiner, L.P.; Islam, T. Multiple sclerosis in Hispanics: A study of clinical disease expression. *Mult. Scler.* **2011**, *17*, 1010–1016. [CrossRef] [PubMed]
27. Ventura, R.E.; Antezana, A.O.; Bacon, T.; Kister, I. Hispanic Americans and African Americans with multiple sclerosis have more severe disease course than Caucasian Americans. *Mult. Scler.* **2017**, *23*, 1554–1557. [CrossRef]
28. Hadjixenofontos, A.; Beecham, A.H.; Manrique, C.P.; Pericak-Vance, M.A.; Tornes, L.; Ortega, M.; Rammohan, K.W.; McCauley, J.L.; Delgado, S.R. Clinical Expression of Multiple Sclerosis in Hispanic Whites of Primarily Caribbean Ancestry. *Neuroepidemiology* **2015**, *44*, 262–268. [CrossRef]
29. Pérez, C.A.; Lincoln, J.A. Racial and ethnic disparities in treatment response and tolerability in multiple sclerosis: A comparative study. *Mult. Scler. Relat. Disord.* **2021**, *56*, 103248. [CrossRef]
30. Pérez, C.A.; Salehbeiki, A.; Zhu, L.; Wolinsky, J.S.; Lincoln, J.A. Assessment of Racial/Ethnic Disparities in Volumetric MRI Correlates of Clinical Disability in Multiple Sclerosis: A Preliminary Study. *J. Neuroimaging* **2021**, *31*, 115–123. [CrossRef]
31. Moutsianas, L.; Jostins, L.; Beecham, A.H.; Dilthey, A.T.; Xifara, D.K.; Ban, M.; Shah, T.S.; Patsopoulos, N.A.; Alfredsson, L.; Anderson, C.A.; et al. Class II HLA interactions modulate genetic risk for multiple sclerosis. *Nat. Genet.* **2015**, *47*, 1107–1113. [CrossRef] [PubMed]
32. Cree, B.A.C.; Reich, D.E.; Khan, O.; De Jager, P.L.; Nakashima, I.; Takahashi, T.; Bar-Or, A.; Tong, C.; Hauser, S.L.; Oksenberg, J.R. Modification of Multiple Sclerosis Phenotypes by African Ancestry at HLA. *Arch. Neurol.* **2009**, *66*, 226–233. [CrossRef] [PubMed]
33. Chi, C.; Shao, X.; Rhead, B.; Gonzales, E.; Smith, J.B.; Xiang, A.H.; Graves, J.; Waldman, A.; Lotze, T.; Schreiner, T.; et al. Admixture mapping reveals evidence of differential multiple sclerosis risk by genetic ancestry. *PLoS Genet.* **2019**, *15*, e1007808. [CrossRef] [PubMed]
34. Nakatsuka, N.; Patterson, N.; Patsopoulos, N.A.; Altemose, N.; Tandon, A.; Beecham, A.H.; McCauley, J.L.; Isobe, N.; Hauser, S.; De Jager, P.L.; et al. Two genetic variants explain the association of European ancestry with multiple sclerosis risk in African-Americans. *Sci. Rep.* **2020**, *10*, 16902. [CrossRef] [PubMed]
35. Isobe, N.; Madireddy, L.; Khankhanian, P.; Matsushita, T.; Caillier, S.J.; Moré, J.M.; Gourraud, P.-A.; McCauley, J.L.; Beecham, A.H.; Piccio, L.; et al. An ImmunoChip study of multiple sclerosis risk in African Americans. *Brain* **2015**, *138*, 1518–1530. [CrossRef] [PubMed]

36. Onuorah, H.-M.; Charron, O.; Meltzer, E.; Montague, A.; Crispino, A.; Largent, A.; Lucas, A.; Freeman, L. Enrollment of Non-White Participants and Reporting of Race and Ethnicity in Phase III Trials of Multiple Sclerosis DMTs: A Systematic Review. *Neurology* **2022**, *98*, e880–e892. [CrossRef]
37. Cree, B.A.C.; Al-Sabbagh, A.; Bennett, R.; Goodin, D. Response to Interferon Beta-1a Treatment in African American Multiple Sclerosis Patients. *Arch. Neurol.* **2005**, *62*, 1681–1683. [CrossRef]
38. Cree, B.A.C.; Pradhan, A.; Pei, J.; Williams, M.J. Efficacy and safety of ocrelizumab vs interferon beta-1a in participants of African descent with relapsing multiple sclerosis in the Phase III OPERA I and OPERA II studies. *Mult. Scler. Relat. Disord.* **2021**, *52*, 103010. [CrossRef]
39. Cree, B.A.C.; Stuart, W.H.; Tornatore, C.S.; Jeffery, D.R.; Pace, A.L.; Cha, C.H. Efficacy of Natalizumab Therapy in Patients of African Descent with Relapsing Multiple Sclerosis: Analysis of AFFIRM and SENTINEL Data. *Arch. Neurol.* **2011**, *68*, 464–468. [CrossRef]
40. Fox, R.J.; Gold, R.; Phillips, J.T.; Okwuokenye, M.; Zhang, A.; Marantz, J.L. Efficacy and Tolerability of Delayed-release Dimethyl Fumarate in Black, Hispanic, and Asian Patients with Relapsing-Remitting Multiple Sclerosis: Post Hoc Integrated Analysis of DEFINE and CONFIRM. *Neurol. Ther.* **2017**, *6*, 175–187. [CrossRef]
41. Chinea, A.; Amezcua, L.; Vargas, W.; Okai, A.; Williams, M.J.; Su, R.; Parks, B.; Mendoza, J.P.; Lewin, J.B.; Jones, C.C. Real World Safety and Effectiveness of Dimethyl Fumarate in Hispanic or Latino Patients with Multiple Sclerosis: 3-Year Results from ESTEEM. *Neurol. Ther.* **2020**, *9*, 495–504. [CrossRef] [PubMed]
42. Williams, M.J.; Amezcua, L.; Okai, A.; Okuda, D.T.; Cohan, S.; Su, R.; Parks, B.; Mendoza, J.P.; Lewin, J.B.; Jones, C.C. Real-World Safety and Effectiveness of Dimethyl Fumarate in Black or African American Patients with Multiple Sclerosis: 3-Year Results from ESTEEM. *Neurol. Ther.* **2020**, *9*, 483–493. [CrossRef]
43. Adler, N.E.; Glymour, M.M.; Fielding, J. Addressing Social Determinants of Health and Health Inequalities. *JAMA J. Am. Med. Assoc.* **2016**, *316*, 1641–1642. [CrossRef]
44. Commission on Social Determinants of Health. *Closing the Gap in a Generation: Health Equity through Action on the Social Determinants of Health: Final Report of the Commission on Social Determinants of Health*; World Health Organization: Geneva, Switzerland, 2008.
45. Saadi, A.; Himmelstein, D.U.; Woolhandler, S.; Mejia, N.I. Racial disparities in neurologic health care access and utilization in the United States. *Neurology* **2017**, *88*, 2268–2275. [CrossRef]
46. Minden, S.L.; Hoaglin, D.C.; Hadden, L.; Frankel, D.; Robbins, T.; Perloff, J. Access to and utilization of neurologists by people with multiple sclerosis. *Neurology* **2008**, *70*, 1141–1149. [CrossRef]
47. Mercado, V.; Dongarwar, D.; Fisher, K.; Salihu, H.M.; Hutton, G.J.; Cuascut, F.X. Multiple Sclerosis in a Multi-Ethnic Population in Houston, Texas: A Retrospective Analysis. *Biomedicines* **2020**, *8*, 534. [CrossRef]
48. Fabius, C.D.; Thomas, K.S.; Zhang, T.; Ogarek, J.; Shireman, T.I. Racial disparities in Medicaid home and community-based service utilization and expenditures among persons with multiple sclerosis. *BMC Health Serv. Res.* **2018**, *18*, 773. [CrossRef] [PubMed]
49. Knighton, A.J.; Savitz, L.; Belnap, T.; Stephenson, B.; VanDerslice, J. Introduction of an Area Deprivation Index Measuring Patient Socioeconomic Status in an Integrated Health System: Implications for Population Health. *EGEMS* **2016**, *4*, 1238. [CrossRef]
50. Pimentel Maldonado, D.A.; Eusebio, J.R.; Amezcua, L.; Vasileiou, E.S.; Mowry, E.M.; Hemond, C.C.; Umeton, R.; Berrios Morales, I.; Radu, I.; Ionete, C.; et al. The impact of socioeconomic status on mental health and health-seeking behavior across race and ethnicity in a large multiple sclerosis cohort. *Mult. Scler. Relat. Disord.* **2022**, *58*, 103451. [CrossRef]
51. Pimentel Maldonado, D.; Moreno, A.; Williams, M.J.; Amezcua, L.; Feliciano, S.; Williams, A.; Machemer, D.; Livingston, T.; LaRocque, M.; Glim, M.; et al. Perceptions and Preferences Regarding Multiple Sclerosis Research Among Racial and Ethnic Groups. *Int. J. MS Care* **2021**, *23*, 170–177. [CrossRef] [PubMed]
52. Hall, W.J.; Chapman, M.V.; Lee, K.M.; Merino, Y.M.; Thomas, T.W.; Payne, B.K.; Eng, E.; Day, S.H.; Coyne-Beasley, T. Implicit Racial/Ethnic Bias Among Health Care Professionals and Its Influence on Health Care Outcomes: A Systematic Review. *Am. J. Public Health* **2015**, *105*, e60–e76. [CrossRef] [PubMed]

biomedicines

MDPI

Article

The Association of Age, Sex, and BMI on Lower Limb Neuromuscular and Muscle Mechanical Function in People with Multiple Sclerosis

Anne Geßner, Maximilian Hartmann, Katrin Trentzsch, Heidi Stölzer-Hutsch, Dirk Schriefer and Tjalf Ziemssen *

Center of Clinical Neuroscience, Neurological Clinic, University Hospital Carl Gustav Carus, TU Dresden, Fetscherstr. 74, 01307 Dresden, Germany; anne.gessner@uniklinikum-dresden.de (A.G.); maximilian.hartmann@uniklinikum-dresden.de (M.H.); katrin.trentzsch@uniklinikum-dresden.de (K.T.); heidi.stoelzer-hutsch@uniklinikum-dresden.de (H.S.-H.); dirk.schriefer@uniklinikum-dresden.de (D.S.)

* Correspondence: tjalf.ziemssen@uniklinikum-dresden.de; Tel.: +49-351-458-4465; Fax: +49-351-458-5717

Abstract: (1) Background: The countermovement jump (CMJ) on a force plate could be a sensitive assessment for detecting early lower-limb muscle mechanical deficits in the early stages of multiple sclerosis (MS). CMJ performance is known to be influenced by various anthropometric, physiological, and biomechanical factors, mostly investigated in children and adult athletes. Our aim was to investigate the association of age, sex, and BMI with muscle mechanical function using CMJ to provide a comprehensive overview of lower-limb motor function in people with multiple sclerosis (pwMS). (2) Methods: A cross-sectional study was conducted with pwMS (N = 164) and healthy controls (N = 98). All participants performed three maximal CMJs on a force plate. Age, sex, and BMI were collected from all participants. (3) Results: Significant age, sex, and BMI effects were found for all performance parameters, flight time, and negative and positive power for pwMS and HC, but no significant interaction effects with the group (pwMS, HC) were detected. The highest significant effects were found for sex on flight time ($\eta^2 = 0.23$), jump height ($\eta^2 = 0.23$), and positive power ($\eta^2 = 0.13$). PwMS showed significantly lower CMJ performance compared to HC in middle-aged (31–49 years), with normal weight to overweight and in both women and men. (4) Conclusions: This study showed that age, sex, and BMI are associated with muscle mechanical function in pwMS and HC. These results may be useful in developing reference values for CMJ. This is a crucial step in integrating CMJ into the diagnostic assessment of people with early MS and developing individualized and effective neurorehabilitative therapy.

Keywords: multiple sclerosis; countermovement jump; muscle mechanical function; neuromuscular function; lower limb assessment

1. Introduction

Multiple sclerosis (MS) is a chronic inflammatory disease characterized by heterogeneity of symptoms and pathological mechanisms [1]. Deficits in neuromuscular function (i.e., the interaction between the nervous and the muscular system) and decrements in mechanical function of the lower-limb muscles (i.e., muscle strength, muscle power, and explosive muscle strength) are key symptoms of the disease as they are associated with impaired activities of daily living and quality of life [2,3]. Neurophysiologically, people with MS (pwMS) show lower voluntary muscle activation in terms of neuromuscular function, as well as increased fatigue attributable to the known MS pathophysiology in the central nervous system [4]. Studies indicate that reduced lower-limb muscle strength and power negatively influence the functional ability of the lower limb in pwMS in walking performance, stair climbing, and balance [3,5]. A decrease in lower-limb muscle strength, power, and rate of force development is frequently observed in pwMS compared to healthy controls (HC), especially during fast dynamic muscle contractions [2]. Muscle mechanical function may therefore serve as a particularly useful outcome for disability as it may be sufficiently sensitive to detect muscle impairment in the early stages of disease and in pwMS presenting with low disability [6].

However, lower-limb muscle mechanical function is not only associated with the degree of disability in MS but also with other factors such as age, sex, and body mass index (BMI). To identify, specify, and monitor sensitive subtle neuromuscular and muscle mechanical deficits, it is crucial to monitor all these confounding factors for the management of optimal disease-modifying and symptomatic treatment. The effect of age on muscle strength in MS can be complex. Various studies have shown that a decrease in muscle strength can be age-related [7,8]. Stagsted et al. show that the combined effects of MS and ageing result in a significant decrease in lower-limb muscle strength, which is associated with a decline in physical function [2]. Regarding BMI, its association with muscle strength or other symptoms in pwMS has not been studied, only the physical composition of muscle mass and body fat [9,10]. BMI increases gradually throughout most of adult life and loss of muscle mass begins between the ages of 30 and 40 and continues into old age [11]. However, lower-limb muscle power has been shown to be positively influenced by BMI more so in men than in women [12]. The proportion of women and men who develop MS and the influence of sex on the course of the disease have been studied. Both the central nervous system and the immune system have been shown to have sex-specific differences, which means that there are many variations in the symptoms that occur. Therefore, further studies investigating the association of sex and MS are needed to understand the sex differences in the incidence and severity of MS [13].

Among the many methods being used to evaluate lower-limb muscle mechanical function, e.g., manual muscle function tests and isokinetic dynamometry, the countermovement jump (CMJ), a vertical maximal jump, presents a new assessment in MS, specifically to measure the decrements of rapid dynamic contractions [2,5,14]. In our previous study, we showed that the CMJ can detect lower-limb motor deficits below the clinical threshold of the Expanded Disability Status Scale (EDSS) in the early stage of MS [14]. This functional assessment of muscle activity combines muscle strength, coordination, and balance and provides a simulation of everyday movements as it is based on the principal of the stretch-shortening cycle (SSC) that occurs during natural movements such as walking [14,15]. In addition, a positive relationship between lower-limb muscle strength and CMJ has been demonstrated in many studies [16–18]. CMJ performance is known to be influenced by various anthropometric, physiological, and biomechanical factors, mostly investigated in children and adult athletes [19–22]. Some studies have focused on the effect of sex on CMJ, finding that males showed significantly higher jumping performance than females [23–25]. Men jump approximately 24 to 27% higher than women [26]. Considering the effect of age, children show an increase and adults a decrease in CMJ performance with increasing age [19].

To date, there have been no studies that have investigated the CMJ in association with age, sex, and BMI in pwMS. Characterization of CMJ in association with age, sex, and BMI is necessary for the individual interpretation of early deficits in neuromuscular and muscle mechanical function and the integration of the CMJ into the diagnostic assessment in pwMS [27,28]; it enables individualized and effective neurorehabilitative therapy strategies for pwMS. Our primary aim in this study was to characterize CMJ performance in pwMS and HC in relation to age, sex, and BMI and to provide reference values for CMJ performance in pwMS.

2. Materials and Methods

2.1. Participants

A cross-sectional study was conducted at the MS Center at the Center of Clinical Neuroscience of the Department of Neurology, University Hospital Carl Gustav Carus, Dresden, Germany. Healthy controls (HC) without any neurological disease, who were age-matched to pwMS, were recruited. Recruitment took place from April 2021 to September 2022.

All participants provided written informed consent for the study. The study received approval from the local ethics committee (BO-EK-320062021). The inclusion criteria for pwMS were as follows: (a) confirmed MS diagnosis; (b) EDSS score between 0 and 3.0; (c) age from 18 to 65 years; (d) ability to walk without aid and rest for ≥500 m; and (e) to perform heel rise, stand on heels, and squats. Exclusion criteria for this study were orthopaedic and surgical conditions that could affect jumping ability, fear of falling while jumping, and current pregnancy.

2.2. Measures and Procedures

2.2.1. Age, Sex, and Body Mass Index

Age, sex, and BMI were collected from all participants. BMI was calculated as weight in kg divided by height in m^2 and classified as normal weight (18–25), overweight (25–30), or obese (>30). As most people are diagnosed with MS between the ages of 20 and 40 [29,30], the following age categories were chosen: young (18–30 years), middle-aged (31–49 years), and old (50–65 years). In terms of sex, the participants were binary classified as male or female.

2.2.2. Expanded Disability Status Scale

Certified raters applied the EDSS to examine the neurological clinical status at pwMS, which is the most commonly used disability scale in MS [31,32]. As part of the examination, it evaluates seven functional systems and ambulation.

2.2.3. Countermovement Jump

On a single force plate, all participants completed three maximal CMJ jumps without arm swing. For all three jumps, the mean values of the individual parameters were used for the statistical analyses. All participants completed a practice jump prior to data collection in order to reduce potential insecurities or errors during the test. Prior to the jumps, the physiotherapist provided verbal and visual instructions to each participant on the correct jumping technique.

For the CMJ, participants were instructed to jump as high as possible with their hands on their hips and legs fully extended during the flight phase of the jump (Figure 1). Participants rested in a standing position for approximately 5 s between jumps. Any CMJs that were inadvertently performed with arms swinging or legs tucked during the flight phase of the jumps were excluded. Jumping trials were performed in socks and everyday clothing.

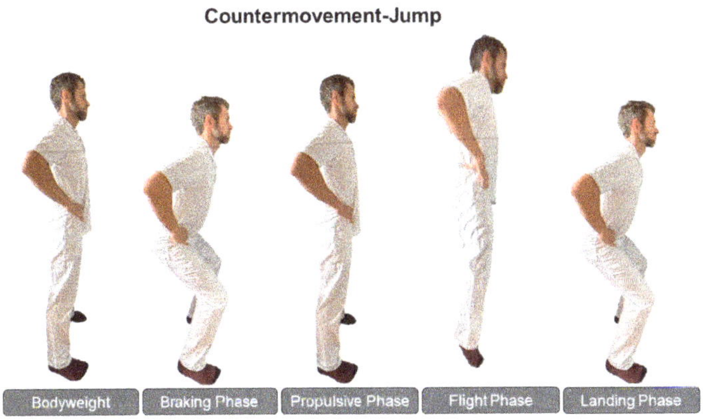

Figure 1. Counter movement jump technique and phases. Bodyweight: the patient stands on the force plate while their body weight is measured. During the braking phase, the patient squats down

until their center of mass reaches its lowest point and their velocity is zero. Propulsive phase: the patient pushes up from the squat and the center of mass velocity becomes positive; flight phase: the time after take-off to the highest point of the center of mass; landing phase: The initial position is reached again when the patient stands still on the force plate, with both feet touching the plate.

2.3. Data Collection

A portable single force plate from AMTI (Advanced Mechanical Technology Inc., Watertown, MA, USA, AccuPower-O) measured the three-dimensional ground reaction forces (Fx, Fy, Fx) and force moments (Mx, My, Mz) during the CMJ at a frequency of 1000 Hz. This force plate, measuring 1016 × 762 × 127 mm (length × width × height), was positioned on a concrete floor and has an internal amplifier. Force plates are the gold standard and a valid instrument with which to record the vertical ground reaction force for vertical jumps [33,34]. AMTI's force plates are strain-gauge-based and have a spring or deformation body. They have the benefits of high measurement accuracy and the ability to compensate for unwanted effects such as temperature dependence of the zero point, bending moment effects, and shear force effects [35]. The participant's body weight was measured using the force plate in the weight phase prior to the start of the braking phase of the CMJ. A threshold value of >5 N from the measured body weight before the jump was used to define the start of the CMJ movement. The end of the countermovement phase was defined as the point when the COM position reached its lowest depth. Temporal, kinetic, and performance jump parameters during the CMJ performance were recorded with a dedicated software for biomechanical analysis (AccuPower Solutions, Version 1.5.4.2082, Watertown, MA, USA). Therefore, not only were strength parameters analyzed but also time-based parameters, as these provide more information about neuromuscular performance [36]. To provide a detailed overview of the overall muscle performance of the lower limb, braking, propulsion, and flight phases were also analyzed. In addition, the parameters used in a previous CMJ study for differentiation between pwMS without motor disability and HC were selected for this study [14]. Table 1 shows a description of the recorded jump parameters according to the jump phases.

Table 1. Countermovement jump parameters measured with the force plate and assignment to jump phases.

Variable Type	Parameters	Unit	CMJ—Phase
Temporal Parameters	Braking Time	s	Braking Phase
	Propulsive Time	s	Propulsive Phase
	Flight Time	s	Flight Phase
Kinetic Parameters	Force at Zero Velocity	N/kg	Braking Phase
	Peak Force	N/kg	Propulsive Phase
	Negative Power	W/kg	Braking Phase
	Positive Power	W/kg	Propulsive Phase
Performance Parameters	Jump Height	cm	Flight Phase
	Flight Time–Contraction Time Ratio	-	Contraction/Flight Phase
	Reactive Strength Index	-	Contraction/Flight Phase

Abbreviations: CMJ = countermovement jump; contraction phase = total of braking and propulsive phase.

2.4. Statistical Analysis

Force values were converted (normalized) to values relative to body weight (N/kg). The distribution of all jump parameters was visually inspected and supplemented with the Shapiro–Wilk test for the assessment of normality. In the evaluation of jump parameters, a descriptive specification of mean values and standard deviations occurred. To evaluate associations of CMJ performance, disease condition (pwMS, HC), age, sex, and BMI, and to quantify differences in jump performance between the associated subgroups (Section 2.2.1), generalized linear models (GLM) were applied. The (continuous) jump parameters served as dependent variables, and fixed main effects were quantified for the following independent variables in each multivariable model: group (pwMS, HC), age (young, middle-aged, old), sex (male, female), BMI (normal weight, overweight, obesity), and the interactions of the group variable with age, sex, and BMI (e.g., age*group, sex*group, and BMI*group). In particular, multiple (nested) GLMs were constructed a priori with a focus on simplicity; starting with a minimal adequate model, including the pre-specified independent variables of interest (basic model 1: group, age, sex, BMI), we progressively added the interaction terms (model 2: model 1 variables and the age*group interaction; model 3: model 1 variables and the sex*group interaction; model 4: model 1 variables and the BMI*group interaction). Thus, model 1 is nested within models 2–4 (and subsequent ones), and accordingly, removal of (insignificant) interaction terms results in simpler models (e.g., basic model 1). Gaussian distribution with an identity link was used for normally distributed jump parameters, and Gamma distribution with a log link function was used for right-skewed jump parameters. Pairwise comparisons (post hoc tests) were conducted, and adjustments were made using the Bonferroni correction to account for multiple group comparisons. Statistical significance was fixed at $p < 0.05$. Effect sizes were determined using eta squared and were interpreted as a measure of effect size as small ($\eta^2 > 0.01$), medium ($\eta^2 > 0.06$), or large ($\eta^2 > 0.14$) [37]. The statistical analyses were performed using IBM Statistical Package for the Social Sciences (SPSS) for Windows, Version 28 (IBM Corp, Armonk, NY, USA).

3. Results

3.1. Participants

A total of 262 study participants (164 pwMS, 98 HC) were eligible for analysis. There was an age distribution of 18 to 64 years among the study participants, with a mean age of 36.29 years (SD ± 9.74) and a mean BMI of 24.59 (SD ± 4.33). In the study cohort, 64.4% were females. Most participants were middle-aged (all: 61.8%; pwMS: 64%; HC: 58.2%) and had normal weight (all: 63.4%; pwMS: 60.4%; HC: 68.4%) (see Table 2). No significant differences for sex, age, and the BMI were found between pwMS and HC. An overview of the participants' characteristics is shown in Table 2.

Table 2. General characteristics of participants. Data are presented as mean (±standard deviation) unless specified otherwise.

		HC (N = 98)	pwMS (N = 164)	p-Value
Sex (female) N (%)		59 (60.2)	110 (67.1)	0.161 [a]
Age (years)		36.60 ± 10.56	36.10 ± 9.25	0.699 [b]
Age Categories	Young (18–30) N (%)	30 (30.6)	44 (26.3)	
	Average Age	25.40 ± 3.26	25.95 ± 3.94	0.527 [b]
	Middle-age (31–49) N (%)	57 (58.2)	105 (64)	
	Average Age	38.56 ± 5.59	37.72 ± 5.50	0.359 [b]
	Old (50–65) N (%)	11 (11.2)	15 (9.1)	
	Average Age	57.00 ± 4.36	54.53 ± 4.17	0.157 [b]
BMI		24.37 ± 3.96	24.71 ± 4.55	0.549 [b]
BMI Categories	Normal weight (18–25) N (%)	69 (68.4)	99 (60.4)	
	Average BMI	22.35 ± 1.76	21.86 ± 1.86	0.086 [b]
	Overweight (25–30) N(%)	43 (26.2)	22 (13.4)	
	Average BMI	26.70 ± 1.33	26.91 ± 1.49	0.587 [b]
	Obesity (30+) N (%)	9 (9.2)	22 (13.4)	
	Average BMI	33.87 ± 3.14	33.25 ± 3.92	0.680 [b]
Disease Duration (years)		n.a	6.87 ± 5.26	-
MS Subtype				
	RRMS (%)	n.a	100%	-

Table 2. *Cont.*

		HC (N = 98)	pwMS (N = 164)	*p*-Value
EDSS (median, IQR)		n.a	1.5 (1.5–2.0)	-
	Pyramidal FSS	-	0 (0–1)	-
	Cerebellar FSS	-	0 (0–0)	-
	Ambulation	-	0 (0–0)	-

Abbreviations: [a] = calculated with chi^2, [b] = calculated with *t*-test, pwMS = people with multiple sclerosis; HC = healthy controls; MS = multiple sclerosis; RRMS = relapsing remitting multiple sclerosis; EDSS = expanded disability status scale; BMI = body mass index; IQR = interquartile range; FSS = functional system score, n.a. = not applicable.

3.2. Effect of Group, Age, Sex, and BMI on CMJ Parameters

The independent variables—age, gender, and BMI (factors)—had significant individual effects on the dependent variables (jumping parameters) (model 1; Table 3); however, each of their combined effects (i.e., the interaction of age*group, sex*group, and BMI*group) was not significant (model 2–4, Table 3). Table 3 shows the results of the associations of CMJ performance (jump parameter), group (pwMS, HC), age, sex, and BMI from the GLM analysis. The results of the contrast (post hoc) tests for group, age, sex, and BMI for model 1 (both MS and HC) are shown in the Figures 2–5.

Table 3. Effect of group, age, BMI, and sex on the CMJ performance.

	Model 1				Model 2	Model 3	Model 4
Parameters (Dependent Variable)	**Group (MS, HC)**	**Age Categories (Young, Middle-Age, Old)**	**BMI Categories (Normal Weight, Overweight, Obesity)**	**Sex Categories (Male, Female)**	**Interaction Group*Age Categories**	**Interaction Group*BMI Categories**	**Interaction Group*Sex Categories**
Braking Time [1,A]	NS -	NS -	NS -	NS -	NS -	NS -	NS -
Propulsive Time [1,A]	NS -	NS -	NS -	NS -	NS -	NS -	NS -
Flight Time [1,B]	$p < 0.001$ * $\eta^2 = 0.0478$	$p < 0.001$ * $\eta^2 = 0.0505$	$p < 0.001$ * $\eta^2 = 0.0828$	$p < 0.001$ * $\eta^2 = 0.2326$	NS -	NS -	NS -
FZV [2,B]	$p < 0.001$ * $\eta^2 = 0.0818$	NS -	$p = 0.002$ * $\eta^2 = 0.0275$	NS -	NS -	NS -	NS -
Peak Force [2,A]	$p < 0.001$ * $\eta^2 = 0.0540$	$p = 0.004$ * $\eta^2 = 0.0233$	NS -	$p < 0.001$ * $\eta^2 = 0.0053$	NS -	NS -	NS -
Negative Power [2,A]	$p < 0.001$ * $\eta^2 = 0.0709$	$p = 0.045$ * $\eta^2 = 0.0133$	$p = 0.004$ * $\eta^2 = 0.0235$	$p < 0.001$ * $\eta^2 = 0.0526$	NS -	NS -	NS -
Positive Power [2,A]	NS -	$p < 0.001$ * $\eta^2 = 0.0381$	$p < 0.001$ * $\eta^2 = 0.0556$	$p < 0.001$ * $\eta^2 = 0.1313$	NS -	NS -	NS -
Jump Height [3,B]	$p < 0.001$ * $\eta^2 = 0.0481$	$p < 0.001$ * $\eta^2 = 0.049$	$p < 0.001$ * $\eta^2 = 0.0802$	$p < 0.001$ * $\eta^2 = 0.2336$	NS -	NS -	NS -
FTCTR [3,B]	$p = 0.005$ * $\eta^2 = 0.0327$	$p = 0.003$ * $\eta^2 = 0.0248$	$p = 0.003$ * $\eta^2 = 0.0248$	$p = 0.006$ * $\eta^2 = 0.0318$	NS -	NS -	NS -
RSI [3,A]	$p < 0.001$ * $\eta^2 = 0.0520$	$p < 0.001$ * $\eta^2 = 0.0403$	$p < 0.001$ * $\eta^2 = 0.0506$	$p < 0.001$ * $\eta^2 = 0.0914$	NS -	NS -	NS -

Results based on the GLM analysis. [1] = temporal parameter; [2] = kinetic parameter; [3] = performance parameter; [A] = Gamma distribution with log link function; [B] = Gaussian distribution with identity link; Model 1 = group, age, sex, and BMI; Model 2 = group, age, sex, BMI, and group*age interaction; Model 3 = group, age, sex, BMI, and group*BMI interaction; Model 4 = group, age, sex, BMI, and group*sex interaction; * = significant effect ($p < 0.005$); $\eta^2 > 0.01$ = small effect; $\eta^2 > 0.06$ = medium effect; $\eta^2 > 0.14$ = large effect. Abbreviations: NS = not significant; FZV = force at zero velocity; RSI = reactive strength index; FTCTR = flight time–contraction time ratio.

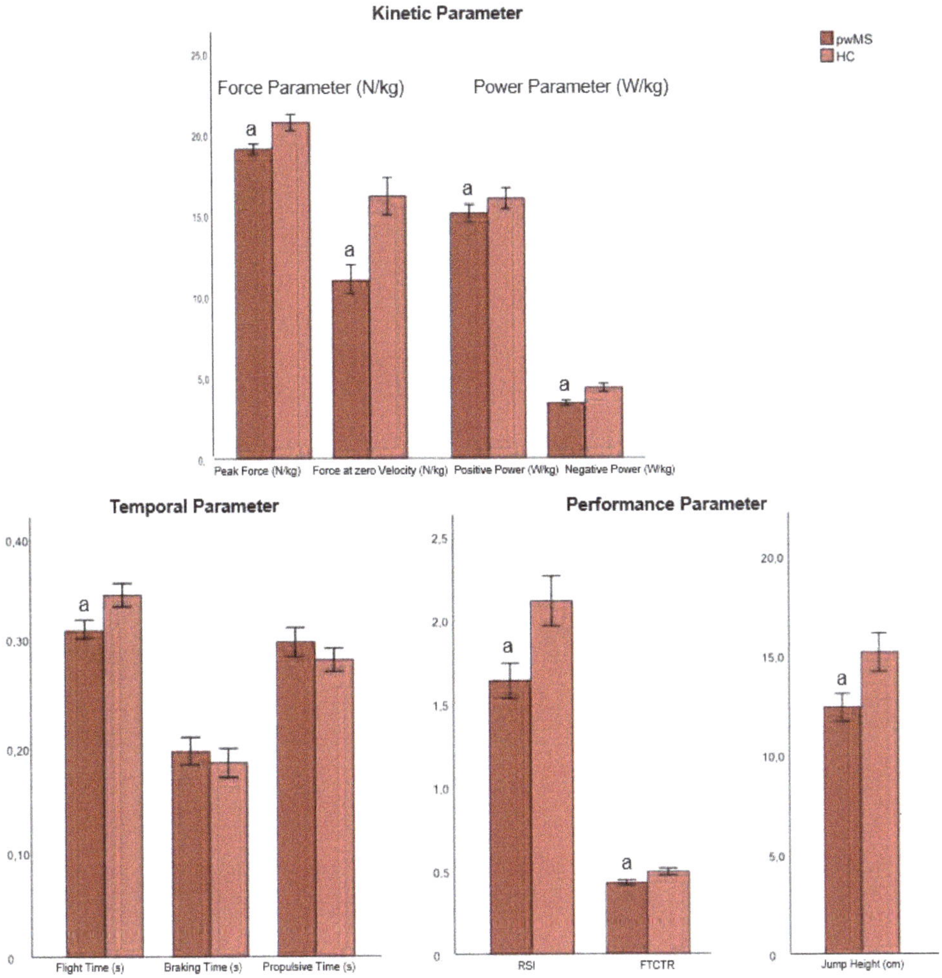

Figure 2. Contrast (post hoc) tests for group (pwMS and HC) on the jumping parameters (means ± SD) (model 1). Abbreviations: a = significant difference with HC ($p < 0.05$); RSI = reactive strength index; FTCTR = flight time–contraction time ratio; RSI and FTCTR have an arbitrary unit.

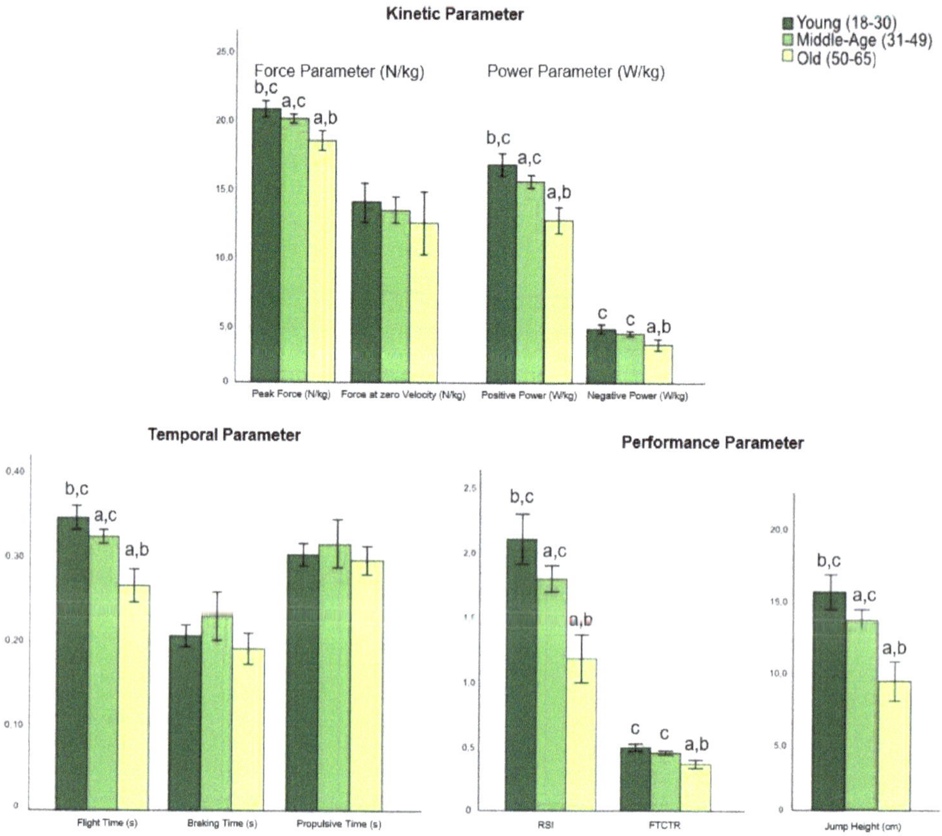

Figure 3. Contrast (post hoc) tests for age (young, middle-age, old) on the jumping parameters (means ± SD) for all participants (both MS and HC) (model 1). Abbreviations: a = significant difference to young ($p < 0.05$); b = significant difference to middle-age ($p < 0.05$); c = significant difference to old ($p < 0.05$); RSI = reactive strength index; FTCTR = flight time–contraction time ratio, RSI and FTCTR have an arbitrary unit.

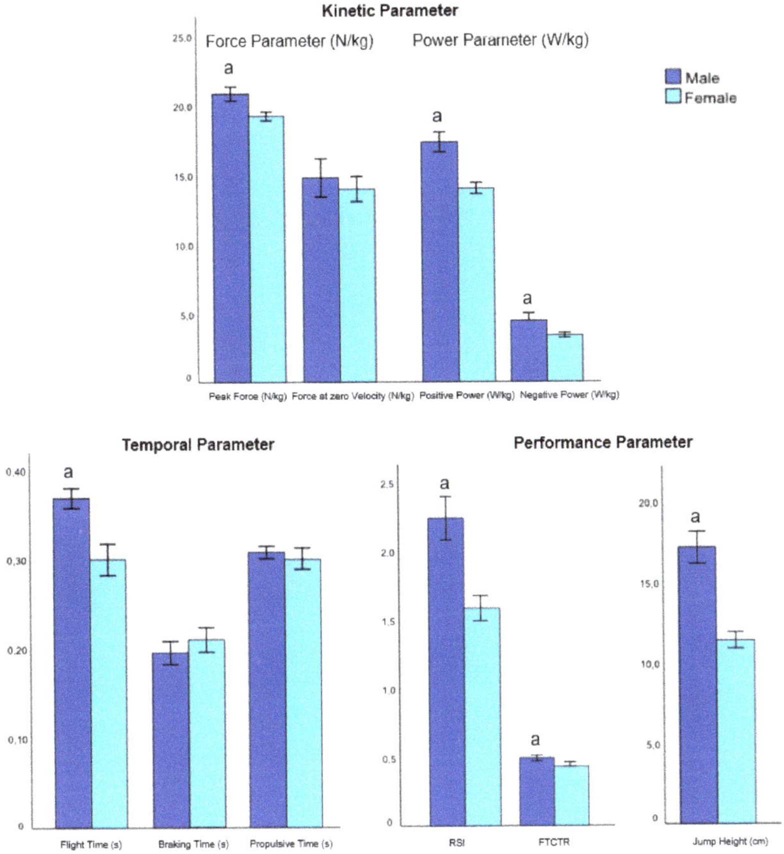

Figure 4. Contrast (post hoc) tests for sex (male, female) on the jumping parameters (means ± SD) for all participants (both MS and HC) (model 1). Abbreviation: a = significant difference with female ($p < 0.05$); RSI = reactive strength index; FTCTR = flight time–contraction time ratio, RSI and FTCTR have an arbitrary unit.

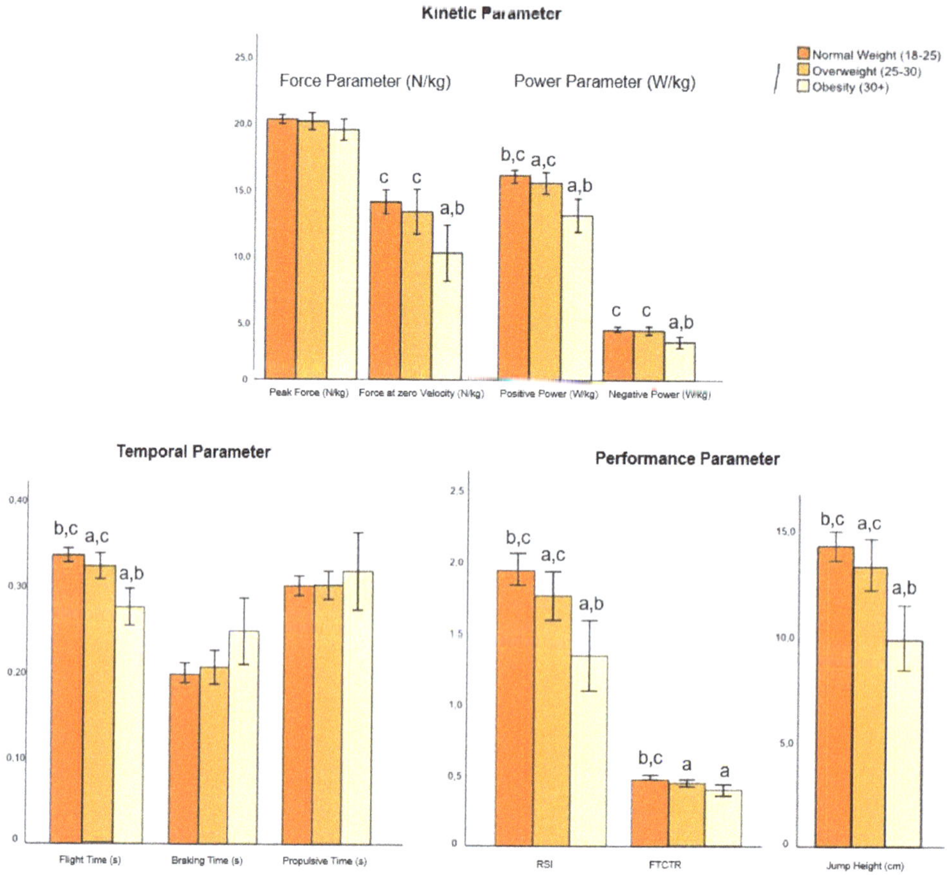

Figure 5. Contrast (post hoc) tests for BMI (normal weight, overweight, obesity) on the jumping parameters (means ± SD) for all participants (both MS and HC) (model 1). Abbreviations: a = significant difference to normal weight ($p < 0.05$); b = significant difference to overweight ($p < 0.05$). c = significant difference to obesity ($p < 0.05$); RSI = reactive strength index; FTCTR = flight time–contraction time ratio; RSI and FTCTR have an arbitrary unit.

3.2.1. Effect of Group

A significant group effect was shown for all performance parameters, force at zero velocity (FZV), peak force, negative power, and flight time, with the highest effect size, with a moderate effect for power and force, in the braking phase (FZV: $\eta^2 = 0.0818$; and negative power: $\eta^2 = 0.0709$) (Tables 3 and S1).

Overall, pwMS had significantly lower peak force in both the braking and propulsive phases compared to HC (see Figure 2). In addition, a significantly lower jump height, reactive strength index (RSI), flight time–contraction time ratio (FTCTR), and negative power, as well a shorter flight time, were observed in the pwMS (see Figure 2). The contrast (post hoc) tests for each group are shown in the Figure 2. Supplementary Table S1 presents a dataset that provides a descriptive analysis of CMJ performance in association to age, sex, and BMI in pwMS and HC.

For young and middle-aged participants (18–49 years), significant group differences (pwMS; HC) were found for almost all jumping parameters (expect braking time, propulsive time and positive power). In contrast, in the 50–65 age, group differences only exist for FTCTR. There were significant group differences in all three BMI categories for flight time and negative power. For FZV, peak force, RSI, and jump height, pwMS and HC with normal weight and overweight are significantly different. In addition, significant group differences are shown for all jump parameters (except braking time, propulsion time, and positive power) for both females and males. The group comparison between pwMS and HC in terms of age, BMI, and sex categories is shown in Table 4.

Table 4. Group comparison between pwMS and HC in terms of age, BMI, and sex.

	Age Categories			BMI Categories			Sex	
	Young 18–30 (pwMS = 44, HC = 30)	Middle-Age 31–49 (pwMS = 105, HC = 57)	Old 50–65 (pwMS = 15, HC = 11)	Normal Weight 18–25 (pwMS = 99, HC = 69)	Overweight 25–30 (pwMS = 43, HC = 22)	Obesity 30+ (pwMS = 22, HC = 9)	Male (pwMS = 54, HC = 39)	Female (pwMS = 110, HC = 59)
Parameters	*p*	*p*	*p*	*p*	*p*	*p*	*p*	*p*
BT [1]	0.097	0.002 *	0.853	0.146	0.141	0.184	0.069	0.133
PT [1]	0.348	0.005 *	0.655	0.010 *	0.233	0.846	0.058	0.309
FT [1]	<0.001 *	<0.001 *	0.174	0.003 *	<0.001 *	0.020 *	<0.001 *	<0.001 *
FZV [2]	<0.001 *	<0.001 *	0.039 *	<0.001 *	<0.001 *	0.057	0.003 *	0.001 *
PF [2]	<0.001 *	<0.001 *	0.506	0.005 *	<0.001 *	0.177	<0.001 *	0.030 *
NP [2]	<0.001 *	<0.001 *	0.064	0.001 *	0.001 *	0.020 *	<0.001 *	0.001 *
PP [2]	0.051	<0.001 *	0.316	0.078	0.047 *	0.114	0.007 *	0.187
JH [3]	<0.001 *	<0.001 *	0.187	0.002 *	<0.001 *	0.029 *	<0.001 *	0.002 *
FTCTR [3]	0.002 *	<0.001 *	0.480	0.012 *	0.003 *	0.233	<0.001 *	0.048 *
RSI [3]	<0.001 *	<0.001 *	0.329	0.007 *	<0.001 *	0.087	<0.001 *	0.011 *

Abbreviations: * = significant ($p < 0.05$); [1] = temporal parameters; [2] = kinetic parameters; [3] = performance parameters; pwMS: people with multiple sclerosis. HC: healthy controls; BMI = body mass index; BT = braking Time; FZV = force at zero velocity; NP = negative power; PF = peak force; PP = positive power; JH = jump height; FT = flight time; FTCTR = flight time–contraction time ratio; RSI = reactive strength index; PT = propulsive time.

3.2.2. Effect of Age

Significant age effects were found for all performance parameters, peak force, negative power, positive power, and flight time (Tables 3 and S1). A significant decrease in jumping performance with increasing age was observed for all participants (pwMS and HC) for peak force, positive power, flight time, RSI, and jump height. Furthermore, a significant decrease in jumping performance was shown between young and old participants as well as between middle-age and old for negative power and FTCTR. The contrast (post hoc) tests for age on the jumping parameters for all participants (both MS and HC) are shown in the Figure 3.

3.2.3. Effect of Sex

For sex, significant effects were found for all performance parameters, i.e., peak force, negative power, positive power, and flight time, with the highest effect for the performance parameter in the flight phase (flight time: $\eta^2 = 0.2326$; and jump height: $\eta^2 = 0.2336$) (Tables 3 and S1). In all participants (pwMS and HC), males showed significantly higher peak force, higher positive and negative power, and longer flight time than females. Additionally, males demonstrated significantly higher jump performance in all performance parameters. The contrast (post hoc) tests for sex on the jumping parameters for all participants (both MS and HC) are shown in the Figure 4.

3.2.4. Effect of BMI

Significant BMI effects were found for positive power, negative power, RSI, FZV, FTCTR, jump height, and flight time (Tables 3 and S1). Similar to sex, jump height ($\eta^2 = 0.0802$) and flight time ($\eta^2 = 0.0828$) had the largest effect size for BMI, with a moderate effect. A significant decrease in jumping performance with increasing BMI was observed for all participants (pwMS and HC) for positive power, flight time, RSI and jump height. Additionally, a significant decrease in jump performance between normal weight and obesity and between overweight and obesity were found for FZV and negative power.

The contrast (post hoc) tests for BMI on the jumping parameters for all participants (both MS and HC) are shown in the Figure 5.

3.2.5. Association of Age, Sex, and BMI on the Jumping Parameters in pwMS

For age in pwMS, a significant decrease in jumping performance was observed between young and old participants, as well as middle-age and old participants, for jump height, flight time, RSI, and positive power (see Supplement Figure S1). FTCTR, peak force, and negative power decreased significantly from middle-age to old age. Comparing the sex differences in jump performance in pwMS, males showed significantly better CMJ performance than females, especially for the kinetic and power parameters (see Supplement Figure S2). For BMI, the pwMS showed a significant decrease in jump performance from normal weight to overweight and from normal weight to obesity for flight time, force at zero velocity, positive power, and all performance parameters (see Supplement Figure S3). The contrast (post hoc) tests for age, sex, and BMI on the jumping parameters for pwMS are shown in the Supplement Figures S1–S3.

4. Discussion

In this study, we analyzed the CMJ performance in HC and pwMS in association with age, sex, and BMI. Furthermore, reference values for the CMJ for both the pwMS and HC were provided. Our study results demonstrated that age, sex, and BMI are associated with the CMJ performance in pwMS and HC. Overall, pwMS demonstrated reduced CMJ performances compared to HC in all performance parameters, i.e., force at zero velocity, peak force, negative power, and flight time. Especially in the middle-age group (age 31–49 years), the pwMS showed significantly lower CMJ performance in all parameters compared to HC. Significant group differences (pwMS; HC) in most parameters were observed for normal weight and overweight (CMJ performance for pwMS < HC). In addition, the pwMS showed reduced CMJ performance in almost all jump parameters (with the exception of braking time, propulsion time, and positive power) for both females and males. Significant age, sex, and BMI effects were found for all performance parameters, flight time, and negative and positive power for pwMS and HC. With increasing age and BMI, CMJ performance decreased and was higher in males (both in pwMS and HC). No significant interaction effects (e.g., age*group, sex*group, and BMI*group) were found. These results suggest that the association of age, sex, and BMI on CMJ performance is almost the same for pwMS and HC and not specific to pwMS. One reason for this could be that the two groups did not differ in terms of age, sex, and BMI (Table 2).

As expected, males showed a higher CMJ performance than females. The highest significant effects were found for sex on flight time ($\eta^2 = 0.23$), jump height ($\eta^2 = 0.23$), and positive power ($\eta^2 = 0.13$). In pwMS, the males jumped 40% higher than females (HC: 38%). Similar results were found in other studies [20,23–25,38]. Sex differences are attributed to the normal growth between males and females. Males typically have a higher percentage of fast twitch (type II) fibers, which are responsible for explosive movements and high muscle strength [39–41]. There are numerous other contributors to differences between the sex, including hormones, chromosomes, and gene-by-environment interactions (e.g., epigenetics) [41]. Besides sex and age, MS also seems to negatively influence the skeletal muscle fiber cross-sectional area, muscle strength, and muscle mass of the lower limbs of mildly affected MS patients, independent of MS type and disease severity [9].

In addition, older pwMS had significantly lower CMJ performance than younger pwMS. These age differences were more pronounced for performance and kinetic parameters than for temporal parameters. Similar results were found where, with advanced age, lower extremity muscle power became reduced to a comparable extent in pwMS and HC [2]. Our finding that old pwMS and HC (50+) do not differ significantly in jumping performance in most parameters (only in FZV) are consistent with Kirkland et al. [42]. They also showed no differences in jumping performance between pwMS and old HC on most measures of jumping, suggesting that the old HC also have some early deficits in neuromuscular control of jumping [42]. In addition to structural, biochemical, and cellular changes, skeletal muscle also undergoes functional changes that negatively affect its mechanical function [43]. Studies have shown that muscle strength may be a more important factor than muscle mass in determining functional limitations and mobility status with age, resulting in a decrease in jumping performance [44]. Vertical jump performance decreases with age due to loss of muscle mass and increase in body fat [45]. It is important to differentiate the normal ageing process, age-related diseases, or an increased degenerative process directly related to the progression of MS. Most often, a combination of these factors leads to the progression of neuromuscular symptoms [46]. To reduce the influence of MS disability and focus on other influencing variables such as age, only MS patients with a low EDSS (<3.0) were included in our study. The median EDSS score of 1.5 in pwMS showed that the MS cohort had only minimal signs in more than one functional system but not obvious disability [31].

The results of a large sarcopenia study showed that power-based measurements, such as leg extension strength dynamometer and the sit-to-stand test, already started to decline at age +50 years. However, power-based parameters such as handgrip strength, habitual gait speed, and lean mass remained unaltered until after the age of +70 years. The cut-off values obtained in this study differ from previous reference data, emphasizing the significance of obtaining updated and local reference materials [7].

Such cut-off values and reference values will also be useful for the CMJ in MS to identify early individual deficits in neuromuscular and muscle mechanical function in the future. Our dataset provides the first CMJ characterization in association with age, sex, and BMI in MS which can used for normative reference in MS. In future studies, a larger MS cohort is needed to generate standardized and reliable normative references that are clinically and scientifically relevant in MS.

Our results showed that a high BMI negatively influenced jumping performance in pwMS. The review by Gianfrancesco and Barcellos also found a significant association between obesity and MS [47]. Thus, obesity at the onset of MS is associated with higher disability scores and a more rapid increase in disability over an observation period of up to 6 years [48]. Obesity is a modifiable risk factor whose influence on disease onset and progression is critical for exercise therapy. Also, the significant group (HC and pwMS) differences, especially in the young participants (between 18 and 30 years), indicate the clinical relevance of the importance of early neurorehabilitation. The CMJ can help detect subtle impairments and provide individualized neurorehabilitation to positively impact functional and neurological reserve [14,49]. The therapeutic benefit of strength training to improve muscle strength and functional capacity is well recognized in pwMS [50]. High-intensity resistance or strength training combined with functional tasks is recommended in this case [51,52].

Several sport-specific studies have shown that high levels of physical activity have a positive effect on jumping performance in adults [19,22]. However, no studies have investigated physical activity in relation to jumping performance in pwMS. This would be important for future studies investigating the association of CMJ performance and physical activity in MS. Based on the knowledge that muscle strength correlates strongly with vertical jump height, it is crucial for further studies to explore this correlation with dynamometer measurements while considering the confounding variables in pwMS [53]. Other confounding variables, which may be a combination of demographic, clinical, and imaging findings, as well as biomarkers, should be investigated in future studies to obtain a complex characterization of mechanical muscle function using the CMJ in pwMS. In addition, longitudinal studies are needed to better understand the influence of the investigated variables and to determine whether the CMJ can be used as a standardized measure of disease progression in MS.

5. Conclusions

In conclusion, the study results showed a significant association between age, sex, and BMI on CMJ performance in pwMS and HC. Our results also suggest that the association of age, sex, and BMI on CMJ performance is almost the same for pwMS and HC. However, pwMS showed significantly lower CMJ performance than HC in middle-age participants (31–49 years), normal weight to overweight, and in both women and men. Characterizing CMJ in association with age, sex, and BMI is useful for identifying individual deficits in neuromuscular and muscle mechanical function in pwMS. These results may be useful in the development of reference jump values and digital twins in order to decisively advance the necessary implementation of individualized neurorehabilitative management of MS at an early stage [27]. In order to determine the causal influence of age, sex, and BMI on mechanical muscle function in pwMS, future studies will need longitudinal data that include other influencing factors such as physical activity and additional assessments such as the dynamometer.

Supplementary Materials: The following supporting information can be downloaded at https://www.mdpi.com/article/10.3390/biomedicines12050971/s1: Table S1: CMJ characteristic in pwMS and HC according to sex, age, and BMI; Figure S1: Association between age and the jumping parameters in pwMS; Figure S2: Association between sex and the jumping parameters in pwMS; Figure S3: Association between BMI and the jumping parameters in pwMS.

Author Contributions: Conceptualization, A.G., M.H., K.T., H.S.-H., D.S. and T.Z.; methodology A.G., M.H., K.T. and D.S.; software, A.G.; validation, A.G. and M.H.; formal analysis, A.G., M.H., K.T., H.S.-H. and D.S.; investigation, A.G. and M.H.; data curation, A.G. and M.H.; writing—original draft preparation, A.G. and M.H.; writing—review and editing, K.T., H.S.-H., D.S. and T.Z.; visualization, A.G.; supervision, K.T., D.S. and T.Z.; project administration, A.G. All authors have read and agreed to the published version of the manuscript.

Funding: This research received no external funding.

Institutional Review Board Statement: This study was conducted in accordance with the Declaration of Helsinki and approved by approved by the local ethics committee (BO-EK-320062021).

Informed Consent Statement: Informed consent was obtained from all subjects involved in the study.

Data Availability Statement: All data produced in the present study are available upon reasonable request to the authors.

Acknowledgments: The authors extend their gratitude to all participants for their time and to Anikó Vágó for recruiting and testing participants.

Conflicts of Interest: The authors declare no conflicts of interest.

References

1. Goldenberg, M.M. Multiple Sclerosis Review. *Pharm. Ther.* **2012**, *37*, 175–184.
2. Stagsted, R.A.W.; Ramari, C.; Skjerbaek, A.G.; Thrue, C.; Dalgas, U.; Hvid, L.G. Lower Extremity Muscle Power—A Critical Determinant of Physical Function in Aging and Multiple Sclerosis. *Exp. Gerontol.* **2021**, *150*, 111347. [CrossRef]
3. Jørgensen, M.L.K.; Dalgas, U.; Wens, I.; Hvid, L.G. Muscle Strength and Power in Persons with Multiple Sclerosis—A Systematic Review and Meta-Analysis. *J. Neurol. Sci.* **2017**, *376*, 225–241. [CrossRef]
4. Mamoei, S.; Hvid, L.G.; Boye Jensen, H.; Zijdewind, I.; Stenager, E.; Dalgas, U. Neurophysiological Impairments in Multiple Sclerosis—Central and Peripheral Motor Pathways. *Acta Neurol. Scand.* **2020**, *142*, 401–417. [CrossRef] [PubMed]
5. Ramari, C.; Hvid, L.G.; de David, A.C.; Dalgas, U. The Importance of Lower-Extremity Muscle Strength for Lower-Limb Functional Capacity in Multiple Sclerosis: Systematic Review. *Ann. Phys. Rehabil. Med.* **2020**, *63*, 123–137. [CrossRef]
6. Taul-madsen, L.; Riemenschneider, M.; Marie-louise, K.J.; Dalgas, U.; Hvid, L.G. Identification of Disability Status in Persons with Multiple Sclerosis by Lower Limb Neuromuscular Function—Emphasis on Rate of Force Development. *Mult. Scler. Relat. Disord.* **2022**, *67*, 104082. [CrossRef] [PubMed]
7. Suetta, C.; Haddock, B.; Alcazar, J.; Noerst, T.; Hansen, O.M.; Ludvig, H.; Kamper, R.S.; Schnohr, P.; Prescott, E.; Andersen, L.L.; et al. The Copenhagen Sarcopenia Study: Lean Mass, Strength, Power, and Physical Function in a Danish Cohort Aged 20–93 Years. *J. Cachexia Sarcopenia Muscle* **2019**, *10*, 1316–1329. [CrossRef]

8. Byrne, C.; Faure, C.; Keene, D.J.; Lamb, S.E. Ageing, Muscle Power and Physical Function: A Systematic Review and Implications for Pragmatic Training Interventions. *Sport. Med.* **2016**, *46*, 1311–1332. [CrossRef] [PubMed]
9. Wens, I.; Dalgas, U.; Vandenabeele, F.; Krekels, M.; Grevendonk, L.; Eijnde, B.O. Multiple Sclerosis Affects Skeletal Muscle Characteristics. *PLoS ONE* **2014**, *9*, e0108158. [CrossRef]
10. Kirmaci, Z.İ.K.; Firat, T.; Özkur, H.A.; Neyal, A.M.; Neyal, A.; Ergun, N. Muscle Architecture and Its Relationship with Lower Extremity Muscle Strength in Multiple Sclerosis. *Acta Neurol. Belg.* **2022**, *122*, 1521–1528. [CrossRef]
11. Wang, Z.; Ying, Z.; Bosy-Westphal, A.; Zhang, J.; Heller, M.; Later, W.; Heymsfield, S.B.; Müller, M.J. Evaluation of Specific Metabolic Rates of Major Organs and Tissues: Comparison Between Nonobese and Obese Women ZiMian. *Obesity* **2012**, *20*, 95–100. [CrossRef] [PubMed]
12. Sartorio, A.; Proietti, M.; Marinone, P.G.; Agosti, F.; Adorni, F.; Lafortuna, C.L. Influence of Gender, Age and BMI on Lower Limb Muscular Power Output in a Large Population of Obese Men and Women. *Int. J. Obes.* **2004**, *28*, 91–98. [CrossRef] [PubMed]
13. Coyle, P.K. What Can We Learn from Sex Differences in MS? *J. Pers. Med.* **2021**, *11*, 1006. [CrossRef] [PubMed]
14. Geßner, A.; Stölzer-Hutsch, H.; Trentzsch, K.; Schriefer, D.; Ziemssen, T. Countermovement Jumps Detect Subtle Motor Deficits in People with Multiple Sclerosis below the Clinical Threshold. *Biomedicines* **2023**, *11*, 774. [CrossRef] [PubMed]
15. Aeles, J.; Vanwanseele, B. Do Stretch-Shortening Cycles Really Occur in the Medial Gastrocnemius? A Detailed Bilateral Analysis of the Muscle-Tendon Interaction During Jumping. *Front. Physiol.* **2019**, *10*, 1504. [CrossRef] [PubMed]
16. Sheppard, J.M.; Cronin, J.B.; Gabbett, T.J.; McGuigan, M.R.; Etxebarria, N.; Newton, R.U. Relative Importance of Strength, Power, and Anthropometric Measures to Jump Performance of Elite Volleyball Players. *J. Strength Cond. Res.* **2008**, *22*, 758–765. [CrossRef] [PubMed]
17. McErlain-Naylor, S.; King, M.; Pain, M.T. homa. G. Determinants of Countermovement Jump Performance: A Kinetic and Kinematic Analysis. *J. Sports Sci.* **2014**, *32*, 1805–1812. [CrossRef]
18. Wisløff, U.; Castagna, C.; Helgerud, J.; Jones, R.; Hoff, J. Strong Correlation of Maximal Squat Strength with Sprint Performance and Vertical Jump Height in Elite Soccer Players. *Br. J. Sports Med.* **2004**, *38*, 285–288. [CrossRef]
19. Focke, A.; Strutzenberger, G.; Jekauc, D.; Worth, A.; Woll, A.; Schwameder, H. Effects of Age, Sex and Activity Level on Counter-Movement Jump Performance in Children and Adolescents. *Eur. J. Sport Sci.* **2013**, *13*, 518–526. [CrossRef]
20. Ntai, A.; Zahou, F.; Paradisis, G.; Smirniotou, A.; Tsolakis, C. Anthropometric Parameters and Leg Power Performance in Fencing. Age, Sex and Discipline Related Differences. *Sci. Sport.* **2017**, *32*, 135–143. [CrossRef]
21. Holden, S.; Boreham, C.; Doherty, C.; Wang, D.; Delahunt, E. Clinical Assessment of Countermovement Jump Landing Kinematics in Early Adolescence: Sex Differences and Normative Values. *Clin. Biomech.* **2015**, *30*, 469–474. [CrossRef] [PubMed]
22. Keiner, M.; Sander, A.; Wirth, K.; Schmidtbleicher, D. Is There a Difference Between Active and Less Active Children and Adolescents in Jump Performance? *J. Strength Cond. Res.* **2013**, *27*, 1591–1596. [CrossRef] [PubMed]
23. Kozinc, Ž.; Žitnik, J.; Smajla, D.; Šarabon, N. The Difference between Squat Jump and Countermovement Jump in 770 Male and Female Participants from Different Sports. *Eur. J. Sport Sci.* **2022**, *22*, 985–993. [CrossRef] [PubMed]
24. Laffaye, G.; Wagner, P.P.; Tombleson, T.I.L. Countermovement Jump Height: Gender and Sport-Specific Differences in the Force-Time Variables. *J. Strength Cond. Res.* **2014**, *28*, 1096–1105. [CrossRef] [PubMed]
25. Siglinsky, E.; Krueger, D.; Ward, R.E.; Caserotti, P.; Strotmeyer, E.S.; Harris, T.B.; Binkley, N.; Buehring, B. Effect of Age and Sex on Jumping Mechanography and Other Measures of Muscle Mass and Function. *J. Musculoskelet. Neuronal Interact.* **2015**, *15*, 301–308. [PubMed]
26. McMahon, J.J.; Rej, S.J.E.; Comfort, P. Sex Differences in Countermovement Jump Phase Characteristics. *Sports* **2017**, *5*, 8. [CrossRef] [PubMed]
27. Voigt, I.; Inojosa, H.; Dillenseger, A.; Haase, R.; Akgün, K.; Ziemssen, T. Digital Twins for Multiple Sclerosis. *Front. Immunol.* **2021**, *12*, 669811. [CrossRef] [PubMed]
28. Ziemssen, T.; Kern, R.; Voigt, I.; Haase, R. Digital Data Collection in Multiple Sclerosis: The MSDS Approach. *Front. Neurol.* **2020**, *11*, 445. [CrossRef] [PubMed]
29. McGinley, M.P.; Goldschmidt, C.H.; Rae-Grant, A.D. Diagnosis and Treatment of Multiple Sclerosis: A Review. *JAMA—J. Am. Med. Assoc.* **2021**, *325*, 765–779. [CrossRef]
30. Hemmer, B.; Bayas, A.; Berthele, A.; Domurath, B.; Faaßhauer, E.; Flachenecker, P.; Gärtner, J.; Gehring, K.; Heesen, C.; Hegen, H.; et al. *Diagnose und Therapie der Multiplen Sklerose, Neuromyelitis-Optica-Spektrum-Erkrankungen und MOG-IgG-Assoziierten Erkrankungen S2k-Leitlinie*; Leitlinien für Diagnostik und Therapie in der Neurologie; Deutsche Gesellschaft für Neurologie: Berlin, Germany, 2023; Available online: https://dgn.org/leitlinie/diagnose-und-therapie-der-multiplen-sklerose-neuromyelitis-optica-spektrum-erkrankungen-und-mog-igg-assoziierten-erkrankungen (accessed on 21 May 2023).
31. Kurtzke, J.F. Rating Neurologic Impairment in Multiple Sclerosis: An Expanded Disability Status Scale (EDSS). *Neurology* **1983**, *33*, 1444–1452. [CrossRef]
32. Inojosa, H.; Schriefer, D.; Ziemssen, T. Clinical Outcome Measures in Multiple Sclerosis: A Review. *Autoimmun. Rev.* **2020**, *19*, 102512. [CrossRef] [PubMed]
33. Vanrenterghem, J.; De Clercq, D.; Van Cleven, P. Necessary Precautions in Measuring Correct Vertical Jumping Height by Means of Force Plate Measurements. *Ergonomics* **2001**, *44*, 814–818. [CrossRef] [PubMed]
34. Buckthorpe, M.; Morris, J.; Folland, J.P. Validity of Vertical Jump Measurement Devices. *J. Sports Sci.* **2012**, *30*, 63–69. [CrossRef] [PubMed]

35. Güllich, A.; Krüger, M. *Sport—Das Lehrbuch Für Das Sportstudium*; 2. Auflage.; Springer Spektrum: Berlin/Heidelberg, Germany, 2013; ISBN 9783662646946.
36. Gathercole, R.; Sporer, B.; Stellingwerff, T.; Sleivert, G. Alternative Countermovement-Jump Analysis to Quantify Acute Neuromuscular Fatigue. *Int. J. Sports Physiol. Perform.* **2015**, *10*, 84–92. [CrossRef] [PubMed]
37. Cohen, J. *Statistical Power Analysis for the Behavioral Science*; Routledge: New York, NY, USA, 1988; 567p. [CrossRef]
38. Bchini, S.; Hammami, N.; Selmi, T.; Zalleg, D.; Bouassida, A. Influence of Muscle Volume on Jumping Performance in Healthy Male and Female Youth and Young Adults. *BMC Sports Sci. Med. Rehabil.* **2023**, *15*, 26. [CrossRef] [PubMed]
39. Haizlip, K.M.; Harrison, B.C.; Leinwand, L.A. Sex-Based Differences in Skeletal Muscle Kinetics and Fiber-Type Composition. *Physiology* **2015**, *30*, 30–39. [CrossRef] [PubMed]
40. Maciejewska-Skrendo, A.; Leznicka, K.; Leońska-Duniec, A.; Wilk, M.; Filip, A.; Cięszczyk, P.; Sawczuk, M. Genetics of Muscle Stiffness, Muscle Elasticity and Explosive Strength. *J. Hum. Kinet.* **2020**, *74*, 143–159. [CrossRef] [PubMed]
41. Landen, S.; Hiam, D.; Voisin, S.; Jacques, M.; Lamon, S.; Eynon, N. Physiological and Molecular Sex Differences in Human Skeletal Muscle in Response to Exercise Training. *J. Physiol.* **2023**, *601*, 419–434. [CrossRef] [PubMed]
42. Kirkland, M.C.; Downer, M.B.; Holloway, B.J.; Wallack, E.M.; Lockyer, E.J.; Buckle, N.C.M.; Abbott, C.L.; Ploughman, M. Bipedal Hopping Reveals Evidence of Advanced Neuromuscular Aging Among People with Mild Multiple Sclerosis. *J. Mot. Behav.* **2017**, *49*, 505–513. [CrossRef]
43. Kragstrup, T.W.; Kjaer, M.; Mackey, A.L. Structural, Biochemical, Cellular, and Functional Changes in Skeletal Muscle Extracellular Matrix with Aging. *Scand. J. Med. Sci. Sport.* **2011**, *21*, 749–757. [CrossRef]
44. Kalyani, R.R.; Corriere, M.; Ferrucci, L. Age-Related and Disease-Related Muscle Loss: The Effect of Diabetes, Obesity, and Other Diseases. *Lancet Diabetes Endocrinol.* **2014**, *2*, 819–829. [CrossRef] [PubMed]
45. Alvero-Cruz, J.R.; Brikis, M.; Chilibeck, P.; Frings-Meuthen, P.; Vico Guzmán, J.F.; Mittag, U.; Michely, S.; Mulder, E.; Tanaka, H.; Tank, J.; et al. Age-Related Decline in Vertical Jumping Performance in Masters Track and Field Athletes: Concomitant Influence of Body Composition. *Front. Physiol.* **2021**, *12*, 643649. [CrossRef] [PubMed]
46. Sanai, S.A.; Saini, V.; Benedict, R.H.B.; Zivadinov, R.; Teter, B.E.; Ramanathan, M.; Weinstock-Guttman, B. Aging and Multiple Sclerosis. *Mult. Scler.* **2016**, *22*, 717–725. [CrossRef] [PubMed]
47. Gianfrancesco, M.; Barcellos, L. Obesity and Multiple Sclerosis Susceptibility: A Review. *J. Neurol. Neuromedicine* **2016**, *1*, 1–5. [CrossRef] [PubMed]
48. Lutfullin, I.; Eveslage, M.; Bittner, S.; Antony, G.; Flaskamp, M.; Luessi, F.; Salmen, A.; Gisevius, B.; Klotz, L.; Korsukewitz, C.; et al. Association of Obesity with Disease Outcome in Multiple Sclerosis. *J. Neurol. Neurosurg. Psychiatry* **2022**, *94*, 57–61. [CrossRef] [PubMed]
49. Riemenschneider, M.; Hvid, L.G.; Stenager, E.; Dalgas, U. Is There an Overlooked "Window of Opportunity" in MS Exercise Therapy? Perspectives for Early MS Rehabilitation. *Mult. Scler. J.* **2018**, *24*, 886–894. [CrossRef] [PubMed]
50. Manca, A.; Dvir, Z.; Deriu, F. Meta-Analytic and Scoping Study on Strength Training in People with Multiple Sclerosis. *J. Strength Cond. Res.* **2019**, *33*, 874–889. [CrossRef] [PubMed]
51. Taul-Madsen, L.; Connolly, L.; Dennett, R.; Freeman, J.; Dalgas, U.; Hvid, L.G. Is Aerobic or Resistance Training the Most Effective Exercise Modality for Improving Lower Extremity Physical Function and Perceived Fatigue in People with Multiple Sclerosis? A Systematic Review and Meta-Analysis. *Arch. Phys. Med. Rehabil.* **2021**, *102*, 2032–2048. [CrossRef] [PubMed]
52. Kjølhede, T.; Vissing, K.; De Place, L.; Pedersen, B.G.; Ringgaard, S.; Stenager, E.; Petersen, T.; Dalgas, U. Neuromuscular Adaptations to Long-Term Progressive Resistance Training Translates to Improved Functional Capacity for People with Multiple Sclerosis and Is Maintained at Follow-Up. *Mult. Scler. J.* **2015**, *21*, 599–611. [CrossRef]
53. Nuzzo, J.L.; McBride, J.M.; Cormie, P.; McCaulley, G.O. Relationship Between Countermovement Jump Performance and Multijoint Isometric and Dynamic Tests of Strength. *J. Strength Cond. Res.* **2008**, *22*, 699–707. [CrossRef]

biomedicines

MDPI

Article

Multiple Sclerosis and *Clostridium perfringens* Epsilon Toxin: Is There a Relationship?

André Huss [1,†], Franziska Bachhuber [1,†], Cécile Feraudet-Tarisse [2], Andreas Hiergeist [3] and Hayrettin Tumani [1,*]

1 Department of Neurology, University Hospital Ulm, 89081 Ulm, Germany; andre.huss@uni-ulm.de (A.H.); franziska.bachhuber@uni-ulm.de (F.B.)
2 CEA, INRAE, Medicines and Healthcare Technologies Department (DMTS), SPI, Paris-Saclay University, 91191 Gif-sur-Yvette, France
3 Institute of Clinical Microbiology and Hygiene, University Medical Center, 93053 Regensburg, Germany
* Correspondence: hayrettin.tumani@uni-ulm.de
† These authors contributed equally to this work.

Abstract: Recent research has suggested a link between multiple sclerosis and the gut microbiota. This prospective pilot study aimed to investigate the composition of the gut microbiota in MS patients, the presence of *Clostridium perfringens* epsilon toxin in the serum of MS patients, and the influence of disease-modifying drugs (DMDs) on epsilon toxin levels and on the microbiota. Epsilon toxin levels in blood were investigated by two methods, a qualitative ELISA and a highly sensitive quantitative ELISA. Neither epsilon toxin nor antibodies against it were detected in the analyzed serum samples. 16S ribosomal RNA sequencing was applied to obtain insights into the composition of the gut microbiota of MS patients. No significant differences in the quantity, diversity, and the relative abundance of fecal microbiota were observed in the gut microbiota of MS patients receiving various DMDs, including teriflunomide, natalizumab, ocrelizumab, and fingolimod, or no therapy. The present study did not provide evidence supporting the hypothesis of a causal relationship between *Clostridium perfringens* epsilon toxin and multiple sclerosis.

Keywords: multiple sclerosis; *Clostridium perfringens*; *C. perfringens* epsilon toxin; microbiota

1. Introduction

Multiple sclerosis (MS) is a chronic inflammatory disease of the central nervous system (CNS) that primarily affects young adults and often leads to accumulating neurological symptoms and disability. Cellular components of the immune system, including B and T lymphocytes, play a pivotal role in the pathogenesis of MS and are the target of current disease-modifying therapies (DMTs). Although the cause of MS is still largely unknown, it has been established that genetic, environmental, and lifestyle risk factors contribute to the complex pathophysiological cascade in MS.

Recent research has suggested a link between MS and the microbiome, particularly the gut microbiota. The microbiota are a collection of microorganisms that live on and inside the human body, including their genome and activity [1]. The gut microbiota encompass the collection of microorganisms that live in the digestive tract. These microorganisms play a critical role in many physiological processes, including digestion, immune function, and metabolism, as well as CNS development and function [2]. As the gut microbiota play an important role in regulating immune function, a disbalance in the gut microbiota may contribute to the pathogenesis of MS.

When comparing the gut microbiota of MS patients and healthy subjects, Thirion and colleagues found substantial microbiome alterations in MS patients that were linked to blood biomarkers of inflammation [3]. In a mouse model of relapsing–remitting, spontaneously developing experimental autoimmune encephalomyelitis (EAE), the presence of non-pathogenic commensal microbiota was a prerequisite for the induction of EAE in mice [4]. Furthermore, in transplantation experiments using microbiota obtained from monozygotic twin pairs discordant for MS, the microbiota from MS-affected twins exhibited a significantly higher propensity for inducing autoimmunity in spontaneous autoimmune encephalitic mice as compared to microbiota derived from their non-MS twin siblings [5].

One specific bacterium that has come into focus in connection with MS is *Clostridium perfringens*. *C. perfringens* is a Gram-positive, spore-forming anaerobic bacterium that is commonly found in the soil and in the intestines of animals, including humans [6,7]. It is known to cause a variety of diseases, including gas gangrene, wound infections, food poisoning, and enterotoxaemia. More recently, it has been suggested that *C. perfringens* may play a role in the development of MS. One of the toxins produced by *C. perfringens* (*C. perfringens* type B and D) is epsilon toxin. This protein toxin is a potent pore-forming neurotoxin that is able to cross the blood–brain barrier [6]. Among other modes of action, in the CNS, epsilon toxin causes blood–brain barrier disruption and has detrimental effects on neurons, oligodendrocytes, and astrocytes [7]. In laboratory studies, epsilon toxin has been shown to cause demyelination, a process that is also observed in MS [8,9].

In 2013, the isolation of *C. perfringens* type B from an MS patient was reported [10]. This finding, together with the known CNS-tropism of *C. perfringens* epsilon toxin, prompted the authors to investigate a potential connection between epsilon toxin and multiple sclerosis. A study in a US population found a higher frequency of immunoreactivity against epsilon toxin in the cerebrospinal fluid and serum when comparing MS patients to healthy controls [10]. Another investigation in a UK population of relapsing–remitting MS, clinically isolated syndrome (CIS), and optic neuritis (ON) patients reported a higher frequency of antibodies against *C. perfringens* epsilon toxin in serum as compared to controls [11].

Teriflunomide is a disease-modifying therapy approved for the treatment of relapsing forms of multiple sclerosis (RRMS). Its mechanism of action involves inhibiting the enzyme dihydroorotate dehydrogenase, which is involved in the synthesis of DNA in rapidly dividing cells, including lymphocytes and mononuclear cells [12]. Teriflunomide has been shown to alter the composition of the gut microbiome in animal studies and may also have an impact on the microbiome [13]. It was hypothesized that teriflunomide might have a direct influence on the bacterial counterpart (O-GlcNAcase) of human dihydroorotate dehydrogenase and acts on the *C. perfringens* population in the intestine.

The aim of this study was to further investigate the gut microbiota in MS patients. Due to the presumed effect of teriflunomide treatment on the gut microbiota, especially on *C. perfringens*, we were further interested in a potential influence of DMTs with teriflunomide on serum epsilon toxin levels.

2. Materials and Methods

2.1. Ethical Approval

This study was conducted in accordance with the tenets of the Declaration of Helsinki and approved by the Ethics Committee of Ulm University (approval number 412/17). All patients provided written informed consent.

2.2. Patients

Forty-one MS patients (27 female, 14 male) with a median age of 42 years (range 19–60 years) were enrolled. Patients visiting for diagnostic or treatment purposes were recruited from the University Hospital Ulm, department of Neurology, and the Specialty Clinic Dietenbronn. Exclusion criteria were CRP values > 1.0 mg/dL, treatment with corticosteroids within the last four weeks, or treatment with mitoxantrone or azathioprine within the last 12 months.

2.3. Sample Collection

Stool samples were self-collected by patients in their home environment using the OMNIgene GUT system, which provides sample stability for up to 60 days at room temperature (Steinbrenner Laborsysteme GmbH, Wiesenbach, Germany, Cat. Nr. OM-200). After receipt, samples were stored at −80 °C until analysis. A total of 37 stool samples were available from 36 patients (due to lack of stool sample returned, incorrect specimen collection, or withdrawn consent in the remaining patients). For this project, no additional collection of blood was performed. Serum samples, collected for diagnostic purposes, were included in the analysis. A total of 38 serum samples were available from 34 patients.

2.4. Microbiome Analysis

Stool samples were shipped to microBIOMix GmbH (Regensburg, Germany) for 16S rDNA-based microbiome analysis [14]. The analysis was performed according to the company's standard procedures. Briefly, DNA was extracted from stool samples, and the V1V3 region of the 16S rRNA gene was amplified. Amplicons were sequenced using the Ion Torrent GeneStudio S5 Plus platform (Thermo Fisher Scientific, Waltham, MA, USA) and the resulting reads were processed as previously described [15,16]. In addition, the total bacterial load was quantified from stool-extracted DNA by real-time PCR quantification of bacterial 16S rRNA copy numbers [17]. Microbiome sequencing data were analyzed in R using the dada2 pipeline. The pairwise adonis test was used to assess statistical differences of beta diversity between treatment groups. Differential abundance analysis was applied to identify statistically different taxonomic features between groups by calculating linear discriminant analysis effect sizes (LefSe) using the lefser package V1.14 [18].

2.5. Epsilon Toxin Analysis: Quantification of and Immunoreactivity against Epsilon Toxin

Serum samples were analyzed for the presence of epsilon toxin using a qualitative sandwich ELISA (Bio-X Diagnostics, Rochefort, Belgium) according to the manufacturer's instructions. Additional positive control samples were included using isolated epsilon toxin from *C. perfringens* (obtained from Institute Pasteur, Paris, France) with a final concentration of 25 and 2.5 ng/mL. Serum samples were furthermore analyzed by Service de Pharmacologie et d'Immunoanalyse (SPI, Gif Sur Yvette Cedex, France), where a highly sensitive immunoassay for the detection of clostridial epsilon toxin in body fluids was recently developed [19]. The limit of detection was defined as the lowest concentration giving an absorbance signal greater than the mean plus 3 standard deviations from negative commercial human control serum replicates (test replicate #1: one commercial human serum (octuplicate); test replicate #2: four different commercial human sera used (tetraplicate for each serum); test replicate #3: triplicate for 5 different commercial human sera). The limit of quantification was defined as the lowest concentration giving an absorbance signal greater than the mean plus 10 standard deviations from negative commercial human control sera replicates (same test). Positive control samples were included with standard curve of isolated epsilon toxin from *C. perfringens* type D strain NCTC2062 (Institute Pasteur, Paris, France) spiked in negative commercial human control sera. All sera were diluted 3-fold in EIA buffer (100 mM potassium phosphate buffer pH 7.4, 0.1% bovine serum albumin, 0.15 M NaCl, and 0.01% sodium azide) containing a final 10% heterophilic blocking reagent. The sandwich ELISA was carried out as previously described [19] with slight modifications: detection was performed with biotinylated PεTX6 (100 µg/mL in EIA buffer for 2 h) followed by 30 min incubation with poly-horseradish peroxidase-labeled streptavidin. After the addition of a tetramethylbenzidine-containing substrate solution for 30 min, 2 M sulfuric acid stopped the reaction and absorbances were read at 450 nm. Furthermore, immunoreactivity towards epsilon toxin was analyzed at SPI by ELISA. Briefly, plates were coated with 5 µg/mL epsilon toxin (Institute Pasteur) and incubated overnight at 4 °C with 100-fold diluted patient sera in 100 mM TrisHCl buffer pH 8.0, 5% milk, 150 mM NaCl, 0.5% tween20, 0.25% CHAPS, and 0.01% sodium azide (Tris-milk buffer). Immunoreactivity towards epsilon toxin was then detected with biotinylated anti-human IgA, IgM, or IgG (IgG1, IgG3, IgG4 or IgG1, IgG2, IgG3, IgG4), monoclonal antibodies, and acetylcholinesterase-labeled streptavidin revealed by Ellman's colorimetric method at 414 nm after 1 h [20]. Limits of detection and quantification were calculated as described above (test replicate #1: one commercial human serum used for negative control (octuplicate); test replicate #2: tetraplicate of five different commercial human control sera).

Ig/epsilon toxin immunocomplexes were investigated at SPI by a sandwich ELISA. Briefly, plates were coated with a mix of 3 murine anti-epsilon toxin monoclonal antibodies (PεTX5, PεTX6 and PεTX7 [19]), incubated for 1h with 30-fold-diluted patient sera in Tris–milk buffer, and detected using peroxidase-coupled goat anti-human antibodies revealed with ABTS diammonium salt at 414 nm after 30 min. Five different commercial human sera were applied as negative control. Each commercial serum was analyzed in quadruplicate. A serum absorbance signal greater than the mean absorbance plus three standard deviations from the negative commercial human control sera was set as the limit of detection.

3. Results

3.1. Microbiome Analysis

For gut microbiome analysis, MS patients were grouped according to the DMT: treatment with teriflunomide ($n = 17$), other therapies (natalizumab, ocrelizumab, or fingolimod, $n = 16$), and no therapy ($n = 4$). The total bacterial load of the intestinal microbiota was assessed by real-time PCR quantification of bacterial 16S rDNA copies. No significant difference in bacterial load was observed between the three different treatment groups (Figure 1).

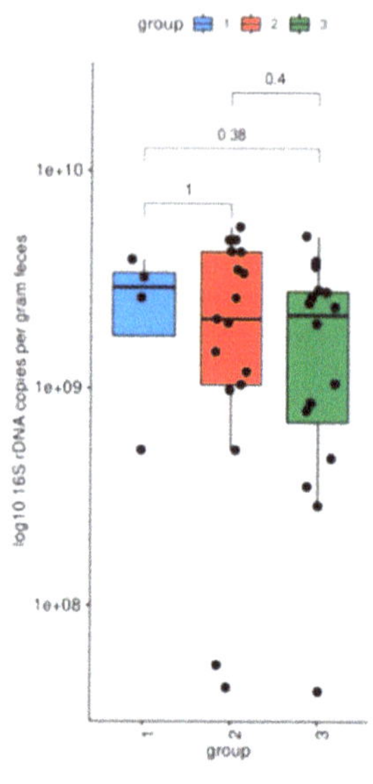

Figure 1. Total bacterial 16S rDNA copies. Group 1 (blue, no therapy); group 2 (red, teriflunomide); group 3 (green, other therapies).

Sequencing analysis of V1V3 regions of 16S rDNA was performed to assess the diversity and distribution of bacterial taxa. All three measures of alpha diversity assessed (Richness, the Inverse Simpson Index, and the Effective Shannon Index) showed no significant differences between the three groups of MS patients (Figure 2). No differences in bacterial compositions between the treatment groups were observed (Supplementary Figure S1). The level of relative abundance of *Clostridiaceae* (where Clostridium perfringens is classified) was very low in all groups. Additionally, no differences in relative abundance of bacteria were observed on the genus level (Supplementary Figure S2).

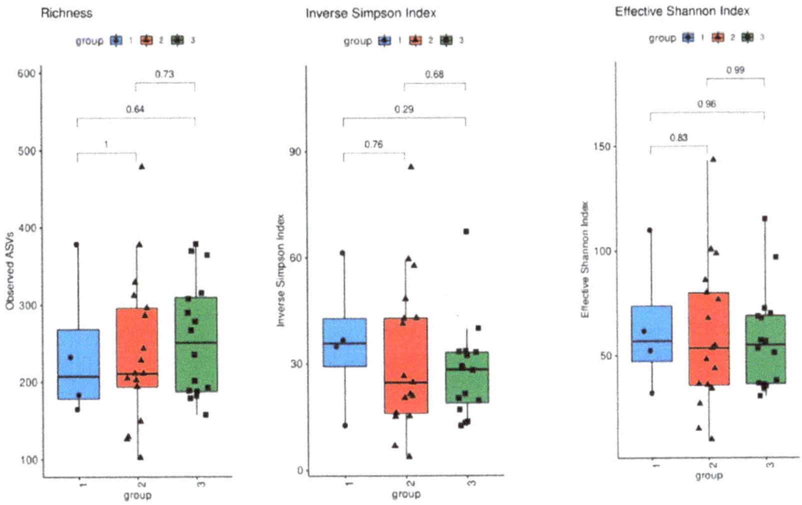

Figure 2. Alpha diversity: V1V3 regions of 16S rDNA. Group 1 (blue, no therapy); group 2 (red, teriflunomide); group 3 (green, other therapies).

Moreover, the evaluation of ordinated Bray–Curtis dissimilarities (Figure 3) and unweighted as well as weighted UNIFrac distances (Figure 4) followed by PERMANOVA analysis revealed no significant difference in beta diversity between the three groups. The evaluation of differential abundance between all groups using linear discriminant analysis (LefSE) revealed no significant features.

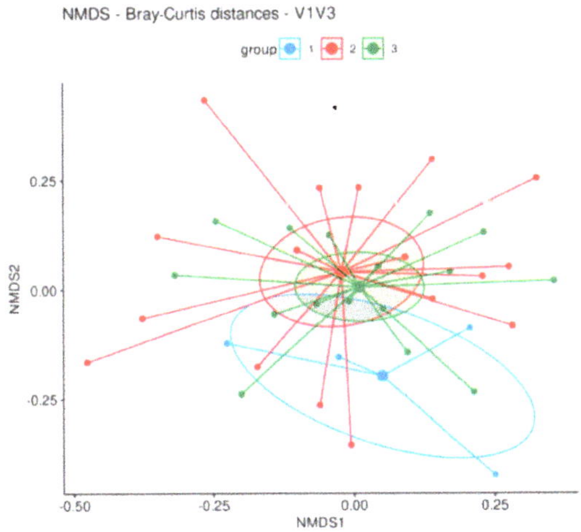

Figure 3. Beta diversity: Bray–Curtis distances. Group 1 (blue dots, no therapy); group 2 (red dots, teriflunomide); group 3 (green dots, other therapies). Large dots indicate the centroid of each group. Ellipses mark the 95 percent confidence intervals around each centroid.

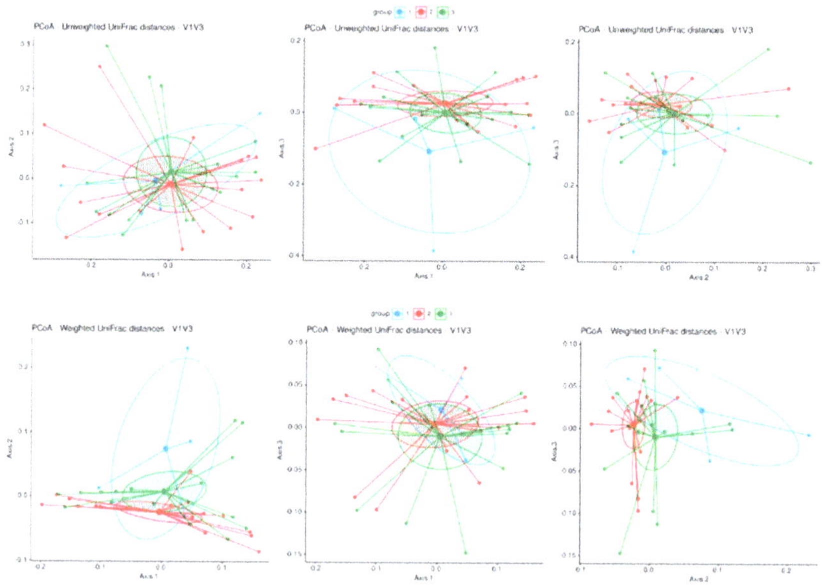

Figure 4. Beta diversity principal coordinate analysis of bacterial bd (including phylogenetic distances): unweighted UNIFrac distance and weighted UNIFrac distance. Group 1 (blue dots, no therapy); group 2 (red dots, teriflunomide); group 3 (green dots, other therapies). Large dots indicate the centroid of each group. Ellipses mark the 95 percent confidence intervals around each centroid.

3.2. Epsilon Toxin in Serum

3.2.1. Direct Detection of Epsilon Toxin

No sample showed a positive signal for epsilon toxin using the commercially available qualitative epsilon toxin assay, while positive control samples spiked with epsilon toxin at concentrations of 25 and 2.5 ng/mL gave strong signals. With the highly sensitive immunoassay [19], no quantifiable levels of epsilon toxin in MS patient serum could be detected. This direct sandwich ELISA reached a limit of detection of 1.1 ± 0.1 pg/mL and limit of quantification around 3.9 ± 0.4 pg/mL and was performed three times in duplicate. Even though some signals were slightly above the limit of detection, no serum with a quantitative positive signal was identified (Supplementary Table S1). As the accessibility of epsilon toxin to detection antibodies is a prerequisite to detection by sandwich ELISA, epsilon toxin complexed with endogenous antibodies in serum could possibly interfere with the direct detection of the toxin in serum by ELISA. Different combinations of physical, chemical, and mechanical approaches for the dissociation of Ig/epsilon toxin immunocomplexes were tested but no irreversible dissociation of immunocomplexes in human serum could be achieved.

3.2.2. Detection of Immunoglobulin/Epsilon Toxin Immunocomplexes

A sandwich ELISA was performed to detect immunocomplexes. The assay was performed twice in duplicate, and one serum sample (1/38, 2.6%) yielded a slightly positive signal in both tests. However, high variability was observed among five commercial human control sera that were applied as negative controls and the addition of variable concentrations of epsilon toxin to patient sera did not result in competition in the ELISA, arguing against a specific detection of Ig/epsilon toxin immunocomplexes in human serum under the analyzed conditions.

3.2.3. Detection of Anti-Epsilon-Toxin Antibodies

Furthermore, immunoassays were performed to detect anti-epsilon toxin antibodies. Four antibody combinations were used to analyze IgG, IgM, and IgA and each test was repeated twice in duplicate. Several signals above the limit of quantification were identified, of which most could not be reproduced in the second test series (Supplementary Table S1). Sera from six MS patients showed reproducible low immunoreactivity against epsilon toxin (4/38, 11%), which was regarded as a non-specific signal, or as part of a polyspecific immune response known to occur in chronic inflammatory diseases of the CNS.

4. Discussion

Microbial dysbiosis and its role in the development of diseases have gained growing interest and it has been suggested that the gut microbiota may play a role in the pathogenesis of MS [5,10,11]. This study aimed to gain further insight into the gut microbiome of MS patients, the presence of Clostridia in it, the occurrence of epsilon toxin in MS patients, and the impact of immune modulatory treatment on both gut microbiota and epsilon toxin levels.

Microbiome analysis, using 16S rRNA sequencing, revealed no significant differences in the quantity, diversity, or composition of the fecal microbiota between MS patients receiving teriflunomide treatment, other therapies, or no therapy. Parameters of alpha and beta diversity were investigated to identify differences in the microbial community structure within individual samples and between the different samples.

The total bacterial load of the gut microbiota was similar between the three groups, indicating that there were no significant differences in the absolute bacterial abundance among the groups. Measures of alpha diversity showed no significant differences in the microbial community structure within individual samples. No significant differences were observed in the relative abundance of specific bacterial families or genera among the groups. Moreover, the evaluation of beta diversity revealed no significant difference between the three groups, suggesting a similar microbial community structure of MS patients who received teriflunomide treatment, other therapies, or no therapy.

The relative abundance of *Clostridiaceae*, where *C. perfringens* is classified, was very low in all groups. It has been suggested that DMTs may reduce the abundance of *C. perfringens* [13]. Most analyzed patients received a DMT. We were especially interested in the impact of teriflunomide treatment on the microbial abundance of Clostridium perfringens and hence on epsilon toxin levels in serum. However, due to the limited number of patients in this pilot study, no statement on the influence of teriflunomide treatment or DMT in general on microbial composition and on the abundance of *C. perfringens* can be made. Taken together, the investigated groups of MS patients were not significantly different regarding their microbiome composition.

Recently, it was suggested that *C. perfringens* epsilon toxin might play a causative role in the etiopathogenesis of multiple sclerosis [10,11]. To confirm an exposure to epsilon toxin in the examined cohort of MS patients, different approaches were considered, including the direct detection of epsilon toxin in serum as well as the demonstration of immunoreactivity to epsilon toxin via the detection of anti-epsilon-toxin antibodies in blood or immunocomplexes made of epsilon toxin and serological antibodies. Previous studies suggested a contribution of *C. perfringens* to the cause of MS based on immunoreactivity to epsilon toxin [10,11]. However, the concomitant polyspecific immune response, which is a hallmark of MS, is not dependent on the presence of a causative antigen and is accompanied by immunoreactivity to a plethora of antigens [21,22]. Identified target antigens include neurotropic viruses and microorganisms as well as various self-antigens [21–24]. The MRZ(-H) reaction, i.e., an intrathecal polyspecific antibody synthesis directed against neurotropic measles, rubella, varicella zoster, and/or herpes simplex viruses is a very specific biomarker for MS and few other chronic inflammatory autoimmune diseases that affect the CNS [25].

As unspecific immunoreactivity against various antigens is known to occur in MS patients and does not necessarily indicate a primary immune response against a disease-related agent, the present study aimed to directly detect epsilon toxin in serum samples. The detection of epsilon toxin has been reported to be challenging, and to the best of our knowledge, there is only one commercially available assay for its detection in human material. Previous studies investigating immunoreactivity to *C. perfringens* epsilon toxin employed conventional Western blot techniques to detect anti-epsilon-toxin antibodies, with a methodological limitation of limited specificity [10,11]. Besides the application of the commercial assay, samples additionally were sent to Service de Pharmacologie et d'Immunoanalyse, where a highly sensitive immunoassay for the detection of epsilon toxin in human biological samples was established and extensively characterized [19]. Among the analyzed samples, there was no evidence for epsilon toxin in MS patient sera. However, it is possible that epsilon toxin is complexed with human serologic antibodies, which could potentially impact or prevent its accessibility to detection by sandwich ELISA.

In addition to the approach of direct epsilon toxin detection, patient samples were tested for the presence of serological antibodies to the toxin. Four antibody pairs were used to detect IgG, IgM, and IgA specific to the toxin. Even though a total of 10/38 samples yielded a positive result in at least one assay, the overlap and especially reproducibility of the results was limited (Supplementary Table S1), and all positive signals were slightly above the determined limit of detection of the respective sandwich ELISAs. Based on the available results, legitimate doubts can be raised on the reproducibility and specificity of the detection of immunoreactivity against epsilon toxin in human serum and results should be interpreted with caution.

As for the direct detection of epsilon toxin in serum, the detection of epsilon toxin-specific immunoglobulins also requires accessibility to detection by the used antibodies, which could be impaired or prevented by the formation of epsilon toxin/immunoglobulin complexes in serum, either in vivo or in vitro. Immunocomplexes were analyzed by sandwich ELISA. Even though one patient sample showed a slightly positive signal in both test replicates, the variations observed in the signals of the commercial human sera applied as negative controls required to assess the specificity of the measured signals in patient samples. For specificity assessment, variable concentrations of epsilon toxin were added to patient sera. As no competition was observed by the hook effect, the results were not in favor of a specific detection of immunocomplexes involving epsilon toxin.

Taken together, the results of this study did not provide evidence supporting the hypothesis of a causal relationship between *C. perfringens* epsilon toxin and MS. In the past, many viral and non-viral agents have been discussed or postulated as possible causes of MS. So far, no infectious agent could be linked to MS pathogenesis in a direct causal relationship. Also, in the currently promising Epstein–Barr virus (EBV) hypothesis, indirect immunological mechanisms are assumed to drive the development of MS [26,27].

The limitations of this study are the small sample size and the small size of its subgroups, especially the number of four untreated MS patients, which does not allow for a comparison between treatment-naïve MS patients and patients receiving DMT. Furthermore, microbiota analysis was restricted to stool samples rather than gastrointestinal samples. Even though it is a common, non-invasive, and user-friendly sampling method, there are several limitations to this approach, as fecal samples are not representative of the comprehensive gut microbiota and bias might be introduced by environmental and pre-analytical factors [28]. The inclusion of both immunoreactivity analysis and direct analysis of epsilon toxin as well as toxin/Ig immunocomplexes is a strength of the study. Additionally, the use of both a commercial and in-house assay for the detection of epsilon toxin in blood enhances the robustness of the investigation.

5. Conclusions

In this pilot study analyzing the gut microbiota and sera of patients with MS, we could not provide evidence supporting the hypothesis of a causal relationship between *Clostridium perfringens* epsilon toxin and MS.

Furthermore, a workflow for gut microbiome analysis and stool self-sampling of patients was developed, paving the way for future studies including more patients. With regard to the analysis of the gut microbiome and serum for the detection of epsilon toxin and anti-epsilon toxin, this study was limited due to its sample size and did not yield significant findings.

Supplementary Materials: The following supporting information can be downloaded at: https://www.mdpi.com/article/10.3390/biomedicines12071392/s1, Figure S1: Family abundance; Figure S2: Genus abundance; Table S1: Serological analyses for the detection of epsilon toxin and epsilon toxin immunoreactivity.

Author Contributions: Conceptualization and design of the study, A.H. (André Huss) and H.T.; acquisition and statistical analysis of the data, A.H. (André Huss), F.B., A.H. (Andreas Hiergeist), C.F.-T., and H.T.; writing—original draft preparation F.B.; writing—review and editing, A.H. (André Huss) and H.T. All authors have read and agreed to the published version of the manuscript.

Funding: This investigator-sponsored study received funding from Sanofi (GZ-2015-11429). The funder had no influence on the study design, data analysis, or interpretation.

Institutional Review Board Statement: This study was conducted in accordance with the Declaration of Helsinki and approved by the Ethics Committee of Ulm University (approval number 412/17, date of approval 15 January 2018).

Informed Consent Statement: Informed consent was obtained from all subjects involved in the study.

Data Availability Statement: Raw data can be provided upon reasonable request by the corresponding author.

Acknowledgments: We would like to express our gratitude towards all patients for their participation in this study. We thank our coworkers at the lab for CSF diagnostics and clinical neurochemistry and the biobank, Ulm, Germany, for excellent technical support. We are also grateful to Dominique Marcé and Elise Yang for expert technical assistance, and Hervé Bernard and Gwenaëlle Le Roux for fruitful discussion at the SPI, Gif sur Yvette, France.

Conflicts of Interest: F.B. declares no conflicts of interest. The funders had no role in the design of this study; in the collection, analyses, or interpretation of data; in the writing of the manuscript; or in the decision to publish the results. A.H. declares no conflicts of interest. H.T. has participated in meetings sponsored by or received honoraria for acting as an advisor/speaker for Alexion, Bayer, Biogen, Bristol-Myers Squibb, Celgene, Diamed, Fresenius, Fujirebio, GlaxoSmithKline, Horizon, Janssen-Cilag, Merck, Novartis, Roche, Sanofi-Genzyme, Siemens, and Teva.

References

1. Berg, G.; Rybakova, D.; Fischer, D.; Cernava, T.; Vergès, M.C.; Charles, T.; Chen, X.; Cocolin, L.; Eversole, K.; Corral, G.H.; et al. Microbiome definition re-visited: Old concepts and new challenges. *Microbiome* **2020**, *8*, 103.
2. Sharon, G.; Sampson, T.R.; Geschwind, D.H.; Mazmanian, S.K. The Central Nervous System and the Gut Microbiome. *Cell* **2016**, *167*, 915–932. [CrossRef]
3. Thirion, F.; Sellebjerg, F.; Fan, Y.; Lyu, L.; Hansen, T.H.; Pons, N.; Levenez, F.; Quinquis, B.; Stankevic, E.; Søndergaard, H.B.; et al. The gut microbiota in multiple sclerosis varies with disease activity. *Genome Med.* **2023**, *15*, 1. [CrossRef] [PubMed]
4. Berer, K.; Mues, M.; Koutrolos, M.; Al Rasbi, Z.; Boziki, M.; Johner, C.; Wekerle, H.; Krishnamoorthy, G. Commensal microbiota and myelin autoantigen cooperate to trigger autoimmune demyelination. *Nature* **2011**, *479*, 538. [CrossRef] [PubMed]
5. Berer, K.; Gerdes, L.A.; Cekanaviciute, E.; Jia, X.; Xiao, L.; Xia, Z.; Liu, C.; Klotz, L.; Stauffer, U.; Baranzini, S.E.; et al. Gut microbiota from multiple sclerosis patients enables spontaneous autoimmune encephalomyelitis in mice. *Proc. Natl. Acad. Sci. USA* **2017**, *114*, 10719–10724. [CrossRef] [PubMed]
6. Smedley, J.G.; Fisher, D.J.; Sayeed, S.; Chakrabarti, G.; McClane, B.A. The enteric toxins of Clostridium perfringens. *Rev. Physiol. Biochem. Pharmacol.* **2004**, *152*, 183–204. [PubMed]

7. Stiles, B.G.; Barth, G.; Barth, H.; Popoff, M.R. Clostridium perfringens Epsilon Toxin: A Malevolent Molecule for Animals and Man? *Toxins* **2013**, *5*, 2138–2160. [CrossRef]
8. Wioland, L.; Dupont, J.L.; Doussau, F.; Gaillard, S.; Heid, F.; Isope, P.; Pauillac, S.; Popoff, M.R.; Bossu, J.L.; Poulain, B. Epsilon toxin from Clostridium perfringens acts on oligodendrocytes without forming pores, and causes demyelination. *Cell. Microbiol.* **2015**, *17*, 369–388. [CrossRef] [PubMed]
9. Linden, J.R.; Ma, Y.; Zhao, B.; Harris, J.M.; Rumah, K.R.; Schaeren-Wiemers, N.; Vartanian, T. Clostridium perfringens Epsilon Toxin Causes Selective Death of Mature Oligodendrocytes and Central Nervous System Demyelination. *mBio* **2015**, *6*, 10–1128. [CrossRef] [PubMed]
10. Rumah, K.R.; Linden, J.; Fischetti, V.A.; Vartanian, T. Isolation of Clostridium perfringens type B in an individual at first clinical presentation of multiple sclerosis provides clues for environmental triggers of the disease. *PLoS ONE* **2013**, *8*, e76359. [CrossRef] [PubMed]
11. Wagley, S.; Bokori-Brown, M.; Morcrette, H.; Malaspina, A.; D'arcy, C.; Gnanapavan, S.; Lewis, N.; Popoff, M.R.; Raciborska, D.; Nicholas, R.; et al. Evidence of Clostridium perfringens epsilon toxin associated with multiple sclerosis. *Mult. Scler. J.* **2019**, *25*, 653–660. [CrossRef] [PubMed]
12. Gold, R.; Wolinsky, J.S. Pathophysiology of multiple sclerosis and the place of teriflunomide. *Acta Neurol. Scand.* **2011**, *124*, 75–84. [CrossRef]
13. Rumah, K.R.; Vartanian, T.K.; Fischetti, V.A. Oral Multiple Sclerosis Drugs Inhibit the In vitro Growth of Epsilon Toxin Producing Gut Bacterium, Clostridium perfringens. *Front. Cell. Infect. Microbiol.* **2017**, *7*, 11. [CrossRef]
14. Hiergeist, A.; Ruelle, J.; Emler, S.; Gessner, A. Reliability of species detection in 16S microbiome analysis: Comparison of five widely used pipelines and recommendations for a more standardized approach. *PLoS ONE* **2023**, *18*, e0280870. [CrossRef]
15. Hiergeist, A.; Gläsner, J.; Reischl, U.; Gessner, A. Analyses of Intestinal Microbiota: Culture versus Sequencing. *ILAR J.* **2015**, *56*, 228–240. [CrossRef] [PubMed]
16. Hiergeist, A.; Reischl, U.; Gessner, A. Multicenter quality assessment of 16S ribosomal DNA-sequencing for microbiome analyses reveals high inter-center variability. *Int. J. Med. Microbiol.* **2016**, *306*, 334–342. [CrossRef]
17. Stämmler, F.; Gläsner, J.; Hiergeist, A.; Holler, E.; Weber, D.; Oefner, P.J.; Gessner, A.; Spang, R. Adjusting microbiome profiles for differences in microbial load by spike-in bacteria. *Microbiome* **2016**, *4*, 28. [CrossRef]
18. Segata, N.; Izard, J.; Waldron, L.; Gevers, D.; Miropolsky, L.; Garrett, W.S.; Huttenhower, C. Metagenomic biomarker discovery and explanation. *Genome Biol.* **2011**, *12*, R60. [CrossRef] [PubMed]
19. Féraudet-Tarisse, C.; Mazuet, C.; Pauillac, S.; Krüger, M.; Lacroux, C.; Popoff, M.R.; Dorner, B.G.; Andréoletti, O.; Plaisance, M.; Volland, H.; et al. Highly sensitive sandwich immunoassay and immunochromatographic test for the detection of Clostridial epsilon toxin in complex matrices. *PLoS ONE* **2017**, *12*, e0181013. [CrossRef]
20. Grassi, J.; Frobert, Y.; Pradelles, P.; Chercuitte, F.; Gruaz, D.; Dayer, J.M.; Poubelle, P.E. Production of monoclonal antibodies against interleukin-1 alpha and -1 beta. Development of two enzyme immunometric assays (EIA) using acetylcholinesterase and their application to biological media. *J. Immunol. Methods* **1989**, *123*, 193–210. [CrossRef]
21. Reiber, H.; Ungefehr, S.; Jacobi, C. The intrathecal, polyspecific and oligoclonal immune response in multiple sclerosis. *Mult. Scler. J.* **1998**, *4*, 111–117. [CrossRef] [PubMed]
22. Brändle, S.M.; Obermeier, B.; Senel, M.; Bruder, J.; Mentele, R.; Khademi, M.; Olsson, T.; Tumani, H.; Kristoferitsch, W.; Lottspeich, F.; et al. Distinct oligoclonal band antibodies in multiple sclerosis recognize ubiquitous self-proteins. *Proc. Natl. Acad. Sci. USA* **2016**, *113*, 7864–7869. [CrossRef] [PubMed]
23. Rostasy, K.; Reiber, H.; Pohl, D.; Lange, P.; Ohlenbusch, A.; Eiffert, H.; Maass, M.; Hanefeld, F. Chlamydia pneumoniae in children with MS: Frequency and quantity of intrathecal antibodies. *Neurology* **2003**, *61*, 125–128. [CrossRef] [PubMed]
24. Villar, L.M.; Sádaba, M.C.; Roldán, E.; Masjuan, J.; González-Porqué, P.; Villarrubia, N.; Espiño, M.; García-Trujillo, J.A.; Bootello, A.; Álvarez-Cermeño, J.C. Intrathecal synthesis of oligoclonal IgM against myelin lipids predicts an aggressive disease course in MS. *J. Clin. Investig.* **2005**, *115*, 187. [CrossRef] [PubMed]
25. Felgenhauer, K.; Reiber, H. The diagnostic significance of antibody specificity indices in multiple sclerosis and herpes virus induced diseases of the nervous system. *Clin. Investig.* **1992**, *70*, 28–37. [CrossRef] [PubMed]
26. Bjornevik, K.; Cortese, M.; Healy, B.C.; Kuhle, J.; Mina, M.J.; Leng, Y.; Elledge, S.J.; Niebuhr, D.W.; Scher, A.I.; Munger, K.L.; et al. Longitudinal analysis reveals high prevalence of Epstein-Barr virus associated with multiple sclerosis. *Science* **2022**, *375*, 296–301. [CrossRef]
27. Soldan, S.S.; Lieberman, P.M. Epstein–Barr virus and multiple sclerosis. *Nat. Rev. Microbiol.* **2022**, *21*, 51–64. [CrossRef]
28. Tang, Q.; Jin, G.; Wang, G.; Liu, T.; Liu, X.; Wang, B.; Cao, H. Current Sampling Methods for Gut Microbiota: A Call for More Precise Devices. *Front. Cell. Infect. Microbiol.* **2020**, *10*, 151. [CrossRef]

biomedicines

MDPI

Article

Diagnoses and Treatment Recommendations—Interrater Reliability of Uroflowmetry in People with Multiple Sclerosis

Anke K. Jaekel [1,2,*], Julia Rieger [1], Anna-Lena Butscher [2], Sandra Möhr [3], Oliver Schindler [4], Fabian Queissert [5], Aybike Hofmann [6], Paul Schmidt [7], Ruth Kirschner-Hermanns [1,2] and Stephanie C. Knüpfer [1,2]

1 Clinic for Urology, University Hospital Bonn, 53127 Bonn, Germany; rkirschnerhermanns@googlemail.com (R.K.-H.); stephanie.knuepfer@ukbonn.de (S.C.K.)
2 Department of Neuro-Urology, Johanniter Rehabilitation Centre Godeshoehe, 53177 Bonn, Germany
3 Clinic for Neurorehabilitation and Paraplegiology, REHAB Basel, 4055 Basel, Switzerland; s.moehr@rehab.ch
4 Clinic for Urology, University Hospital Ulm, 89070 Ulm, Germany
5 Clinic for Urology, University Hospital Münster, 48149 Münster, Germany
6 Clinic St. Hedwig, Department of Paediatric Urology, University Medical Center Regensburg, 93053 Regensburg, Germany
7 Statistical Consulting for Science and Research, Berlin Statistical Consulting for Science and Research, 13086 Berlin, Germany
* Correspondence: a.k.jaekel@gmail.com

Abstract: Background: Uroflowmetry (UF) is an established procedure in urology and is recommended before further investigations of neurogenic lower urinary tract dysfunction (NLUTD). Some authors even consider using UF instead of urodynamics (UD). Studies on the interrater reliability of UF regarding treatment recommendations are rare, and there are no relevant data on people with multiple sclerosis (PwMS). The aim of this study was to investigate the interrater reliability (IRR) of UF concerning diagnosis and therapy in PwMS prospectively. Methods: UF of 92 PwMS were assessed by 4 raters. The diagnostic criteria were normal findings (NFs), detrusor overactivity (DO), detrusor underactivity (DU), detrusor–sphincter dyssynergia (DSD) and bladder outlet obstruction (BOO). The possible treatment criteria were as follows: no treatment (NO), catheter placement (CAT), alpha-blockers, detrusor-attenuating medication, botulinum toxin (BTX), neuromodulation (NM), and physiotherapy/biofeedback (P/BF). IRR was assessed by kappa (κ). Results: κ of diagnoses were NFs = 0.22; DO = 0.17; DU = 0.07; DSD = 0.14; and BOO = 0.18. For therapies, the highest κ was BTX = 0.71, NO = 0.38 and CAT = 0.44. Conclusions: There is a high influence of the individual rater. UD should be subject to the same analysis and a comparison should be made between UD and UF. This may have implications for the value of UF in the neuro-urological management of PwMS, although at present UD remains the gold standard for the diagnostics of NLUTD in PwMS.

Keywords: multiple sclerosis; bladder disorder; neurogenic; bladder

1. Introduction

Uroflowmetry (UF) has been a well-established diagnostic procedure in urology for many years [1]. It is used to diagnose functional disorders of the lower urinary tract in children and adults [2,3]. In this non-invasive urodynamic procedure, a urinary flow rate per time is determined using various technical principles and a flow curve is recorded while voiding urine [4]. Finally, the post-void residual (PVR) is measured by sonography of the bladder [5]. Conclusions can be drawn about the existing type of anatomical or functional disorders of the lower urinary tract from the various forms of UF curves, the micturition volume, the strength of the urine flow, and PVR [4]. The advantages of UF are its simplicity, non-invasiveness, and short duration [1].

The procedure is indicated for both neurogenic and non-neurogenic functional disorders of the lower urinary tract. It is recommended in various urological guidelines [2,3,5].

For neurogenic lower urinary tract dysfunction (NLUTD) in people with multiple sclerosis (PwMS), so far there are no explicit guideline recommendations for UF. Nevertheless, individual authors recommend uroflowmetry, even as a substitute for urodynamics [6], which is the gold standard in the diagnostics of NLUTD [7]. Others only recommend urodynamics for PwMS in the case of treatment failure or prior to surgical treatment [8]. These recommendations are based on the fact that urodynamics (UD), associated with high effort and invasiveness, have ultimately no impact on the treatment outcome. Therefore, neuro-urological expert committees discuss whether UF can play a role in reducing the need for invasive UD [9].

Recommendations for the standardised performance and reporting of uroflowmetry were published by the International Continence Society in 2002 [4]. Due to the involvement of the autonomic nervous system in micturition, there are many factors influencing uroflowmetry: the environment, the patient's compliance and current situation, the micturition position, and the voiding volume [10,11]. Clear recommendations on how to perform UF were defined: a minimum bladder-filling volume should be maintained, the person should void in their usual posture, and information on the subjective representativeness of the examination should be obtained [4,12].

Another significant factor influencing UF is the rater-related individual interpretation of the examination. The rater develops a treatment proposal from his/her subjective perspective by the inclusion of clinical information, bladder diaries (BDs), and questionnaires [13].

The extent to which a measurement procedure is dependent on the influence of the examiner can be measured using reliability [14]. Interrater reliability (IRR) measures the agreement of the assessment between different raters. There are a variety of studies on IRR of UF in children and adults with different study designs [15–17]. So far, there has been no study on the IRR of UF in PwMS that relates not only to the uroflow curve itself, but also to the underlying diagnosis and treatment recommendation.

To assess the long-term significance of UF in comparison to UD regarding NLUTD in PwMS, our intention was to assess the IRR of UF regarding suspected diagnosis and treatment recommendations. We also analysed the IRR of the suspected diagnosis from medical history and BDs.

2. Patients and Methods

This study included all PwMS who had been presented to the neuro-urology department of an inpatient neurological rehabilitation centre for further diagnosis of NLUTD between 2017 and 2022 and who met the following requirements: written informed consent for prospective evaluation of their data, detailed urological history, a completed BD with documented drinking and micturition volumes in ml over 2 days, and uroflowmetry that was performed according to the standards of the International Continence Society. Ninety-two PwMS met these criteria. Inclusion in this study was independent of the clinical course or severity of the disease. Exclusion criteria were invalid uroflowmetry with a micturition volume of <150 mL, a BD that could not be analysed due to invalid or illegible documentation, and the absence of an informed consent form.

All UF examinations were conducted by a highly experienced neuro-urological team consisting of 2 physicians and 3 nurses. The UF was indicated after the patient had undergone an initial consultation with the physician. The examination was scheduled on a different date than the initial consultation. The UF examination procedure was explained in detail in advance. All of the participants were scheduled for UF in the same standardised time slot with a filled bladder. The examination was conducted, according to the preference of the PwMS, in a sitting or standing position in a closed quiet toilet suitable for the disabled. The measurement was performed using an MMS Nexam Pro Urodynamic System (Laborie/Medical Measurement Systems B.V., Enschede, The Netherlands) after the participants had expressed a strong desire to void urine. The measurement of PVR was performed by transabdominal sonography with a GE LOGIQ S7 Pro (GE Ultrasound Korea Inc. Seongnam-si, Korea).

Four experienced neuro-urologists were recruited as raters. They received the following data: diagnoses of the participants, a summarised medical history, information on gender, summarised information from BDs, graphics of the UF curves with information on voided volume in ml, PVR in ml, and maximum urinary flow in ml/s. The raters were asked to assign the individual uroflowmetry findings to the most appropriate diagnostic category, considering the clinical information and the BDs, and to select a corresponding treatment recommendation. A standardised evaluation form was used for this purpose. The answering options listed in the form are shown in Figure 1. All raters were blinded to the original clinical findings.

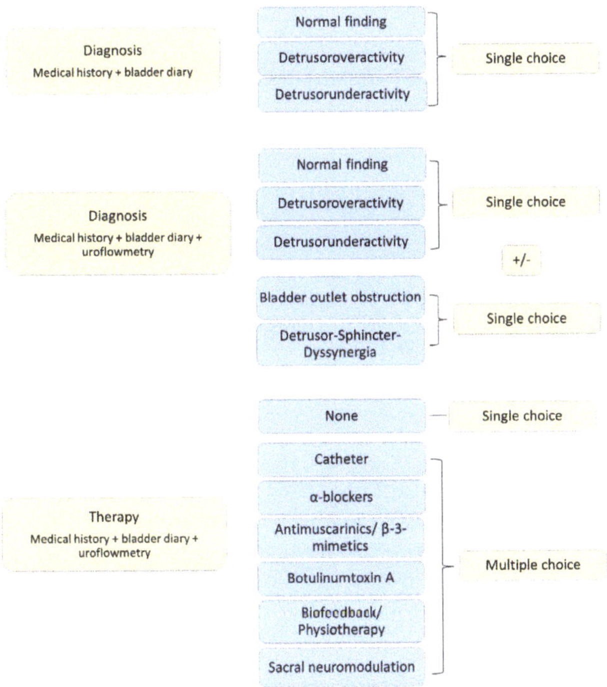

Figure 1. Visualisation of the potential answers on the evaluation form. "+/−"—a combination of both single choices is optional, but not mandatory.

The primary endpoint was the IRR regarding the following items:

- (A) Suspected diagnosis from medical history and BDs;
- (B) Suspected diagnosis from medical history, BDs, and UF;
- (C) Therapy suggestion from medical history, BDs, and UF.

For all primary endpoints, the agreement between 2 raters was determined using Cohen's kappa (κ_C) and the agreement between all raters was assessed using Fleiss' kappa (κ_F). For the primary endpoints B and C, the answers could be obtained using multiple-choice assessment (see Figure 1). The possibility of multiple-choice assessment resulted in the following analyses:

Analysis A: *IRR for the suspected diagnoses from the medical history and BDs;*

Analysis B-1: *IRR for each single suspected diagnosis from medical history, BDs, and UF;*

Analysis B-2: *IRR for the combined suspected diagnoses from medical history, BDs, and UF;*

Analysis C-1: *IRR for each single therapy suggestion from medical history, BDs, and UF;*

Analysis C-2: *IRR for the combined therapy suggestions from medical history, BDs, and UF.*

On a scale of 0.0–1.0, a kappa statistic of 0–0.2 indicates slight agreement, 0.21–0.4 indicates fair agreement, 0.41–0.6 indicates moderate agreement, 0.61–0.8 indicates substantial agreement, and 0.81–1.0 indicates nearly perfect agreement [18].

All analyses were performed with the statistical programming language R (R Core Team 2019) (R version 4.2.2 (09 March 2024) [19].

The study was conducted in accordance with the Declaration of Helsinki and approved by the Ethics Committee for ethical approval (EK 313/13-University Hospital Bonn).

3. Results

3.1. Patient and Disease Characteristics

The study included 92 PwMS, of which 64 (69.6%) were female and 28 (30.4%) male. Of these, 9 PwMS (9.8%) showed the primary progressive, 69 PwMS (75.0%) showed the relapsing–remitting, and 14 PwMS (15.2%) showed the secondary progressive form of MS. Bladder emptying was spontaneous in 89 cases (96.7%); in 1 case (1.1%), it required triggering; and it was conducted in 2 cases (2.2%) by residual urine catheterisation after spontaneous micturition. The descriptive analysis of the demographic variables is shown in Table 1.

Table 1. Descriptive analysis of the demographic variables.

	Mean (SD)	Median (IQR)	Min; Max	Missing N (%)
Age of patients in years	47.5 (9.4)	48 (40.8; 55.2)	25; 72	0 (0)
Duration of MS in months	118.7 (96.7)	102.5 (35.8; 168.2)	1; 445	0 (0)
Expanded Disability Status Scale	3.9 (1.4)	4 (2.9; 4.5)	1,5; 8	12 (13.04)

Of the 92 PwMS, 20 (21.7%) had no urological symptoms at the time of the analysis, 3 (3.3%) had symptoms lasting 1–6 months, 1 (1.1%) for 6–12 months, 15 (16.3%) for 1 to 2 years, 15 (16.3%) for 3 to 5 years, 12 (13%) for 6–10 years, and 5 (5.4%) over 10 years. Overall, 21 PwMS (22.8%) did not specify the duration of urological symptoms. An overview of the distribution and type of urological symptoms is shown in Table 2.

Table 2. Overview of the urinary symptoms of the included PwMS (number of PwMS (N) = 92, no missings).

Neurogenic Lower Urinary Tract Symptoms	Yes N (%)	No N (%)
Staged micturition/interrupted urine flow	18 (19.6)	74 (80.4)
Initiation delay	11 (12)	81 (88)
Weak urine stream	11 (12)	81 (88)
Residual urine sensation	18 (19.6)	74 (80.4)
Desire to press	15 (16.3)	77 (83.7)
Drizzle	5 (5.4)	87 (94.6)
Urinary retention	1 (1.1)	91 (98.9)
Nocturia	37 (40.2)	55 (59.8)
Pollakiuria	45 (48.9)	47 (51.1)
Urgency	52 (56.5)	40 (43.5)
Incontinence	50 (54.3)	42 (45.7)

3.2. Interrater Reliability of the Suspected Diagnoses

3.2.1. Analysis A

For the suspected diagnosis from medical history and BDs, the raters had 3 options: normal findings (NF), detrusor overactivity (DO) and detrusor underactivity (DU) for single selection. The paired comparisons for each singular suspected diagnosis were as follows.

for NFs, $\kappa_C = 0.24$ to $\kappa_C = 0.58$; for DO, $\kappa_C = 0.23$ to $\kappa_C = 0.54$; and for DU, $\kappa_C = -0.02$ to $\kappa_C = 0.17$ (Figure 2). The paired comparison between the raters for all suspected diagnoses showed Cohens' kappa values of 0.25 to 0.54 and thus fair-to-moderate agreement [18] (Figure 3). The results of the comparison of all raters (Fleiss' kappa) are shown in Figures 2 and 3. DU achieved the lowest IRR.

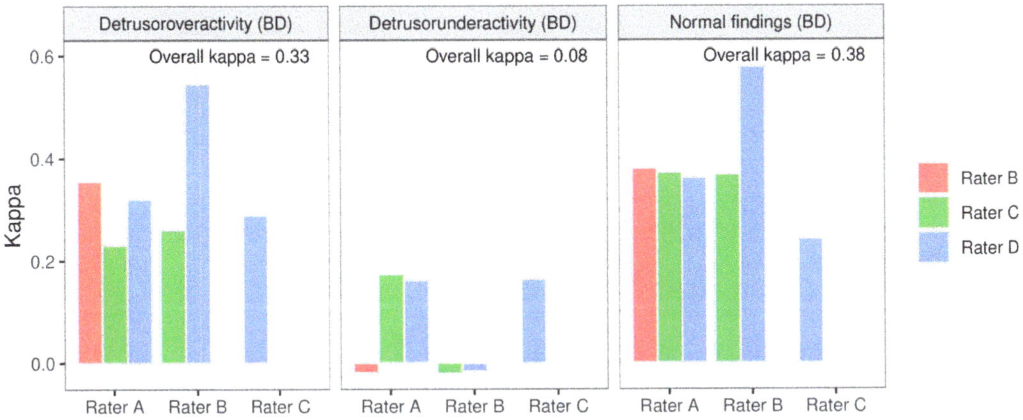

Figure 2. Interrater reliability of single suspected diagnoses from anamnesis and bladder diary between the raters paired and overall.

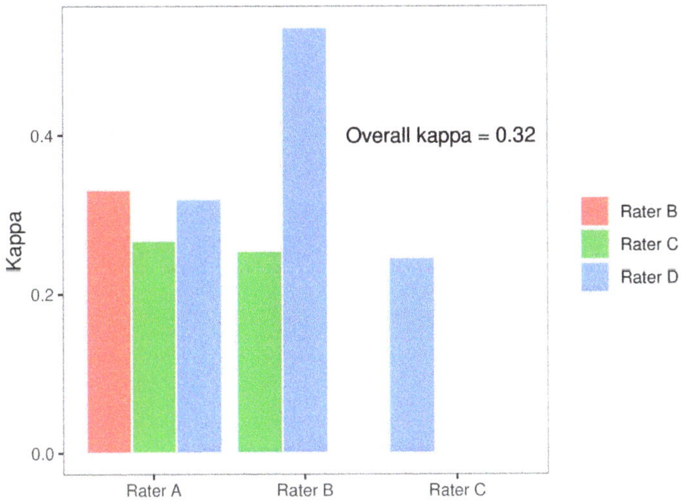

Figure 3. Interrater reliability of all suspected diagnoses from anamnesis and bladder diary between the raters paired and overall.

3.2.2. Analysis B

The raters had 5 options for the suspected diagnosis from medical history, BDs, and UF. In addition to NFs, DO, DU, bladder outlet obstruction (BOO), and detrusor–sphincter–dyssynergia (DSD) could be selected. This resulted in multiple-choice answers and thus 14 combinations for suspected diagnoses. The IRR was notably lower for combinations compared to the individual diagnoses with a maximum $\kappa_C = 0.19$. Figure 4 shows the paired interrater reliability of the single suspected diagnoses (analysis B-1). As in analysis A, the diagnosis DU achieved the lowest IRR. Table 3 shows the paired interrater reliability of the combinations for suspected diagnoses (analysis B-2).

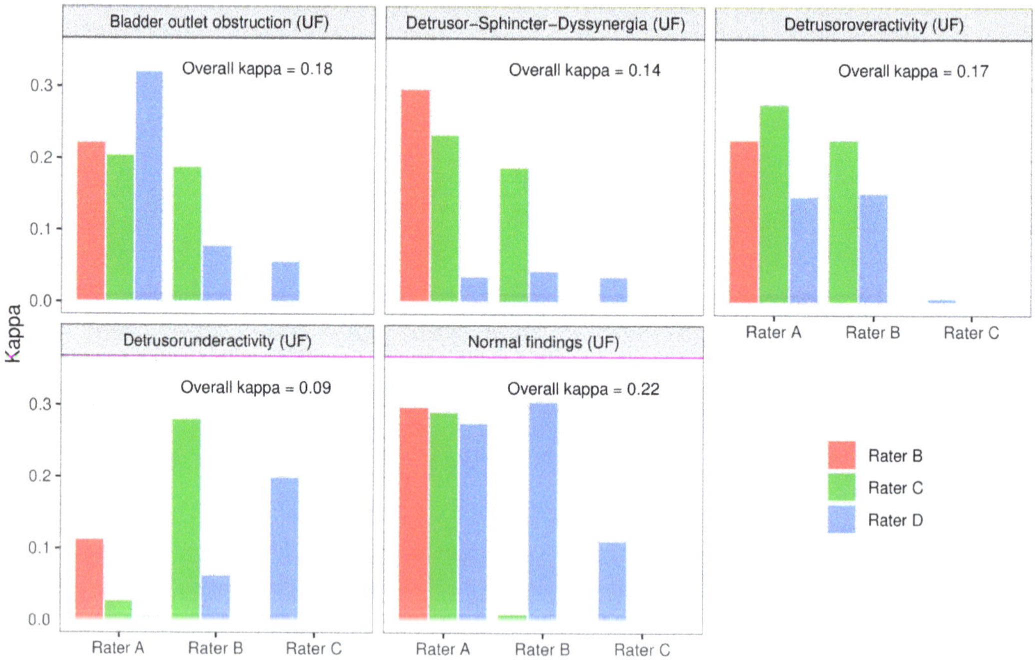

Figure 4. Interrater reliability of the single suspected diagnoses between the paired raters and overall (analysis B-1).

Table 3. Overview of interrater reliability of combined suspected diagnoses between the raters paired and overall (analysis B-2).

Paired Interrater Reliability of the Combined Suspected Diagnoses			
		Match rate in % Cohen's kappa 95% CI	
Rater	B	C	D
A	30.4% 0.19 0.09; 0.28	22.8% 0.13 0.04; 0.22	23.9% 0.14 0.06; 0.23
B		22.8% 0.12 0.03; 0.21	21.7% 0.1 0.01; 0.19
C			25% 0.09 0; 0.18
Fleiss' kappa 0.12			

A uniform consensus with 100% agreement between all raters was found for the diagnoses NO, DU, BOO, and DSD in one data set each and for DO in 8 data sets.

3.3. Interrater Reliability of the Therapy Suggestions (Analysis C)

The IRR of the therapy suggestions from UF was determined to be analogous to the suspected diagnoses for each of the seven predefined therapy suggestions and for the therapy combinations that occurred. For the several treatment suggestions considered, NO

$\kappa_C = 0.38$, KAT $\kappa_C = 0.45$, and BTX $\kappa_C = 0.71$ showed the highest IRR between the rater pairs. We revealed the lowest IRR for NM $\kappa_C = -0.06$ and P/BF $\kappa_C = 0.07$ (Figure 5).

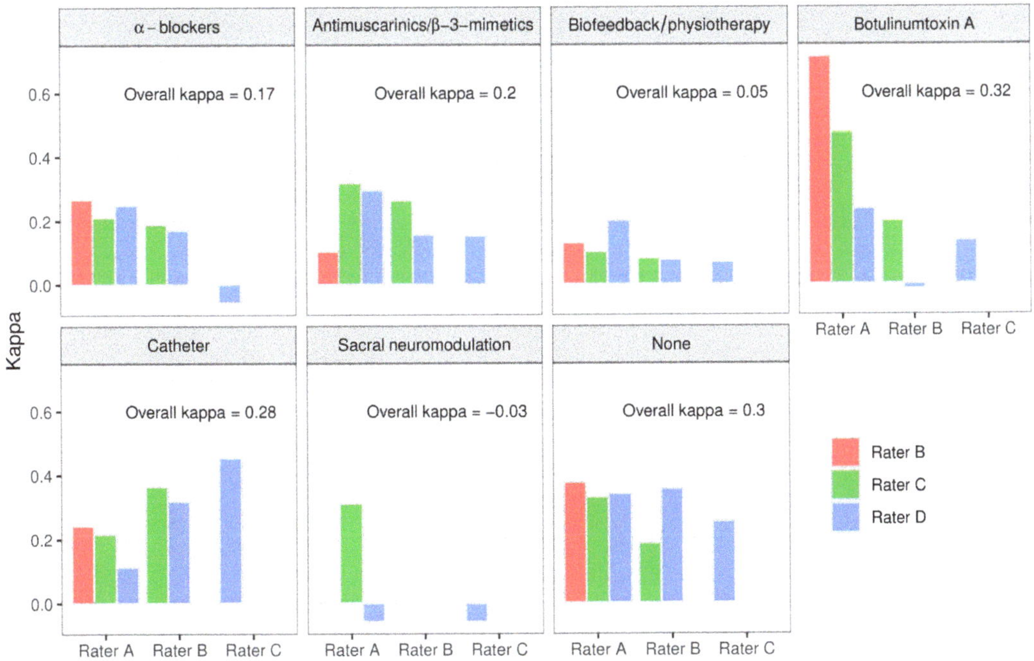

Figure 5. Interrater reliability of the single therapy suggestions between the raters paired and overall.

The possibility of therapy combinations resulted in a variety of selected combinations. The combined treatment suggestions showed a remarkably low agreement with a Fleiss' kappa of 0.08. The best agreement in this subanalysis was achieved by the therapy suggestion "no therapy" with a $\kappa_F = 0.31$. Table 4 provides an overview of the IRR between the rater pairs for combinations of treatment suggestions.

Table 4. Overview of the interrater reliability between the rater pairs for combinations of treatment suggestions (analysis C-2).

Paired Interrater Reliability of the Combined Therapy Suggestions			
		Match rate in % Cohen's kappa 95% CI	
Rater	B	C	D
A	15.2% 0.09 0.02; 0.16	17.4% 0.1 0.03; 0.16	19.6% 0.1 0.02; 0.18
B		17.4% 0.09 0.02; 0.17	10.9% 0.05 0.0; 0.11
C			17.4% 0.1 0.03; 0.17
Fleiss' kappa 0.08			

4. Discussion

In everyday urological practice, it is often impossible to examine PwMS regarding NLUTD using video urodynamics. Although the examination represents the gold standard in the diagnostics of NLUTD [7], it is invasive, associated with side effects [20], costly, and limited in availability [21]. Compared to persons with traumatic or congenital damage of the spinal cord, NLUTD in PwMS results in less damage to the upper urinary tract [22] and not every PwMS is initially affected by NLUTD [23]. Therefore, the rationalised work-up of the NLUTD in PwMS is continually the subject of various expert panels and guideline recommendations [23]. However, a standardised recommendation and predictor for the presence of NLUTD—reviewed in prospective longitudinal studies—have not yet been clearly identified. At the same time, multiple sclerosis results in a high financial and personnel burden on the healthcare system [24] and leads to a severe loss in the quality of life of those affected [23]. To address all those needs, it is essential to develop a sufficient and less costly screening/preselection procedure [9]. In light of these facts, there is a growing interest in UF as a non-invasive, straightforward urodynamic procedure [1,6]. UF is widely available in urological practices and together with medical history and BDs it is often the basis of treatment decisions in daily practice. Therefore, the aim of our work was to analyse the IRR of UF not only regarding the suspected diagnosis, but also the derived clinical consequences. To this end, we had 4 neuro-urologically experienced raters assess 92 data sets based on medical history, BDs, and UF from PwMS regarding predefined suspected diagnoses and therapy suggestions.

For the diagnoses from medical history, BDs, and UF, we obtained a fair agreement with kappa values of 0.32 (κ_C) and 0.2 (κ_F), respectively, for the singular consideration of the diagnoses, both between the rater pairs and in the overall rater comparison. However, many kappa values were lower, especially when combinations of diagnoses were considered. For the singular analyses of the treatment suggestions, the kappa values tended to be slightly higher. Particularly in the treatment suggestions "catheter", "botulinum toxin" and "none", the kappa between the rater pairs was up to 0.71 and was 0.32 in the overall comparison of all raters. When looking at treatment combinations, the IRR fell significantly to values below 0.2 for slight agreement. The fewer options were available, the higher was the raters' agreement.

This is a methodological problem: the more choices available to raters, the lower is the probability of deciding for the same result. This is particularly the case when the decisions are not dichotomous, e.g., pathological or non-pathological, but are based on an individual interpretation by the rater. Gacci et al. [16], involving over 100 urologists specialised in functional urology, were able to show that there is a high IRR when curves and numerical uroflowmetry results are categorised as normal or abnormal. When a diagnosis was included, the IRR in the same group of investigators fell to a κ value of up to <0.1, except for the diagnosis "no abnormalities", where substantial agreement (0.7) was still achieved. This could be because the decision in favour of or against a therapy is still based on a dichotomous decision-making process. The study by van de Beek et al. [25] showed analogous results as early as 1997, whereby the diagnosis "normal findings" also showed the best IRR.

In paediatric urological studies, the IRR of UF also showed similar results. Chang and Yang, 2008, showed a regularly substantial κ (0.68–0.81) in the differentiation of normal vs. pathological findings; in the assessment of specific, pathological waveforms, the IRR was $\kappa = 0.07$ for the same investigators [26]. As soon as an interpretative aspect was included in the diagnosis, the IRR dropped considerably.

The study by Faasse et al. [15] also focussed on the assessment of the UF curve shape in children. The IRR of uroflow EMG was analysed and a specific selection of diagnoses was specified in the study design. Working according to fixed diagnostic criteria, this was a single selection. An agreement of $\kappa = 0.33$ up to a maximum of 0.74 was demonstrated between the rater pairs. The slightly lower kappa values observed in our work in comparison to those reported in the studies mentioned before can be attributed to the fact that, in addition to the querying specific curve shapes, several diagnostic suggestions may also be applicable. In our study, the storage function of the bladder could be assessed using normal findings, detrusor overactivity, and detrusor underactivity, as well as the micturition phase with DSD or BOO. This resulted in many combinations, despite the predefined answers in the form. However, these answers reflect the complexity of the diagnostic and decision-making process that results from UF in daily practice: a clear idea of the underlying diagnosis is essential to determining treatment recommendations. A simple yes/no decision as to whether a pathological condition exists is not sufficient.

The low IRR for DU was noticeable in all our results. On the one hand, we believe that this is due to the poor differentiability between DU and BOO in UF for both genders [27–30], as the shape of the curve and the measured uroflow parameters can be identical for both diagnoses. On the other hand, the clinical definition and diagnosis of DU and detrusor hypocontractility [30–34] are still not finally clarified. Additional indices and parameters are constantly being tested [28,29,31] in order to reliably differentiate the diagnosis of DU with non-invasive measures. These aspects have a negative influence on the consistency of the raters, which influences κ_C [14]. Another aspect of information that has an impact on κ_C is the prevalence of a trait. The less frequently a characteristic is actually present or the less frequently it is estimated to be present, the lower κ_C is [14]. We are unable to assess the influence of the prevalence of the diagnoses in our current study at this time, as we have not correlated the diagnoses with the urodynamic results. This will be the subject of a further study in which the IRR of UD and UF will be compared.

In summary, various authors consider the diagnostic value of UF to be insufficient [13] or as limited [15–17] due to the IRR achieved. Some authors consider UF to be a good screening tool between normal and abnormal micturition [26]. However, all authors see the need for standardisation in the reporting of the curves [15–17,26].

In our opinion, in its current form UF can be an adjunct to the management of NLUTD in PwMS, e.g., act as a follow-up during therapy compared to a pre-treatment assessment. However, the design of all previous studies on IRR does not allow the conclusion that having a limited IRR is also detrimental to the affected patient. The reasons for decisions are not included and could provide reasonable explanations for different decisions. Each rater has an individual horizon of experience and follow-up strategies. The IRR would need to be combined with an outcome measure of treatment success to be able to make statements about the question of unfavourable treatment success with a low IRR.

In the future, artificial intelligence-supported, learning algorithms based on UD studies could be used to refine the diagnostic value of UF for PwMS. These would need to be designed to allow dichotomous decisions to be made as a small detail of the whole, leading to a more complex diagnostic or therapeutic decision. Parameters with a high degree of selectivity and impact on the therapy decision must be identified for this purpose. The first artificial intelligence-assisted approaches to the diagnosis of detrusor underactivity in men are already available [32]. Choo et al. have developed algorithms for the reporting of uroflowmetry in men and women using artificial intelligence [35]. However, the curve so far can only be assessed as normal or pathological, and the results are compared with the judgements of urological specialists and not with underlying urodynamics. Incorporating uroflowmetry with other clinical predictors, working according to the methodology demonstrated by Ito et al. [36], could offer another comprehensive approach to estimating the necessity for additional diagnostics for NLUTD in PwMS. Therefore, further investigations are needed to correlate the results of UD with non-invasive diagnostics and clinical treatment outcomes in PwMS.

5. Conclusions

The suspected suggested diagnosis and treatment suggestions from UF are subject to a high level of individual influence by the raters. If there are several differential diagnoses and therapies to choose from, as it occurs in the daily use of UF, interrater reliability decreases considerably. This results in a variety of possible treatment decisions. To evaluate the possible long-term relevance of UF in addition to UD, the current gold standard in diagnostics of NLUTD in PwMS, UD should be subjected to the same analysis. The results of this analysis then should be compared with those of the UF. According to our study, the standardisation of UF findings based on a dichotomous decision-making algorithm could help to improve the consistency of the assessment.

6. Limitations

Our study had some limitations. The main limitation was that the findings were based on medical records. The raters did not have the real patients in front of them. The influence of the patient's constitution, such as physical or mental limitations, and the effect on the decision of the rater was therefore completely absent. Furthermore, the data originate from a neurological inpatient rehabilitation clinic, which has an influence on the type of PwMS participating, as more severe or advanced cases requiring rehabilitation are usually treated in these institutions (selection bias). In summary, all raters had the same conditions, and the focus of this study was on interrater reliability and not on the most correct result for the patient.

Author Contributions: Conceptualization, A.K.J. and R.K.-H.; methodology, A.K.J., S.C.K. and A.H.; software, J.R.; validation, J.R. and A.K.J.; formal analysis, P.S.; investigation, S.M., F.Q., O.S. and A.K.J.; resources, A.-L.B.; data curation, A.-L.B. and J.R.; writing—original draft preparation, A.K.J.; writing—review and editing, A.H.; visualization, P.S. and J.R.; supervision, S.C.K.; project administration, S.C.K.; funding acquisition, R.K-H. All authors have read and agreed to the published version of the manuscript.

Funding: The primary funding was provided by the German charity fund 'Förderverein zur Kontinenzforschung und Kontinenzaufklärung e. V.', Karmeliterhöfe, Karmeliterstr. 10, 52064 Aachen, Germany, grant number 2023/05. This work was supported by the Open Access Publication Fund of the University of Bonn.

Institutional Review Board Statement: This study was conducted in accordance with the Declaration of Helsinki and approved by the Ethics Committee for ethical approval (EK 313/13-University Hospital Bonn).

Informed Consent Statement: Informed consent was obtained from all the subjects involved in this study.

Data Availability Statement: The data presented in this study are available on request from the corresponding author. The data are not publicly available due to privacy.

Conflicts of Interest: The authors declare no conflicts of interest.

References

1. Gammie, A.; Rosier, P.; Li, R.; Harding, C. How can we maximize the diagnostic utility of uroflow?: ICI-RS 2017. *Neurourol. Urodyn.* **2018**, *37*, S20–S24. [CrossRef] [PubMed]
2. Radmayr, C.; Bogaert, G.; Bujons, A.; Burgu, B.; Castagnetti, M.; 't Hoen, L.A.; O'Kelly, F.; Pakkasjärvi, N.A.; Quadackers, J.; Rawashdeh, Y.F.H.; et al. *EAU Guidelines on Paediatric Urology*; EAU Guidelines Office: Arnhem, The Netherlands, 2023. Available online: https://uroweb.org/guidelines/paediatric-urology (accessed on 6 March 2024).
3. Cornu, J.N.; Gacci, M.; Hashim, H.; Herrmann, T.R.M.; Malde, S.; Netsch, C.; De Nunzio, C.; Rieken, M.; Sakalis, V.; Tutolo, M. *EAU Guidelines on Managemnt of Non-Neurogenic Male LUTS*; EAU Guidelines Office: Arnhem, The Netherlands, 2023. Available online: https://uroweb.org/guidelines/management-of-non-neurogenic-male-luts (accessed on 6 March 2024).
4. Schäfer, W.; Abrams, P.; Liao, L.; Mattiasson, A.; Pesce, F.; Spangberg, A.; Sterling, A.M.; Zinner, N.R.; Kerrebroeck, P.V. Good urodynamic practices: Uroflowmetry, filling cystometry, and pressure-flow studies. *Neurourol. Urodyn.* **2002**, *21*, 261–274. [CrossRef] [PubMed]
5. Harding, C.K.; Lapitan, M.C.; Arlandis, S.; Bø, K.; Cobussen-Boekhorst, H.; Costantini, E.; Groen, J.; Nambiar, A.K.; Omar, M.I.; Peyronnet, B.; et al. *EAU Guidelines on Management of Non-Neurogenic Female LUTS*; EAU Guidelines Office: Arnhem, The Netherlands, 2023. Available online: https://uroweb.org/guidelines/non-neurogenic-female-luts (accessed on 6 March 2024).
6. El Helou, E.; Sarkis, J.; Mjaess, G.; Zalaket, J.; Mouawad, C.; Sayegh, N.; Ghattas, S.; Azar, C.; El Helou, J.; Abboud, H.; et al. Urodynamics in patients with multiple sclerosis: Is it necessary? A randomized-controlled trial. *Scand. J. Urol.* **2021**, *55*, 161–168. [CrossRef] [PubMed]

7. Blok, B.; Castro-Diaz, D.; Del Popolo, G.; Groen, J.; Hamid, R.; Karsenty, G.; Karsenty, T.M.; Musco, S.; Padilla-Fernández, B.; Pannek, J. *EAU Guidelines on Neuro-Urology*; EAU Guidelines Office: Arnhem, The Netherlands, 2023. Available online: https://uroweb.org/guidelines/neuro-urology (accessed on 6 March 2024).
8. Fowler, C.J.; Panicker, J.N.; Drake, M.; Harris, C.; Harrison, S.C.W.; Kirby, M.; Lucas, M.; Macleod, N.; Mangnall, J.; North, A.; et al. A UK consensus on the management of the bladder in multiple sclerosis. *Postgrad. Med. J.* **2009**, *85*, 552–559. [CrossRef]
9. Gammie, A.; Speich, J.E.; Damaser, M.S.; Gajewski, J.B.; Abrams, P.; Rosier, P.F.W.M.; Arlandis, S.; Tarcan, T.; Finazzi Agrò, E. What developments are needed to achieve less-invasive urodynamics? ICI-RS 2019. *Neurourol. Urodyn.* **2020**, *39* (Suppl. S3), S36–S42. [CrossRef]
10. Rosier, P.F.W.M.; Schaefer, W.; Lose, G.; Goldman, H.B.; Guralnick, M.; Eustice, S.; Dickinson, T.; Hashim, H. International Continence Society Good Urodynamic Practices and Terms 2016: Urodynamics, uroflowmetry, cystometry, and pressure-flow study. *Neurourol. Urodyn.* **2017**, *36*, 1243–1260. [CrossRef]
11. Dönmez, M.İ.; Özkent, M.S.; Hamarat, M.B.; Kocalar, M. Through the zipper or pants down: Does it change uroflowmetry parameters in healthy males? *Low. Urin. Tract Symptoms* **2022**, *14*, 341–345. [CrossRef]
12. Gammie, A.; Drake, M.J. The fundamentals of uroflowmetry practice, based on International Continence Society good urodynamic practices recommendations. *Neurourol. Urodyn.* **2018**, *37*, S44–S49. [CrossRef] [PubMed]
13. Netto, J.M.B.; Hittelman, A.; Lambert, S.; Murphy, K.; Collette-Gardere, T.; Franco, I. Interpretation of uroflow curves: A global survey measuring inter and intra rater reliability. *Neurourol. Urodyn.* **2020**, *39*, 826–832. [CrossRef]
14. Wirtz, M.; Kutschmann, M. Analyse der Beurteilerübereinstimmung für kategoriale Daten mittels Cohens Kappa und alternativer Masse. *Rehabilitation* **2007**, *46*, 370–377. [CrossRef]
15. Faasse, M.A.; Nosnik, I.P.; Diaz-Saldano, D.; Hodgkins, K.S.; Liu, D.B.; Schreiber, J.; Yerkes, E.B. Uroflowmetry with pelvic floor electromyography: Inter-rater agreement on diagnosis of pediatric non-neurogenic voiding disorders. *J. Pediatr. Urol.* **2015**, *11*, 198.e1–198.e6. [CrossRef] [PubMed]
16. Gacci, M.; Del Popolo, G.; Artibani, W.; Tubaro, A.; Palli, D.; Vittori, G.; Lapini, A.; Serni, S.; Carini, M. Visual assessment of uroflowmetry curves: Description and interpretation by urodynamists. *World J. Urol.* **2007**, *25*, 333–337. [CrossRef] [PubMed]
17. Liu, Y.-B.; Yang, S.S.; Hsieh, C.-H.; Lin, C.-D.; Chang, S.-J. Inter-Observer, Intra-Observer and Intra-Individual Reliability of Uroflowmetry Tests in Aged Men: A Generalizability Theory Approach. *Low. Urin. Tract Symptoms* **2014**, *6*, 76–80. [CrossRef] [PubMed]
18. Landis, J.R.; Koch, G.G. The Measurement of Observer Agreement for Categorical Data. *Biometrics* **1977**, *33*, 159. [CrossRef]
19. R Core Team. *R: A Language and Environment for Statistical Computing*; R Foundation for Statistical Computing: Vienna, Austria, 2020. Available online: https://www.R-project.org/ (accessed on 9 March 2024).
20. Klingler, H.C.; Madersbacher, S.; Djavan, B.; Schatzl, G.; Marberger, M.; Schmidbauer, C.P. Morbidity of the evaluation of the lower urinary tract with transurethral multichannel pressure-flow studies. *J. Urol.* **1998**, *159*, 191–194. [CrossRef] [PubMed]
21. Baunacke, M.; Leuchtweis, I.; Kaufmann, A.; Schmidt, M.; Groeben, C.; Borkowetz, A.; Eisenmenger, N.; Thomas, C.; Huber, J. Decreasing Number of Urodynamics in Urological and Gynaecological Clinics Reflects Decreased Importance for Surgical Indications: German Population-Based Data from 2013 to 2019. *Urol. Int.* **2022**, *106*, 1068–1074. [CrossRef] [PubMed]
22. Musco, S.; Padilla-Fernández, B.; Del Popolo, G.; Bonifazi, M.; Blok, B.F.M.; Groen, J.; 't Hoen, L.; Pannek, J.; Bonzon, J.; Kessler, T.M.; et al. Value of urodynamic findings in predicting upper urinary tract damage in neuro-urological patients: A systematic review. *Neurourol. Urodyn.* **2018**, *37*, 1522–1540. [CrossRef] [PubMed]
23. Aharony, S.M.; Lam, O.; Corcos, J. Evaluation of lower urinary tract symptoms in multiple sclerosis patients: Review of the literature and current guidelines. *Can. Urol. Assoc. J.* **2017**, *11*, 61–64. [CrossRef] [PubMed]
24. Paz-Zulueta, M.; Parás-Bravo, P.; Cantarero-Prieto, D.; Blázquez-Fernández, C.; Oterino-Durán, A. A literature review of cost-of-illness studies on the economic burden of multiple sclerosis. *Mult. Scler. Relat. Disord.* **2020**, *43*, 102162. [CrossRef]
25. Van de Beek, C.; Stoevelaar, H.J.; McDonnell, J.; Nijs, H.; Casparie, A.F.; Janknegt, R.A. Interpretation of Uroflowmetry Curves by Urologists. *J. Urol.* **1997**, *157*, 164–168. [CrossRef]
26. Chang, S.-J.; Yang, S.S.D. Inter-observer and intra-observer agreement on interpretation of uroflowmetry curves of kindergarten children. *J. Pediatr. Urol.* **2008**, *4*, 422–427. [CrossRef] [PubMed]
27. Lee, K.S.; Song, P.H.; Ko, Y.H. Does uroflowmetry parameter facilitate discrimination between detrusor underactivity and bladder outlet obstruction? *Investig. Clin. Urol.* **2016**, *57*, 437–441. [CrossRef] [PubMed]
28. Chow, P.-M.; Hsiao, S.-M.; Kuo, H.-C. Identifying occult bladder outlet obstruction in women with detrusor-underactivity-like urodynamic profiles. *Sci. Rep.* **2021**, *11*, 23242. [CrossRef] [PubMed]
29. Arevalo-Vega, D.; Ponce, L.; Valdevenito, J.P.; Gallegos, H.; Dell'Oro, A.; Santis-Moya, F.; Calvo, C.I. Defining bladder outlet obstruction and detrusor underactivity in females with overactive bladder: Are we forgetting about the free uroflowmetry? *Neurourol. Urodyn.* **2023**, *42*, 1255–1260. [CrossRef] [PubMed]
30. Ahmed, A.; Farhan, B.; Vernez, S.; Ghoniem, G.M. The challenges in the diagnosis of detrusor underactivity in clinical practice: A mini-review. *Arab J. Urol.* **2016**, *14*, 223–227. [CrossRef] [PubMed]
31. Oelke, M.; Rademakers, K.L.J.; Van Koeveringe, G.A. Unravelling detrusor underactivity: Development of a bladder outlet resistance-Bladder contractility nomogram for adult male patients with lower urinary tract symptoms. *Neurourol. Urodyn.* **2016**, *35*, 980–986. [CrossRef] [PubMed]

32. Matsukawa, Y.; Kameya, Y.; Takahashi, T.; Shimazu, A.; Ishida, S.; Yamada, M.; Sassa, N.; Yamamoto, T. Characteristics of uroflowmetry patterns in men with detrusor underactivity revealed by artificial intelligence. *Int. J. Urol.* **2023**, *30*, 907–912. [CrossRef]
33. Lee, J.; Yoo, S.; Cho, M.C.; Jeong, H.; Choo, M.S.; Son, H. Significance of a decrease in the proportion of detrusor muscle to bladder wall for non-invasive diagnosis of detrusor underactivity in men with lower urinary tract symptoms. *Sci. Rep.* **2022**, *12*, 5237. [CrossRef]
34. Osman, N.I.; Chapple, C.R.; Abrams, P.; Dmochowski, R.; Haab, F.; Nitti, V.; Koelbl, H.; Van Kerrebroeck, P.; Wein, A.J. Detrusor underactivity and the underactive bladder: A new clinical entity? A review of current terminology, definitions, epidemiology, aetiology, and diagnosis. *Eur. Urol.* **2014**, *65*, 389–398. [CrossRef]
35. Choo, M.S.; Ryu, H.Y.; Lee, S. Development of an Automatic Interpretation Algorithm for Uroflowmetry Results: Application of Artificial Intelligence. *Int. Neurourol. J.* **2022**, *26*, 69–77. [CrossRef]
36. Ito, H.; Sakamaki, K.; Young, G.J.; Blair, P.S.; Hashim, H.; Lane, J.A.; Kobayashi, K.; Clout, M.; Abrams, P.; Chapple, C.; et al. Predicting prostate surgery outcomes from standard clinical assessments of lower urinary tract symptoms to derive prognostic symptom and flowmetry criteria. *Eur. Urol. Focus* **2024**, *10*, 197–204. [CrossRef] [PubMed]

biomedicines

MDPI

Article

Decreased Expression of the EAAT5 Glutamate Transporter at Photoreceptor Synapses in Early, Pre-Clinical Experimental Autoimmune Encephalomyelitis, a Mouse Model of Multiple Sclerosis

Ali El Samad †, Julia Jaffal †, Dalia R. Ibrahim, Karin Schwarz and Frank Schmitz *

Institute of Anatomy, Department of Neuroanatomy, Medical School Homburg, Saarland University, 66421 Homburg, Germany; ali.elsamad.94@hotmail.com (A.E.S.); juliajaffal8@gmail.com (J.J.); daliaibrahim93@outlook.com (D.R.I.); karin.schwarz@uks.eu (K.S.)

* Correspondence: frank.schmitz@uks.eu

† These authors contributed equally to this work.

Abstract: Background: Multiple sclerosis is a frequent neuroinflammatory and neurodegenerative disease of the central nervous system that includes alterations in the white and gray matter of the brain. The visual system is frequently affected in multiple sclerosis. Glutamate excitotoxicity might play a role in disease pathogenesis. Methodology: In the present study, we analyzed with qualitative and quantitative immunofluorescence microscopy and Western blot analyses whether alterations in the EAAT5 (SLC1A7) glutamate transporter could be involved in the previously observed alterations in structure and function of glutamatergic photoreceptor ribbon synapses in the EAE mouse model of MS. EAAT5 is a presynaptic glutamate transporter located near the presynaptic release sites. Results: We found that EAAT5 was strongly reduced at the photoreceptor synapses of EAE retinas in comparison to the photoreceptor synapses of the respective control retinas as early as day 9 post-immunization. The Western blot analyses demonstrated a decreased EAAT5 expression in EAE retinas. Conclusions: Our data illustrate early alterations of the EAAT5 glutamate transporter in the early pre-clinical phase of EAE/MS and suggest an involvement of EAAT5 in the previously observed early synaptic changes at photoreceptor synapses. The precise mechanisms need to be elucidated by future investigations.

Keywords: multiple sclerosis; EAE; retina; photoreceptor synapse; EAAT5 (SLC1A7); glutamate transporter

1. Introduction

Multiple sclerosis (MS) is a chronic autoimmune disease of the central nervous system (CNS). Neuroinflammation and neurodegeneration play an important role in MS. The disease results in axonal fiber tract damage/demyelination in the white matter [1–4]. Alterations in MS are not restricted to the white matter of the CNS but are present also in the gray matter of the CNS (e.g., [5–9]). Gray matter alterations include abnormalities of synapses and synapse networks as well as neurodegeneration and were observed in different brain regions of MS patients and in animal models of MS (for review, [10–13]).

It is well known that glutamate levels are elevated in MS, e.g., in the cerebrospinal fluid of MS patients, suggesting that glutamate excitotoxicity and possibly dysfunctions of glutamatergic synaptic signaling might play a role in the pathogenesis of MS ([14–18]; for review, see [12,19–23]). Multiple sources from neurons, glial- and immune cells could contribute to elevated extracellular glutamate levels [12,22–24].

The visual system is frequently affected in MS and inflammation of the optic nerve (optic neuritis) is an early symptom in MS. In animal models of MS, retinal changes included degeneration of retinal ganglion cells and alterations in synapse structure and function that could be inflammation-driven (e.g., [12,25–28]). Changes in photoreceptor synapses occurred early in the pre-clinical phase of EAE before obvious alterations in the optic nerve [25–27]. The molecular mechanisms of these early synaptic changes are not completely understood.

In previous studies ([25–27]; for review, [13]), we observed alterations of photoreceptor synapses in the EAE mouse model of MS on day 9 after injection. Photoreceptor synapses are continuously active glutamatergic ribbon synapses that contain presynaptic ribbons as eponymous structural specialization [29]. Synaptic ribbons are anchored to the presynaptic release sites and bind large numbers of glutamatergic synaptic vesicles to promote continuous synaptic vesicle exocytosis. RIBEYE is a main and unique component of synaptic ribbons [30–32]. In general, glutamate transporters remove glutamate released by synaptic transmission from the synaptic cleft and transport glutamate either into neuronal cells or glial cells to prevent glutamatergic excitotoxicity [12,33,34].

In the present study, we investigated whether an imbalance of glutamate homeostasis caused by alterations of glutamate transporters could possibly contribute to photoreceptor synapse pathology in EAE retinas. Five families of glutamate transporters have been cloned and functionally characterized [33–40]. In our analyses, we focused on the EAAT5 (SLC1A7) glutamate plasma membrane transporter that is strongly expressed in the retina [40–46]. EAAT5 is known to be localized in close vicinity of the presynaptic release sites of ribbon synapses [41–46]. We analyzed EAAT5 expression in the retina of MOG/CFA-injected EAE mice (9 days after injection) in comparison to control-injected mice. We found that EAAT5 expression at the presynaptic release site of photoreceptor synapses is strongly decreased in EAE mice in comparison to control mice, suggesting that malfunctions of glutamate transporters/glutamate clearance could contribute to the previously observed synapse pathology in EAE.

2. Materials and Methods

2.1. Animals

All procedures concerning laboratory animals were reviewed and approved by the local animal authorities (Tierschutzbeauftragte der Universität des Saarlandes and Landesamt für Verbraucherschutz; Geschäftsbereich 3; 66115 Saarbrücken, Germany; GB 3-2.4.2.2-25-2020). Female C57BL/6J mice older than 10 weeks and with a body weight between 20 g and 25 g were used for EAE induction, as previously described [25–27,47]. Mice were kept on a 10 h light–14 h dark cycle and provided with standard food and water ad libitum.

2.2. Antibodies (Tables 1 and 2)

Table 1. Primary antibodies.

Antibody	Source	References	Dilution
EAAT5 (immunogen affinity-purified rabbit polyclonal) *	Abcam; Cambridge, UK; ab230217	n.a.	1:200 (IF) 1:500 (WB)
RIBEYE(B) (mouse monoclonal, clone 2D9)	Lab-made	[25,48]	1:1000 (IF)
Actin (mouse monoclonal antibody, clone C4)	Millipore; Molsheim, France; #1501R	[49]	1:1000 (IF) 1:1000 (WB)
6xHis, HexaHis-tag (mouse monoclonal antibody, clone 1B7G5)	Proteintech; Planegg-Martinsried, Germany; #66005-1-Ig	[50]	1:5000 (WB)

* EAAT5 is a 559 amino acid (aa) long protein in mice (NP_666367.3, GI:1597486091) with a predicted running position at ≈65 kDa in the Western blot (WB) analyses. The affinity-purified rabbit polyclonal EAAT 5 antibody (abcam) was raised against a fusion protein corresponding to amino acid (aa) 100–250 of human EAAT5 (O00341). The specificity of the antibody was verified by a fusion protein that we generated from recombinant synthetic DNA (see below).

Table 2. Secondary antibodies.

Antibody	Source	Dilution
Chicken anti-rabbit-Alexa488	Invitrogen, Molecular Probes, Karlsruhe, Germany; A-21441	1:1000 (IF)
Donkey anti-rabbit-Alexa488	Invitrogen, Molecular Probes, Karlsruhe, Germany; A-21206	1:1000 (IF)
Donkey anti-mouse-Alexa568	Invitrogen, Molecular Probes, Karlsruhe, Germany; A-10037	1:1000 (IF)
Goat anti-rabbit-horseradish peroxidase (HRP)	Sigma; Taufkirchen, Germany; A6154	1:5000 (WB)
Goat anti-mouse-horseradish peroxidase (HRP)	Sigma; Taufkirchen, Germany; A3673	1:5000 (WB)

Abbreviations: IF, immunofluorescence microscopy; WB, Western blot.

2.3. Methods

2.3.1. Induction of EAE in Female Mice

Experimental autoimmune encephalomyelitis (EAE) was induced by immunizing 10–12 week old female C57BL/6J mice (20–25 g body weight) with $MOG_{35–55}$ peptide of mouse myelin oligodendrocyte glycoprotein as previously described [25–27,51]. MS is a disease that predominantly affects young female adults in humans. For the EAE model, we also used only female mice, as most of the EAE studies do (e.g., [25–27,52–54]). Mice were either injected with a ready-to-go emulsion from Hooke Laboratories ($MOG_{35–55}$/CFA Emulsion PTX, Hooke Laboratories, Lawrence, MA, USA; #EK-2110; 1 mg MOG peptide/mL of emulsion) or with lab-made emulsions. For the preparation of lab-made MOG/CFA suspensions, $MOG_{35–55}$ peptide was dissolved in sterile water (2 mg/mL) and emulsified in a one-to-one ratio with complete Freund adjuvant (CFA), that is composed of incomplete Freund adjuvant (iCFA, Sigma; #F5506) to which 10 mg/mL inactivated *Mycobacterium tuberculosis* were added (Fisher Scientific; Schwerte, Germany; 10218823). For control emulsion (CFA), complete Freund adjuvant was emulsified in a one-to-one ratio with sterile water. A total of 200 µL of the respective emulsion (either MOG/CFA (experimental group) or CFA (control group)) was subcutaneously administered in the axillary and groin region of the mice. Blood–brain barrier permeability was enhanced by two intraperitoneal injections of 200 ng pertussis toxin (PTX) from *B. pertussis* (List Biological Laboratories, Campbell, CA, USA; #181). The first one on the day of immunization (60 min after application of emulsion) and the second one on the subsequent day (16–20 h after immunization). Five independent immunizations, each composed of CFA-injected control animals and MOG/CFA-injected experimental animals, were performed for immunofluorescence microscopy and 5 independent immunizations, each composed of CFA-injected control animals and MOG/CFA-injected experimental animals, were performed for Western blot analyses. In these injections, animals were randomly allocated to the respective groups (i.e., control group or experimental group) and housed in the same cage.

2.3.2. Cloning of pET28a-EAAT5

In brief, cDNA encoding amino acids 100–250 of human EAAT5 were cloned into the vector pET-28a via Gibson assembly [55]. For this purpose, pET-28a vector was linearized by restriction digest with *NheI* and *XhoI*. The insert was provided as a synthetic DNA construct (gBlock, Integrated DNA Technologies (IDT), Coralville, IA, USA). The gBlock contained 34 nucleotides of overlapping vector sequences at both ends. At 5′ end of the gBlock vector sequence was followed by a *NheI* restriction site, a STREP-Tag II and the sequence encoding amino acids 100-250 of human EAAT5. The 3′ end of the gBlock was completed with 34 nucleotides of vector sequence, including the *XhoI* restriction site. In the resulting recombinant vector, EAAT5 is expressed as fusion protein containing a N-terminal hexa-His-Tag, followed by a thrombin cutting side and the STREP-Tag II. At the C-terminal end, the resulting fusion protein contains a second hexa-His-tag. Gibson assembly was performed according to the manufacturer's protocol using the Gibson assembly cloning kit (New England Biolabs, Frankfurt am Main, Germany).

2.3.3. Cloning of pET28a-Cre (Control Protein)

Fusion protein comprising the membrane permeable HIV TAT peptide followed in frame by Cre recombinase was cloned into the vector pET-28a via Gibson assembly [55]. For this, the vector was linearized by restriction digest using *NheI* and *XhoI*. The insert was provided as synthetic DNA construct (gBlock, Integrated DNA Technologies (IDT), Coralville, IA, USA). The gBlock contained 34 nucleotides of overlapping vector sequences at both ends. The 5′ end of the gBlock vector sequence was followed by a *NheI* restriction site, a STREP-Tag II, and the sequence encoding the TAT-Cre fusion protein. The 3′ end of the gBlock was completed by 34 nucleotides of vector sequence. In the resulting cloned vector, TAT-Cre is expressed as fusion protein containing a N-terminal hexa-His-Tag, followed by a thrombin cutting side and the STREP-Tag II. Gibson assembly was performed according to the manufacturer's protocol using the Gibson assembly cloning kit (New England Biolabs; Frankfurt am Main, Germany).

2.3.4. Fusion Protein Expression and Purification

Fusion protein expression was conducted in BL21 T7 Express bacteria. Transformed bacteria were grown in LB medium supplemented with 2% glucose and kanamycin (final concentration 10 µg/mL) at 37 °C until they reached OD_{600} = 0.8. Expression of fusion protein was induced by adding IPTG to a final concentration of 0.1 mM. After 5 h of induction with IPTG (at RT), bacteria were harvested by centrifugation. The bacterial pellet was washed several times with ice cold PBS and was finally resuspended in imidazole lysis buffer (300 mM NaCl, 50 mM NaH_2PO_4, 2.5 mM imidazole, pH 8.0) supplemented with lysozyme (1 mg/mL). After 30 min incubation of ice, followed by sonication, the bacterial lysate was cleared by centrifugation (10,000× *g*; 30 min 4 °C). Cleared lysate was incubated with Ni-NTA agarose overnight on an overhead rotator at 4 °C to allow binding of fusion protein to the Ni-NTA matrix (1 mL of Ni-NTA matrix/500 mL of bacterial culture). Next, lysate-Ni-NTA mixture was loaded into a column and flow thru was collected for SDS-Page analysis. The column was than washed with 5 bed volumes of washing buffers containing increasing concentrations of imidazole, starting with 10 mM imidazole (300 mM NaCl, 50 mM NaH_2PO_4, 10 mM imidazole, pH 8.0), followed by washes with 20 mM imidazole (300 mM NaCl, 50 mM NaH_2PO_4, 20 mM imidazole, pH 8.0) and 250 mM imidazole (300 mM NaCl, 50 mM NaH_2PO_4, 250 mM imidazole, pH 8.0). To elute the bound fusion protein, 6 mL of elution buffer (300 mM NaCl, 50 mM NaH_2PO_4, 400 mM imidazole, pH 8.0) were applied to the column and flow thru was collected in 0.5 mL fractions. EAAT5 fusion protein was enriched in faction 8–10 as assessed by SDS-PAGE and Western blotting.

2.3.5. Pre-Absorption of EAAT5 Antibody for Immunolabeling Experiments

Pre-absorption blocking experiments were performed to verify the specificity of EAAT5 antibody (Abcam, ab230217, Table 1). First, we determined the suitable working dilution (1:200, Table 1) of the EAAT5 antibody, which results in an antibody protein concentration of ~167 nM. The corresponding EAAT5 blocking fusion protein against which EAAT5 antibody was raised, as well as an unrelated fusion protein (HexaHIS-tagged Cre recombinase) were mixed with the EAAT5 antibody in a molar ratio of 5:1 in different tubes (an experimental tube and control tube). Both tubes were incubated on a rotator overnight at 4 °C. On the following day, both tubes were centrifuged at 30,000 rpm (Biofuge Stratos centrifuge, #3331 rotor; ThermoFisher; Waltham, MA, USA) for 5 min. The supernatants were employed for immunostaining experiments. Different semi-thin sections were co-immunolabeled simultaneously. One was incubated with mouse monoclonal RIBEYE antibody 2D9 and the EAAT5 antibody that was pre-absorbed with EAAT5 fusion protein as described above. In parallel, another section was double immunostained with EAAT5 antibody pre-absorbed with the unrelated fusion protein (HexaHIS-tagged Cre) along with anti-RIBEYE antibody 2D9. The antibodies against RIBEYE served as reference immunosignals. Both incubations were performed overnight at 4 °C. On the next day, sections were washed multiple times with PBS to remove unbound primary antibodies and were subsequently incubated with the corresponding fluorescent conjugated secondary antibody for 2 h at RT (see Table 2). Binding of the EAAT5 rabbit polyclonal antibody was detected with donkey anti-rabbit immunoglobulins conjugated to Alexa 488 and binding of the mouse monoclonal RIBEYE antibody (clone 2D9) was detected with donkey anti-mouse immunoglobulins conjugated to Alexa 568. Lastly, the sections were washed five times (5 min each) with PBS and mounted in n-propyl gallate (NPG) antifade solution, as previously described [25,30,56–59]. Negative control incubations were performed under the same conditions as described above, but in the absence of the primary antibody to check for non-specific fluorescence signals, e.g., by autofluorescence.

2.3.6. Immunolabeling of Retinal Sections

Immunofluorescence microscopy was performed on semi-thin retinal resin sections from MOG/CFA-injected EAE mice and CFA-injected control mice, as previously described [25–27]. For this purpose, eyes were isolated from the respective mice within 5 min post-mortem. The anterior eyecup was removed as described [25–27,60]. The posterior eyecup with the attached retina was flash-frozen in liquid-nitrogen-cooled isopentane and freeze-dried in a vacuum generated by a DUO 004B vacuum pump (Arthur-Pfeiffer Vakuumtechnik, Wetzlar, Germany), as previously described [25–27,48,56,57,60]. During lyophilization, the samples were cooled with liquid nitrogen for ~two days. After that, the samples were equilibrated to room temperature and infiltrated for ~48 h with Epon resin, as described [25–27,60]. Infiltration with Epon resin was performed the first 12 h at 28 °C in an overhead rotator at 2rpm to ease infiltration of the samples with Epon. Afterwards, the infiltration with Epon resin was continued at RT. After infiltration with Epon resin, samples were polymerized for 2 days at 60 °C. From the hardened tissue blocks, 0.5 μm thin (semi-thin) sections were cut with a Reichert ultramicrotome using a diamond knife (Diatome; Nidau, Switzerland) to generate standardized sections of identical thickness. Sections were collected on glass coverslips. The Epon resin was removed from the semi-thin sections and processed for immunocytochemistry, as previously described [25–27,48,56,57,60]. The sections were processed for double-immunolabeling with the indicated antibodies and incubated overnight at 4 °C in the indicated optimized primary antibody dilutions (see Table 1). In each experiment, a reference (CFA) and experimental samples (MOG/CFA) were processed simultaneously under identical conditions. The next day, sections were washed several times with PBS to remove unbound primary antibodies and subsequently incubated with the corresponding fluorophore-conjugated secondary antibodies (Table 2) for 1 h at room temperature (RT). Finally, sections were washed again several times with PBS and were embedded in NPG-antifade, as described [25,48,56–58,61].

2.3.7. Confocal Microscopy and Quantitative Analyses of Immunosignals

Confocal microscopy was performed with a Nikon A1R confocal microscope (Düsseldorf, Germany), as previously described [25,56–59]. Images were acquired with a 60×/1.40 N.A. oil objective under the control of NIS Elements software (NIS Elements AR 3.2, 64 bit; Düsseldorf, Germany). In the individual experiments, image acquisition from MOG/CFA- and CFA-samples was performed under identical conditions by using the re-use image settings option in the NIS Elements software. Image acquisition and analyses were performed in a blinded manner with the experimenter not knowing whether the samples were from CFA- or MOG/CFA-injected mice. CFA- and MOG/CFA-injected samples from each embedding were imaged under identical conditions using the re-use option of the NIS Elements software. Five independent experiments were performed for each experimental group. For quantification, an identical rectangular ROI was used for both samples and placed along the OPL that could be unambiguously identified by the actin and EAAT5 immunosignals. ROIs were managed with the Analyze-Tools-ROI Manager of ImageJ. EAAT5 and actin immunosignals were simultaneously recorded. Actin signals served as a reference signal to correct for potential differences in section thickness. Actin is particularly suitable as a reference protein because actin turned out to remain unchanged between CFA- and MOG/CFA-injected samples [25]. Fluorescence intensities of both proteins were measured as integrated density. EAAT5 immunosignal integrated densities were normalized to the corresponding actin integrated density values. The arithmetic mean values of CFA were set to 100% and the MOG/CFA values were related to them. Integrated density values were analyzed with Microsoft Excel. Statistical analyses were performed with GraphPad Prism 10 (version 10.2.3), see below.

2.3.8. Statistical Analyses of Immunofluorescence Signals

Statistical analyses were performed with GraphPad 10 (version 10.2.3). Based on our experience and previously performed a priori sample size estimations ($\alpha \leq 0.05$; effect size Cohen's d = 0.8; power = 0.8) using G*Power Version 3.1.9.6 [62], a total of 5 independent immunizations, each composed of CFA-injected control animals and MOG/CFA-injected experimental animals, were performed. In these injections, animals were randomly allocated to the respective groups (i.e., control group or experimental group) and housed in the same cage. For quantification, samples were randomly drawn from these five independent injections and analyzed by immunofluorescence. First, we tested whether data from these individual experiments could be pooled. For this purpose, we determined whether the reference/control group (CFA) from the independent individual experiments differed significantly from each other. To decide this, we determined whether data were normally distributed using the Shapiro–Wilk test. Not all data were normally distributed. Next, we used Kruskal–Wallis ANOVA and post hoc Dunn tests to compare the different CFA reference groups from the individual experiments. The values of the individual CFA reference (control) animals did not differ significantly from each other in the different independent experiments. Therefore, we pooled the data for further analysis. Pooled data from CFA and MOG/CFA samples were analyzed for statistical differences by the non-parametric Mann–Whitney *U* test. Differences were considered statistically different with $p < 0.05$. Post hoc analysis of data obtained for immunofluorescence data showed a power of 0.985 with an effect size Hedges' g = 0.953835 and $\alpha = 0.0001$ [63].

2.3.9. Miscellaneous Procedures

Western Blot (WB) Analyses

The specificity of EAAT5 antibody was analyzed by Western blot (WB) with retinal lysates from wild-type mice. Retinal lysate was prepared as described next. In order to analyze possible changes in the global expression of EAAT5 in EAE retinas in comparison to control retinas, retina extracts from MOG/CFA-injected EAE mice and CFA-injected control mice were prepared in ice-cold RIPA lysis buffer containing 150 mM NaCl, 50 mM Tris, pH 7.4, 1% NP-40, 0.5% sodium deoxycholate, 0.1% SDS, and cOMPLETE EDTA-free protease inhibitor cocktail (Roche; COEDTAF-RO). An Ultra Turrax T8A (IKA Labortechnik; Staufen im Breisgau, Germany) was used to homogenize the retinas for 1–2 s. After this step, the retinal lysate was kept in the RIPA lysis buffer for 20 min on ice (with gentle agitation) and then centrifuged at 13,000 rpm for 30 min (at 4 °C). The pellet was discarded while the supernatant was collected in a new tube, mixed 1:1 (*v*/*v*) with SDS Laemmli buffer and heated for 10 min to 96 °C. Protein quantification was performed with the Amidoblack method [64]. For this purpose, 5 µL of protein sample dissolved in SDS-Laemmli buffer and BSA standards were spotted on cellulose acetate membranes, air dried, and stained with an Amido Black 10B solution (0.5% (*w*/*v*) Amido Black 10B in methanol (45%, *v*/*v*)/water (45% *v*/*v*)/10% acetic acid (10%, *v*/*v*)) for 10 min at RT. Next, the cellulose acetate sheets were washed three times with 1 mL wash solution (47.5% each of methanol and water, and 5% glacial acetic acid) (5 min each). The stained cellulose acetate sheets were then dried again at RT and the individual samples were cut apart. The individual samples were transferred into separate test tubes (2 mL Eppendorf cups) and dissolved in 1 mL dissolution solution (80% (*v*/*v*) formic acid, 10% (*v*/*v*) acetic acid and 10% (*w*/*v*) trichloro acetic acid). For complete dissolution, the membrane pieces were incubated at 50 °C under constant shaking for 30 min followed by measuring the absorbance of the resulting solution at 620 nm using a UV/Visible spectrophotometer (Pharmacia-Pfizer, New York, NY, USA). Protein concentrations were determined by comparing the absorbance values to a BSA standard curve. We applied 30 μg of protein of the retinal lysates on each lane and separated by 10% acrylamide SDS-PAGE. After SDS-PAGE, proteins were electro-transferred from the resolving gel to nitrocellulose membrane at 50 volts for 6.5 h at 4 °C. On the next day, the membrane with the electro-transferred proteins was washed several times with PBS and incubated with 5% (*w*/*v*) non-fatty dry milk in PBS for 1 hr at room temperature (RT) to block non-specific binding sites and incubated with the primary antibody dilutions indicated in Table 1 (on a shaker, overnight at 4 °C). After this, the membrane was washed several times with PBS to remove unbound primary antibody and incubated in the corresponding secondary antibody conjugated with horseradish peroxidase (HRP) with the antibody dilutions as given in Table 2 with gentle shaking (for 2 h at RT). Later, membranes were washed three times (10 min each) to remove unbound secondary antibody. Antibody binding was visualized by chemiluminescence (ECL) acquired by Bio-Rad Gel Doc imaging systems (Bio-Rad ChemiDoc™ MP Imaging System and Bio-Rad ChemiDoc™ XRS Imaging System; Feldkirchen, Germany). For re-probing of WB membranes, membranes were incubated with 0.2 M glycine and 0.1% SDS, pH 2.2, in H_2O (stripping buffer) for 20 min at room temperature with mild shaking to remove bound antibodies. Then, the membrane was washed 3 times (10 min each) with TBST (Tris-buffered saline with 0.1% (*w*/*v*) Tween® 20 detergent) to remove the stripping buffer. Afterwards, the membrane was incubated with 5% (*w*/*v*) non-fatty dry milk in PBS for 1 h (RT) to saturate non-specific protein binding sites. After that, the membrane was probed with the mouse monoclonal anti-actin primary antibody (clone C4 at the dilution given in Table 1). Binding of mouse monoclonal actin antibody was detected with the corresponding secondary antibody (Table 2) and visualized via ECL, as described above.

Quantification of WB Bands and Statistical Analyses

Image Studio Lite software (Li-Cor, version 5.2) was employed to analyze the band chemoluminescence signal corresponding to the global expression of EAAT5 protein present in whole retinal lysate samples from independent experiments. Five independent experiments were analyzed on pairs of retinal lysates from CFA and MOG/CFA mice. Using the analysis option of the Image Studio Lite software (Li-Cor, version 5.2), a rectangular ROI was drawn specifically around the targeted band to measure the chemoluminescence pixel intensity sum corrected for area and background (signal value). The band intensity of the EAAT5 target protein was normalized to the reference protein (actin) band intensity in the same lane to correct for possible loading differences. Actin was shown to remain unchanged between MOG/CFA- and CFA-injected samples [25]. For statistical analysis, the normalized EAAT5 band intensity values of each CFA sample were set to 100% and the corresponding MOG/CFA normalized EAAT5 band intensity value was related to it. Next, these normalized data were exported and statistically analyzed using GraphPad prism 10. MOG/CFA values were normally distributed according to Shapiro–Wilk tests. Therefore, one sample *t*-test was used for statistical difference analysis and $p < 0.05$ was considered a significant difference. Values were calculated and plotted as arithmetic means and standard errors of the mean (S.E.M.) with GraphPad prism 10. All individual values were depicted.

3. Results

In the present study, we analyzed the expression of the glutamate transporter EAAT5 in photoreceptor synapses of the outer plexiform layer (OPL) in the mouse retina by immunofluorescence microscopy. We compared retinas from MOG/CFA-injected EAE mice with retinas from CFA-injected control mice on day 9 after injection. For immunocytochemistry, we used an antigen affinity-purified polyclonal antibody against EAAT5.

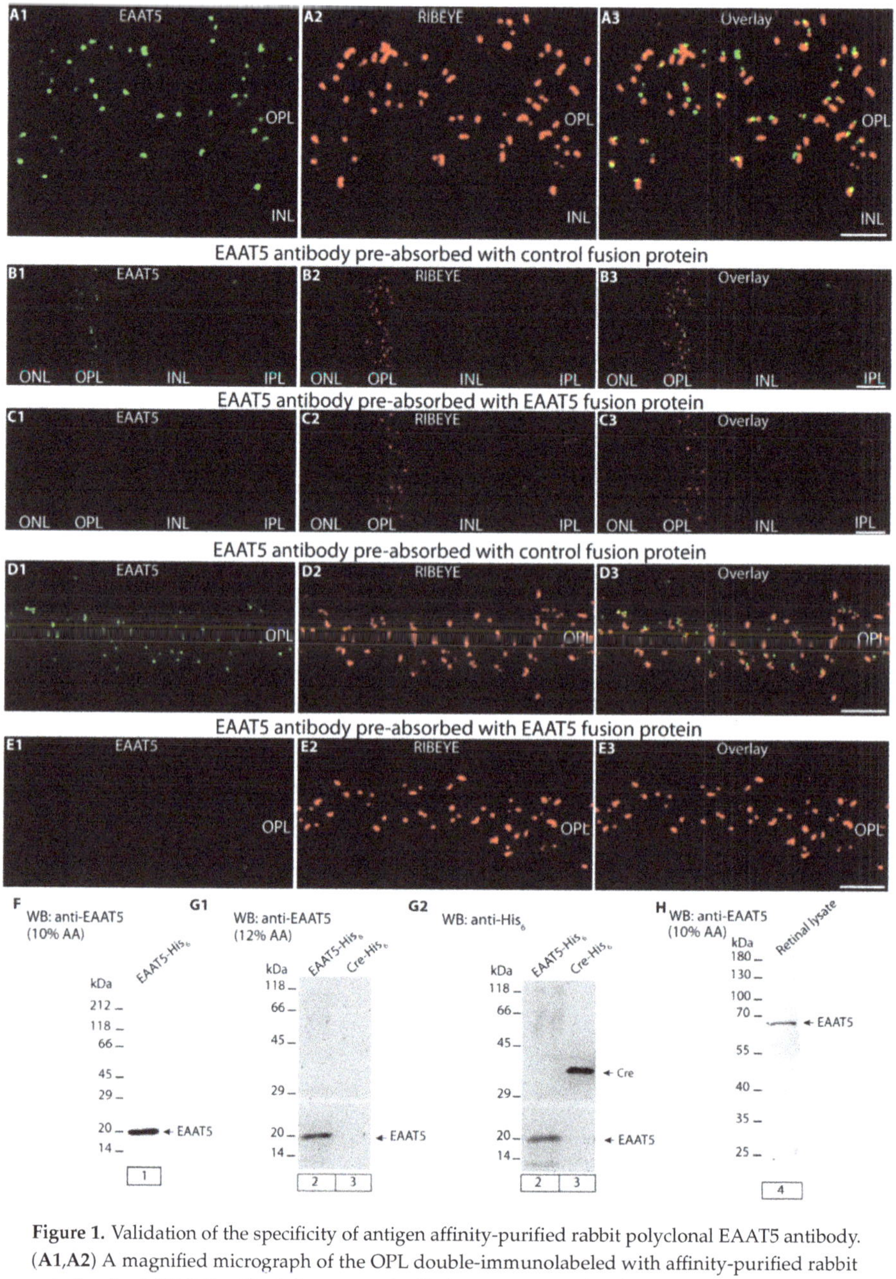

Figure 1. Validation of the specificity of antigen affinity-purified rabbit polyclonal EAAT5 antibody. (**A1,A2**) A magnified micrograph of the OPL double-immunolabeled with affinity-purified rabbit polyclonal anti-EAAT5 antibody in green and with the mouse monoclonal anti-RIBEYE (2D9) antibody in red, respectively. (**A3**) A merged image for both antibodies in the OPL of photoreceptor synapses. (**B1–E3**) The pre-absorption experiments of EAAT5 signals performed on 0.5 µm-thin (semi-thin) wild-type retina sections. (**B1,D1**) The EAAT5 antibody was pre-absorbed with either an unrelated control fusion protein or (**C1,E1**) with the EAAT5 fusion protein against which the antibody was raised. (**B2,C2,D2,E2**) The RIBEYE immunosignals were unaffected by blocking with either fusion protein. (**B3,C3,D3,E3**) The signals from the respective red and green channels were overlaid. (**F–H**) Western

blots (WB) analyses of the EAAT5 antibody that was generated against EAAT5 fusion protein. (**F,G1**) The EAAT5 antibody detects a ~20 kDa band in lane 1 and 2 corresponding to the EAAT5 fusion protein. (**G1**) Lane 3 containing Cre control fusion protein did not show a band/reactivity with the EAAT5 antibody thus demonstrating the specificity of the antigen affinity-purified polyclonal EAAT5 antibody. (**G2**) shows anti-HexaHIS antibody incubation of the very same blot strip in G1, manifesting the loading of both EAAT5 and Cre control fusion protein. (H) single band ≈ 65 kDa is detected in retina lysate from wild-type mice by EAAT5 antibody. Abbreviations: OPL, outer plexiform layer. Scale bars: 5 µm.

The EAAT5 antibody produced strong punctate signals in the OPL near the presynaptic release sites of photoreceptor synapses (Figure 1A1–A3). The presynaptic release sites were immunolabeled with mouse monoclonal antibodies against RIBEYE (clone 2D9) (Figure 1A2,A3). RIBEYE is the main component of synaptic ribbons [30–32]. This punctate EAAT5 immunosignal near the presynaptic release sites was expected because a very similar immunolabeling pattern was previously observed for EAAT5 in the mouse retina [46].

In addition to a strong EAAT5 immunosignal in the OPL, we also observed a punctate EAAT5 immunolabeling pattern in the inner plexiform layer (IPL) (Figure 1B1,B3) that represents EAAT5 in the presynaptic terminals of rod bipolar cells, as previously reported by another group [46].

The EAAT5 immunosignals in the OPL and IPL were completely abolished if the EAAT5 antibody was pre-absorbed with the EAAT5 fusion protein against which it was raised (Figure 1C1,C3,E1,E3). The RIBEYE immunosignals were un-affected by the pre-absorption of the EAAT5 antibody with the EAAT5 fusion protein (Figure 1C2,E2). The EAAT5 immunosignals (as well as the RIBEYE immunosignals) remained unaffected if the EAAT5 antibody was pre-absorbed with an irrelevant HIS-tagged fusion protein (Figure 1B1–B3,D1–D3) demonstrating the specificity of the immunolabeling data in the pre-absorption experiment.

In Western blot analyses, the EAAT5 antibody detected the recombinant, bacterially expressed EAAT5 fusion protein it was raised against (Figure 1F, lane 1; Figure 1G1, lane 2) but not the Cre control fusion protein (Figure 1G1, lane 2), further indicating the specificity of the antibody. In Figure 1G2, both fusion proteins from the same blot as shown in Figure 1G1 were incubated with anti-HexaHIS monoclonal antibody to visualize both proteins and to document the loading of the EAAT5 fusion protein and Cre control protein on the WB membrane. The EAAT5 antibody detected a protein band at the expected running position of ≈65 kDa in wild-type mouse retinal lysates (Figure 1H).

We used the affinity-purified rabbit polyclonal EAAT5 antibody, that has been validated by the experiments shown in Figure 1, to analyze the expression of EAAT5 in photoreceptor synapses in the OPL from MOG/CFA-injected EAE mice in comparison to photoreceptor synapses in the OPL of CFA-injected littermate control mice by immunohistochemistry (Figure 2). In photoreceptor synapses in the OPL of MOG/CFA-injected EAE mice (Figure 2B1–B3,D1–D3), the EAAT5 immunosignals were strongly reduced in comparison to photoreceptor synapses in the OPL of CFA-injected littermate control mice (Figure 2A1–A3,C1–C3) as evaluated by qualitative (Figure 2A1–A3,B1–B3,C1–C3,D1–D3) and quantitative immunocytochemistry (Figure 2E1,E2). In these immunolabelling analyses, the retinal sections were co-immunolabelled with antibodies against EAAT5 and actin (Figure 2A1–A3,B1–B3,C1–C3,D1–D3). Actin served as reference protein for the visualization of retinal layers (including the OPL) as well as for the quantification/normalization of the EAAT5 immunosignals (Figure 2E1,E2). Actin is a suitable reference protein for this purpose because actin was shown to remain unchanged in EAE at this stage [25].

The global expression of EAAT5 protein, as judged by the Western blot analyses (Figure 3), was also decreased in the retinas from MOG/CFA-injected EAE mice in comparison to CFA-injected control mice at day 9 after injection.

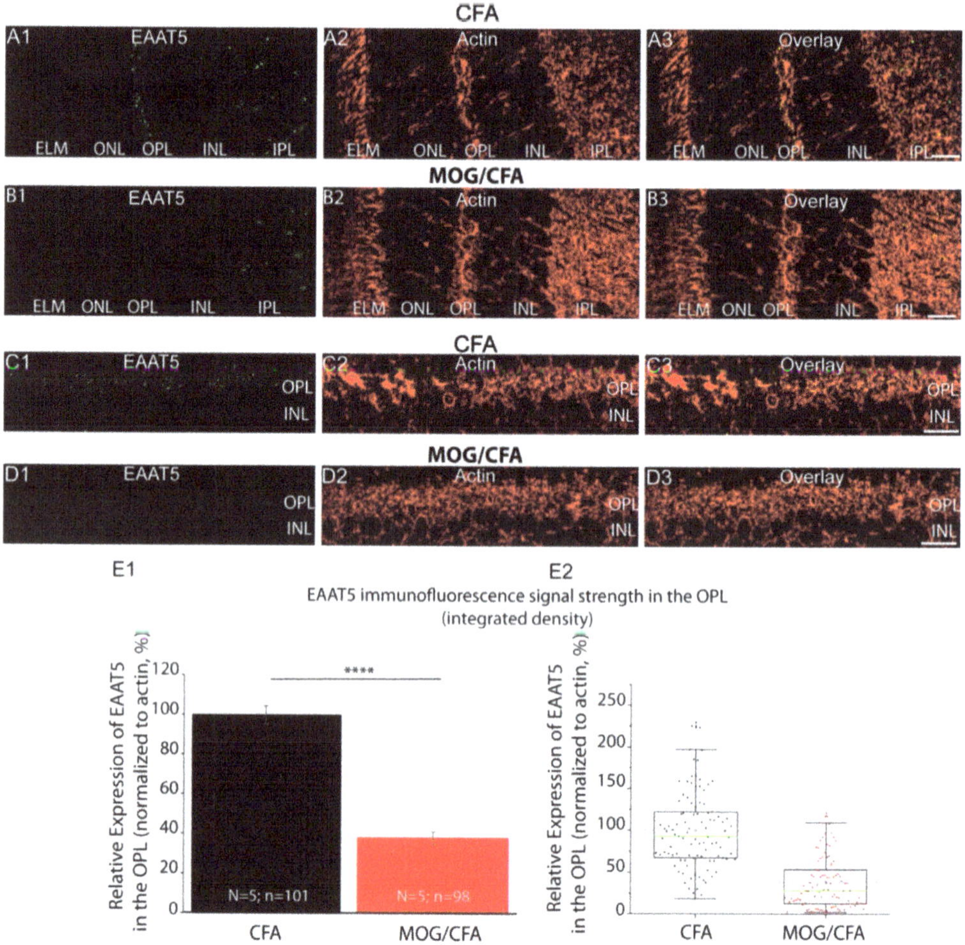

Figure 2. EAAT5 immunofluorescence signals are strongly reduced in photoreceptor synapses in OPL from MOG/CFA-injected EAE mice in comparison to CFA-injected control mice. (**A1–D3**) Double immunolabeling of 0.5 µm-thin (semi-thin) retina sections from CFA-injected control mice and MOG/CFA-injected EAE mice (day 9 post injection) with mouse monoclonal antibody against actin (clone C4, in red channel) and rabbit polyclonal antibody against EAAT5 (in green channel). Immunosignals from respective green and red channels were superimposed in (**A3**,**B3**,**C3**,**D3**). (**C1–D3**) Zoomed view of OPL that is double immuno-labeled with EAAT5 and RIBEYE antibodies. (**E1**) Histogram depicts mean fluorescence intensities (%) of EAAT5 immunosignals of controls (CFA) and EAE mice (MOG/CFA) in OPL. Values in (**E1**) are means ± S.E.M. (****, $p \leq 0.0001$). (**E2**) Box and whisker diagram shows distribution of individual values from (**E1**). Boxes mean and median values denoted by horizontal dashed blue line and solid green line, respectively. Boxes illustrate 25th–75th percentiles of data points, and whiskers represent 1.5 times of interquartile range (IQR). Statistical significance was determined with Mann–Whitney U-test (for details, see Methods Section 2.3). Abbreviations: CFA, complete Freund's adjuvant; EAE, experimental autoimmune encephalomyelitis; MOG, myelin oligodendrocyte protein; N, number of mice; n, number of confocal images analyzed to quantify integrated densities of fluorescence signals from retinal sections; OPL, outer plexiform layer; S.E.M., standard error of mean. Scale bars: 5 µm.

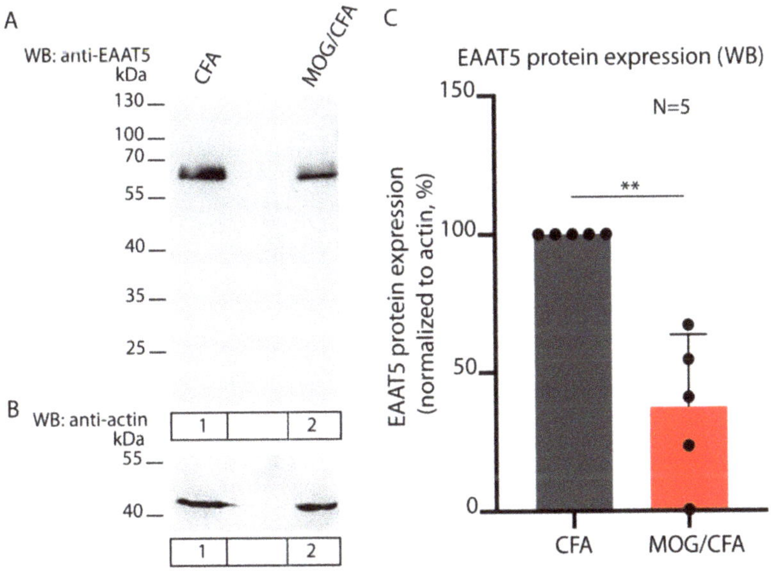

Figure 3. The Western blot (WB) analyses of the total EAAT5 expression in the retinal lysates of MOG/CFA-injected EAE mice and CFA-injected control mice on day 9 after injection. (**A**) The EAAT5 antibody detects EAAT5 at the expected running position of ≈65 kDa in the WB analyses of retinal lysates from CFA-injected control mice and MOG/CFA-injected EAE mice (lanes 1 and 2, respectively). (**B**) shows the same WB membrane as shown in (A) but re-probed with an antibody against actin. Actin (at ≈43 kDa) served as loading control. (**C**) summarizes the results from 5 independent Western blot experiments in which EAAT5 expression was analyzed in retinas from CFA- and MOG/CFA-injected mice (as normalized EAAT5 expression, normalized to the loading control (actin)). CFA control group values were assigned to 100% for better assessment of the relative differences between CFA-injected control mice and MOG/CFA-injected EAE mice. Values in (**C**) are means ± S.E.M. One sample *t*-test was used to determine the statistical significance (*p*-value). Abbreviations: WB, Western blot; CFA, complete Freund's adjuvant; EAE, experimental autoimmune encephalomyelitis; MOG, myelin oligodendrocyte protein; S.E.M., standard error of the mean; N, number of experiments; **, $p < 0.01$.

4. Discussion

Multiple sclerosis (MS) is a chronic neuroinflammatory disease of the CNS in which pro-inflammatory cytokines are up-regulated [22]. Pro-inflammatory cytokines were previously reported to cause down-regulation of glutamate transporters in various regions of the CNS (e.g., [45,65–69]; for review, [10,13,70,71]). In some studies, though, an enhanced expression of glutamate transporters was found (e.g., [72]). Of note, a glutamate transporter polymorphism has been observed to be associated with higher glutamate concentrations in relapsing multiple sclerosis, pointing to an important contribution of glutamate transporters in the pathogenesis of MS [73,74].

Glutamate transporters, in general, remove glutamate released by synaptic transmission from the synaptic cleft and physiologically transport glutamate back into neuronal cells or glial cells to prevent glutamatergic excitotoxicity [12,33,34,38,75,76]. Dysfunctional glutamate uptake could lead to glutamate spillover of glutamate from synaptic sites to extrasynaptic sites (for review, [12,75,77]). Binding of glutamate to extrasynaptic glutamate receptors leads to functional impairment and finally cell death via multiple mechanisms and pathways ([78–80]; for review, [12,81–83]). The mechanisms of glutamatergic excitotoxicity include neurons and glial cells ([80,84]; for review, [12,77,82]).

In the present study, we focused on the EAAT5 glutamate transporter. EAAT5 is located in the presynaptic terminals of retinal neurons, i.e., photoreceptors and bipolar cells, in close proximity to the presynaptic glutamate release sites that are characterized by synaptic ribbons [42–44,46].

In the current work, we demonstrated that the presynaptic glutamate transporter EAAT5 is strongly down-regulated in photoreceptor synapses of MOG/CFA-injected EAE mice in comparison to photoreceptor synapses from CFA-injected control mice. Down-regulation of EAAT5 in photoreceptor synapses was demonstrated by qualitative and quantitative immunofluorescence microscopy. In EAE, we observed a strong decrease in EAAT5 at photoreceptor synapses close to the presynaptic ribbons. A decreased expression of EAAT5 was also demonstrated by the Western blot analyses of whole retinal lysates. The physiological consequences of the strongly decreased expression of EAAT5 at photoreceptor ribbon synapses in EAE remain to be elucidated by future investigations. Clearly, the EAAT5 transporter is close to the presynaptic release site and contributes to high temporal resolution of synaptic signaling in the retina as judged by electrophysiological analyses [46]. Interestingly, visual performance/frequence sensitivity is also compromised in EAE as measured by optometry [25]. The decreased expression of EAAT5 determined in this study could contribute to that phenomenon. EAAT5 as a presynaptic glutamate transporter has a large glutamate-gated chloride conductance that could function as a presynaptic feedback inhibitor that improves temporal resolution of synaptic transmission via its glutamate-gated chloride channel function and its impact on presynaptic membrane potential [35,39,41,44,46,85–90]. The lack or lower activity of this EAAT5-based feedback mechanism in EAE photoreceptor synapses could contribute to the decreased visual performance in EAE mice (decreased frequence sensitivity) in previously published optometry experiments on MOG/CFA-injected EAE mice [25].

Whether a decreased expression of EAAT5 in EAE photoreceptor synapses as observed in the present study is relevant to prevent a possible spillover of glutamate from the synaptic cleft to extra-synaptic sites remains to be investigated. Recent analyses showed that EAAT5 is a low-capacity glutamate transporter that is rapidly saturated ([44,91–93]; for review, [94]). Therefore, glutamate transporters other than EAAT5 could have a stronger impact on a possible spillover of glutamate from synaptic to extrasynaptic sites, particularly at higher rates of vesicular glutamate release at the synapse. It remains to be elucidated whether other glutamate transporters are also decreased at EAE photoreceptor synapses. Recently, it was shown that the GLAST (EAAT1, SLC1A3) glutamate transporter plays an important role in protecting retinal ganglion cells from glutamatergic excitotoxicity in EAE [24]. The GLAST glutamate transporter is a high-capacity glutamate transporter in the retina [95,96] and could also exert an important function to prevent spillover of glutamate from synaptic to extrasynaptic sites at photoreceptor synapses in EAE. This must be investigated by future studies.

Outlook

In the present study, we showed alterations of the glutamate transporter EAAT5 in the mouse model of multiple sclerosis and demonstrated that the EAAT5 glutamate transporter is less enriched at photoreceptor synapses of MOG/CFA-injected EAE mice in comparison to CFA-injected control mice. EAAT5 is a low-capacity glutamate transporter operating in close vicinity to presynaptic release sites at which exocytosis of glutamatergic synaptic vesicles occurs. EAAT5 is also expressed at the presynaptic terminals of retinal bipolar cells. Retinal bipolar cells are structurally and functionally much more diverse than photoreceptor synapses. Future analyses will show whether the EAAT5 transporter is also compromised at retinal bipolar cell ribbon synapses. The recently generated EAAT5 knockout [46] is an ideal tool to further analyze the functional role of EAAT5 in multiple sclerosis disease development and progression. It will be important to analyze whether other glutamate transporters are affected in EAE, including high-capacity glutamate transporters, that could possibly contribute to photoreceptor synapse pathology. Interestingly, a recent study demonstrated that the GLAST/EAAT1 glutamate is also downregulated in the inner retina in the EAE animal model of MS and that AAV-mediated overexpression of GLAST/EAAT1 protects retinal ganglion cells from cell death [74]. These findings suggest an important role of glutamate transporters for the pathogenesis of multiple sclerosis, and the analyses of glutamate transporters in EAE/MS could help to develop new therapeutic strategies for the treatment of the disease.

Author Contributions: A.E.S. performed experiments and analyzed data; J.J. performed experiments and analyzed data; D.R.I. analyzed data and supported methodology; K.S. performed experiments and analyzed data; F.S. performed experiments, analyzed data, and designed the study; J.J., A.E.S. and F.S. wrote the paper draft. All authors have read and agreed to the published version of the manuscript.

Funding: The work of the authors was supported by a grant from the Dr. Rolf M. Schwiete foundation (grant 2021-022).

Institutional Review Board Statement: The study was conducted according to the guidelines of the Declaration of Helsinki and approved by the Institutional Review Board (Landesamt für Verbraucherschutz, Geschäftsbereich 3; 66115 Saarbrücken, Germany; GB 3-2.4.1.1-K110/180-07).

Informed Consent Statement: Not applicable.

Data Availability Statement: All data are presented in the main manuscript and the manuscript figures.

Acknowledgments: The authors appreciate the skillful technical assistance of Gabi Kiefer and Sabine Schmidt.

Conflicts of Interest: The authors declare no conflicts of interest.

References

1. Korn, T. Pathophysiology of multiple sclerosis. *J. Neurol.* **2008**, *255* (Suppl. S6), 2–6. [CrossRef] [PubMed]
2. Yamout, B.I.; Alroughani, R. Multiple sclerosis. *Sem. Neurol.* **2018**, *38*, 212–225.
3. Filippi, M.; Bar-Or, A.; Piehl, F.; Preziosa, P.; Solari, A.; Vukusic, S.; Rocca, M.A. Multiple Sclerosis. *Nat. Rev.* **2018**, *4*, 43. [CrossRef]
4. Dobson, R.; Giovannoni, G. Multiple sclerosis—A review. *Eur. J. Neurol.* **2019**, *26*, 27–40. [CrossRef] [PubMed]
5. Pirko, I.; Lucchinetti, C.F.; Sriram, S.; Bakshi, R. Gray matter involvement in multiple sclerosis. *Neurology* **2007**, *68*, 634–642. [CrossRef]
6. Fisher, E.; Lee, J.C.; Nakamura, K.; Rudick, R.A. Gray matter atrophy in multiple sclerosis: A longitudinal study. *Ann. Neurol.* **2008**, *64*, 255–265. [CrossRef]
7. Vercellino, M.; Masera, S.; Lorenzatti, M.; Condello, C.; Merola, A.; Mattioda, A.; Tribolo, A.; Capello, E.; Mancardi, G.L.; Mutani, R.; et al. Demyelination, inflammation, and neurodegeneration in multiple sclerosis deep gray matter. *J. Neuropathol. Exp. Neurol.* **2009**, *68*, 489–502. [CrossRef]
8. Chard, D.; Miller, D. Grey matter pathology in clinically early multiple sclerosis: Evidence from magnetic resonance imaging. *J. Neurol. Sci.* **2009**, *282*, 5–11. [CrossRef]
9. Dutta, R.; Trapp, B.D. Mechanisms of neuronal dysfunction and degeneration in multiple sclerosis. *Prog. Neurobiol.* **2011**, *93*, 1–12. [CrossRef]
10. Mandolesi, G.; Gentile, A.; Musella, A.; Fresegna, D.; DeVito, F.; Bulitta, S.; Sepman, H.; Marfia, G.A.; Centonze, D. Synaptopathy connects inflammation and neurodegeneration in multiple sclerosis. *Nat. Rev. Neurol.* **2015**, *11*, 711–724. [CrossRef]
11. Stampanoni Bassi, M.; Mori, F.; Buttari, F.; Marfia, G.A.; Sancesario, A.; Centonze, D.; Iezzi, E. Neurophysiology of synaptic functioning in multiple sclerosis. *Clin. Neurophysiol.* **2017**, *128*, 1148–1157. [CrossRef] [PubMed]
12. Fairless, R.; Bading, H.; Diem, R. Pathophysiological ionotropic glutamate signaling in neuroinflammatory disease as a therapeutic target. *Front. Neurosci.* **2021**, *15*, 741280. [CrossRef] [PubMed]
13. Schwarz, K.; Schmitz, F. Synapse dysfunctions in multiple sclerosis. *Int. J. Mol. Sci.* **2023**, *24*, 1639. [CrossRef] [PubMed]
14. Stover, J.F.; Pleines, U.E.; Morganti-Kossmann, M.C.; Kossmann, T.; Lowitsch, K.; Kempski, O.S. Neurotransmitters in cerebrospinal fluid reflect pathological activity. *Eur. J. Clin. Investig.* **1997**, *27*, 1038–1043. [CrossRef]
15. Pitt, D.; Werner, P.; Raine, C.S. Glutamate excitotoxicity in a model of multiple sclerosis. *Nat. Med.* **2000**, *6*, 67–70. [CrossRef]
16. Sarchielli, P.; Greco, L.; Floridi, A.; Gallai, V. Excitatory amino acids and multiple sclerosis: Evidence from cerebrospinal fluid. *Arch. Neurol.* **2003**, *60*, 1082–1088. [CrossRef]
17. Werner, P.; Pitt, D.; Raine, C.S. Multiple sclerosis: Altered glutamate homeostasis in lesions correlates with oligodendrocyte and axonal damage. *Ann. Neurol.* **2003**, *50*, 169–180. [CrossRef]
18. Srinivasan, R.; Sailasuta, N.; Hurd, R.; Nelson, S.; Pelletier, D. Evidence of elevated glutamate in multiple sclerosis using magnetic resonance spectroscopy at 3T. *Brain* **2005**, *128*, 1016–1025. [CrossRef]
19. Kostic, M.; Zivkovic, N.; Stojanovic, I. Multiple sclerosis and glutamate excitotoxicity. *Rev. Neurosci.* **2013**, *24*, 71–88. [CrossRef]

20. Stojanovic, I.R.; Kostic, M.; Ljubisavljevic, S. The role of glutamate and its receptors in multiple sclerosis. *J. Neural Transm.* **2014**, *1121*, 945–955. [CrossRef]
21. Macrez, R.; Stys, P.K.; Vivien, D.; Lipton, S.A.; Docagne, F. Mechanisms of glutamate toxicity in multiple sclerosis. *Lancet Neurol.* **2016**, *15*, 1089–1101. [CrossRef] [PubMed]
22. Levite, M. Glutamate, T cells and multiple sclerosis. *J. Neural Transm.* **2017**, *124*, 775–798. [CrossRef] [PubMed]
23. Kuzmina, U.S.; Zainullina, L.F.; Vakhitov, V.A.; Bakhtiyarova, K.Z.; Vakhitova, Y.V. The role of glutamate in the pathogenesis of multiple sclerosis. *Neurosci. Behav. Physiol.* **2020**, *50*, 669–675. [CrossRef]
24. Boccuni, I.; Fairless, R. Retinal glutamate neurotransmission: From physiology to pathophysiological mechanisms of retinal ganglion cell degeneration. *Life* **2022**, *12*, 638. [CrossRef]
25. Dembla, M.; Kesharwani, A.; Natarajan, S.; Fecher-Trost, C.; Fairless, R.; Williams, S.K.; Flockerzi, V.; Diem, R.; Schwarz, K.; Schmitz, F. Early auto-immune targeting of photoreceptor synapses in mouse models of multiple sclerosis. *EMBO Mol. Med.* **2018**, *10*, e8926. [CrossRef]
26. Mukherjee, A.; Katiyar, R.; Dembla, E.; Dembla, M.; Kumar, P.; Belkacemi, A.; Jung, M.; Beck, A.; Flockerzi, V.; Schwarz, K.; et al. Disturbed presynaptic Ca^{2+} signaling in photoreceptors in the EAE mouse model of multiple sclerosis. *iScience* **2020**, *23*, 101830. [CrossRef]
27. Kesharwani, A.; Schwarz, K.; Dembla, E.; Dembla, M.; Schmitz, F. Early changes in exo- and endocytosis in the EAE mouse model of multiple sclerosis correlate with decreased synaptic ribbon size and reduced ribbon-associated vesicle pools in rod photoreceptor synapses. *Int. J. Mol. Sci.* **2021**, *22*, 10789. [CrossRef]
28. Cordano, C.; Werneburg, S.; Abdelhak, A.; Bennett, D.J.; Beaudry-Richard, A.; Duncan, G.J.; Oertel, F.C.; Boscardin, W.J.; Yiu, H.H.; Jabassini, N.; et al. Synaptic injury in the inner plexiform layer of the retina is associated with progression in multiple sclerosis. *Cell Rep. Med.* **2024**, *5*, 101490. [CrossRef]
29. Moser, T.; Grabner, C.P.; Schmitz, F. Sensory processing at ribbon synapses in the retina and the cochlea. *Physiol. Rev.* **2020**, *100*, 103–144. [CrossRef]
30. Schmitz, F.; Königstorfer, A.; Südhof, T.C. RIBEYE, a component of synaptic ribbons: A protein's journey through evolution provides insight into synaptic ribbon function. *Neuron* **2000**, *28*, 857–872. [CrossRef]
31. Zenisek, D.; Horst, N.K.; Merrifield, C.; Sterling, P. Visualizing synaptic ribbons in the living cell. *J. Neurosci.* **2004**, *24*, 9752–9759. [CrossRef] [PubMed]
32. Maxeiner, S.; Luo, F.; Tan, A.; Schmitz, F.; Südhof, T.C. How to make a synaptic ribbon: RIBEYE deletion abolishes ribbons in retinal synapses and disrupts neurotransmitter release. *EMBO J.* **2016**, *35*, 1098–1114. [CrossRef] [PubMed]
33. Danbolt, N.C. Glutamate uptake. *Prog. Neurobiol.* **2001**, *65*, 1–105. [PubMed]
34. Kanner, B.I. Structure and function of sodium-coupled GABA and glutamate transporters. *J. Membr. Biol.* **2006**, *213*, 89–100. [CrossRef]
35. Machtens, J.P.; Kortzak, D.; Lansche, C.; Leinenweber, A.; Kilian, P.; Begemann, B.; Zachariae, U.; Ewers, D.; de Groot, B.L.; Briones, R.; et al. Mechanisms of anion conduction by coupled glutamate transporters. *Cell* **2015**, *160*, 542–553. [CrossRef]
36. Martinez-Lozada, Z.; Guillem, A.M.; Robinson, M.G. Transcriptional regulation of glutamate transporters: From extracellu lar signals to transcription factors. *Adv. Pharmacol.* **2016**, *76*, 103–145.
37. Fahlke, C.; Kortzak, D.; Machtens, J.P. Molecular physiology of EAAT anion channels. *Pflugers Arch.* **2016**, *468*, 491–502. [CrossRef]
38. Rose, C.R.; Ziemens, D.; Untiet, V.; Fahlke, C. Molecular and cellular physiology of sodium-dependent glutamate transporters. *Brain Res. Bull.* **2018**, *136*, 3–16. [CrossRef]
39. Alleva, C.; Machtens, J.P.; Kortzak, D.; Weyand, I.; Fahlke, C. Molecular basis of coupled transport and anion conduction in excitatory amino acid transporters. *Neurochem. Res.* **2022**, *47*, 9–22. [CrossRef]
40. Kovermann, P.; Engels, M.; Müller, F.; Fahlke, C. Cellular physiology and pathophysiology of EAAT anion channels. *Front. Cell. Neurosci.* **2022**, *15*, 815279. [CrossRef]
41. Arriza, J.L.; Eliasof, S.; Kavanaugh, M.P.; Amara, S.G. Excitatory amino acid transporter 5, a retinal glutamate transporter coupled to a chloride conductance. *Proc. Natl. Acad. Sci. USA* **1997**, *94*, 4155–4160. [CrossRef] [PubMed]
42. Pow, D.; Barnett, N.L. Developmental expression of excitatory amino acid transporter 5: A photoreceptor and bipolar cell glutamate transporter in rat retina. *Neurosci. Lett.* **2000**, *280*, 21–24. [CrossRef] [PubMed]
43. Fyk-Kolodziej, B.; Qin, P.U.; Dzhagaryan, A.; Pourcho, R.G. Differential cellular and subcellular distribution of glutamate transporters in the cat retina. *Vis. Neurosci.* **2004**, *21*, 551–565. [CrossRef] [PubMed]
44. Wersinger, E.; Schwab, Y.; Sahel, J.P.; Rendon, A.; Pow, D.V.; Picaud, S.; Roux, M.J. The glutamate transporter EAAT5 works as a presynaptic receptor in mouse rod bipolar cells. *J. Physiol.* **2006**, *577*, 221–234. [CrossRef]
45. Lee, D.H.; Seubert, S.; Huhn, K.; Brecht, L.; Rötger, C.; Waschbisch, A.; Schlachetzki, J.; Klausmeyer, A.; Melms, A.; Wiese, S.; et al. Fingolimod effects in neuroinflammation: Regulation of astroglial glutamate transporters? *PLoS ONE* **2017**, *12*, e0171552. [CrossRef]
46. Gehlen, J.; Aretzweiler, C.; Maturaga, A.; Fahlke, C.; Müller, F. Excitatory amino acid transporter 5 improves temporal resolution in the retina. *eNeuro* **2021**, *8*, ENEURO.0406-21.2021. [CrossRef]
47. Fairless, R.; Williams, S.K.; Hoffmann, D.B.; Stojic, A.; Hochmeister, S.; Schmitz, F.; Storch, M.K.; Diem, R. Preclinical retinal neurodegeneration in a model of multiple sclerosis. *J. Neurosci.* **2012**, *32*, 5585–5597. [CrossRef]

48. Shankhwar, S.; Schwarz, K.; Katiyar, R.; Jung, M.; Maxeiner, S.; Südhof, T.C.; Schmitz, F. RIBEYE B-domain is essential for RIBEYE A-domain stability and assembly of synaptic ribbons. *Front. Mol. Neurosci.* **2022**, *15*, 838811. [CrossRef]
49. Lessard, J.L. Two monoclonal antibodies to actin: One muscle selective and one generally reactive. *Cell Motil. Cytoskelet.* **1988**, *10*, 349–362. [CrossRef]
50. Long, L.; Wei, J.; Lim, S.A.; Raynor, J.L.; Shi, H.; Connely, J.P.; Wang, H.; Guy, C.; Xie, B.; Chapman, N.M.; et al. CRISPR screens unveil signal hubs for nutrients licensing of T cell immunity. *Nature* **2021**, *600*, 308–313. [CrossRef]
51. Robinson, A.P.; Harp, C.T.; Noronha, A.; Miller, S.D. The experimental autoimmune encephalomyelitis (EAE) model of MS: Utility for understanding disease pathophysiology and treatment. *Handb. Clin. Neurol.* **2014**, *122*, 173–189. [PubMed]
52. Voskuhl, R.R.; Gold, S.M. Sex-related factors in multiple sclerosis: Genetic, hormonal and environmantal contributions. *Nat. Rev. Neurol.* **2015**, *8*, 255–263. [CrossRef] [PubMed]
53. McCombe, P.A.; Greer, J.M. Effects of biological sex and pregnancy in experimental autoimmune encephalomyelitis: It's complicated. *Front. Immunol.* **2022**, *13*, 1059833. [CrossRef] [PubMed]
54. Rahn, E.J.; Iannitti, T.; Donahue, R.R.; Taylor, B.K. Sex differences in a mouse model of multiple sclerosis: Neuropathic pain behavior in females but not males and protection from neurological deficits during proestrus. *Biol. Sex Diff.* **2014**, *5*, 4. [CrossRef]
55. Gibson, D.G.; Young, L.; Chuang, R.Y.; Venter, J.C.; Hutchison, C.A.; Smith, H.O. Enzymatic assembly of DNA molecules up to several hundred kilobases. *Nat. Methods* **2009**, *6*, 343–345. [CrossRef]
56. Wahl, S.; Katiyar, R.; Schmitz, F. A local, periactive zone endocytic machinery at photoreceptor synapses in close vicinity to synaptic ribbons. *J. Neurosci.* **2013**, *33*, 10278–10300. [CrossRef]
57. Wahl, S.; Magupalli, V.G.; Dembla, M.; Katiyar, R.; Schwarz, K.; Köblitz, L.; Alpadi, K.; Krause, E.; Rettig, J.; Sung, C.H.; et al. The disease protein Tulp1 is essential for periactive zone endocytosis in photoreceptor ribbon synapses. *J. Neurosci.* **2016**, *36*, 2473–2493. [CrossRef]
58. Dembla, M.; Wahl, S.; Katiyar, R.; Schmitz, F. ArfGAP3 is a component of the photoreceptor synaptic ribbon complex and forms a NAD(H)-regulated/redox-sensitive complex with RIBEYE that is important for endocytosis. *J. Neurosci.* **2014**, *34*, 5245–5260. [CrossRef]
59. Eich, M.L.; Dembla, E.; Wahl, S.; Dembla, M.; Schwarz, K.; Schmitz, F. The calcineurin-binding, activity-dependent splice variant dynamin1xb is highly enriched in synapses in various regions of the central nervous system. *Front. Mol. Neurosci.* **2017**, *10*, 230. [CrossRef]
60. Suiwal, S.; Dembla, M.; Schwarz, K.; Katiyar, R.; Jung, M.; Carius, Y.; Maxeiner, S.; Lauterbach, M.A.; Lancaster, C.R.D.; Schmitz, F. Ciliary proteins repurposed by the synaptic ribbon: Trafficking myristoylated proteins at the synaptic ribbon. *Int. J. Mol. Sci.* **2022**, *23*, 7135. [CrossRef]
61. Dembla, E.; Dembla, M.; Maxeiner, S.; Schmitz, F. Synaptic ribbons foster active zone stability and illumination-dependent active zone enrichment of RIM2 and Cav1.4 in photoreceptor synapses. *Sci. Rep.* **2020**, *10*, 5957. [CrossRef] [PubMed]
62. Faul, F.; Erdfelder, E.; Lang, A.G.; Buchner, A. G*Power 3: A flexible statistical power analysis program for the social, behavioral, and biomedical sciences. *Behav. Res. Methods* **2007**, *39*, 175–191. [CrossRef] [PubMed]
63. Hedges, L. Distribution theory for Glass's estimator of effect size and related estimators. *J. Educ. Stat.* **1981**, *6*, 107–128. [CrossRef]
64. Dieckmann-Schuppert, A.; Schnittler, H.J. A simple assay for quantification of protein in tissue sections, cell cultures, and cell homogenates, and of protein immobilized on solid surfaces. *Cell Tiss. Res.* **1997**, *288*, 119–126. [CrossRef]
65. Pitt, D.; Nagelmeier, I.E.; Wilson, H.C.; Raine, C.S. Glutamate uptake by oligodendrocytes: Implications for excitotoxicity in multiple sclerosis. *Neurology* **2003**, *61*, 1113–1120. [CrossRef]
66. Vercellino, M.; Merola, A.; Piacentino, C.; Votta, B.; Capello, E.; Mancardi, G.L.; Mutani, R.; Giordana, M.T.; Cavalla, P. Altered glutamate reuptake in relapsing-remitting and secondary progressive multiple sclerosis cortex: Correlation with microglia infiltration, demyelination, and neuronal and synaptic damage. *J. Neuropathol. Exp. Neurol.* **2007**, *66*, 732–739. [CrossRef]
67. Mandolesi, G.; Musella, A.; Gentile, A.; Grasselli, G.; Haji, N.; Sepman, H.; Fresegna, D.; Bullitta, S.; De Vito, F.; Musumeci, G.; et al. Interleukin-1β alters glutamate transmission at Purkinje cell synapses in a mouse model of multiple sclerosis. *J. Neurosci.* **2013**, *33*, 12105–12121. [CrossRef]
68. Mandolesi, G.; Gentile, A.; Musella, A.; Centonze, D. IL-1β dependent cerebellar synaptopathy in a mouse model of multiple sclerosis. *Cerebellum* **2015**, *14*, 19–22. [CrossRef]
69. Potenza, N.; Mosca, N.; Mondola, P.; Damiano, S.; Russo, A.; De Felice, B. Human miR-26a-5p regulates the glutamate transporter SLC1A1 (EAAT3) expression: Relevance in multiple sclerosis. *Biochim. Biophys. Acta Mol. Bas. Dis.* **2018**, *1864*, 317–323. [CrossRef]
70. Todd, A.C.; Hardingham, G.E. The regulation of astrocytic glutamate transporters in health and neurodegenerative diseases. *Int. J. Mol. Sci.* **2020**, *21*, 9607. [CrossRef]
71. Sheng, L.; Luo, Q.; Chen, L. Amino acid solute carrier transporters in inflammation and autoimmunity. *Drug Metab. Dispos.* **2022**, *50*, 1228–1237. [CrossRef] [PubMed]
72. Vallejo-Illaramandi, A.; Domercq, M.; Perez-Cerda, F.; Ravid, R.; Matute, C. Increased expression and function of glutamate transporters in multiple sclerosis. *Neurobiol. Dis.* **2006**, *21*, 154–164. [CrossRef]
73. Pampliega, O.; Domercq, M.; Villoslada, P.; Sepulcre, J.; Rodriguez-Antiguedad, A.; Matute, C. Association of an EAAT2 polymorphism with higher glutamate concentration in relapsing multiple sclerosis. *J. Neuroimmunol.* **2008**, *195*, 194–198. [CrossRef] [PubMed]

74. Boccuni, I.; Bas-Orth, C.; Bruehl, C.; Draguhn, A.; Fairless, R. Glutamate transporter contribution to retinal ganglion cell vulnerability in a rat model of multiple sclerosis. *Neurobiol. Dis.* **2023**, *187*, 106306. [CrossRef] [PubMed]
75. Izumi, Y.; Shimamoto, K.; Benz, A.M.; Hammerman, S.B.; Olney, J.W.; Zorumski, C.F. Glutamate transporters and retinal excitotoxicity. *Glia* **2002**, *39*, 58–68. [CrossRef]
76. Vandenberg, R.J.; Ryan, R.M. Mechanisms of glutamate transport. *Physiol. Rev.* **2013**, *93*, 1621–1657. [CrossRef]
77. Bading, H. Therapeutic targeting of the pathological triad of extrasynaptic NMDA receptor signaling in neurodegenerations. *J. Exp. Med.* **2017**, *214*, 569–578. [CrossRef]
78. Hardingham, G.E.; Arnold, F.J.; Bading, H. Nuclear calcium signalling controls CREB-mediated gene expression triggered by synaptic activity. *Nat. Neurosci.* **2001**, *4*, 261–267. [CrossRef]
79. Hardingham, G.E.; Arnold, F.J.; Bading, H. A calcium microdomain near NMDA receptors: On switch for ERK-dependent synapse-to-nucleus communcation. *Nat. Neurosci.* **2001**, *4*, 565–566. [CrossRef]
80. Hardingham, G.E.; Fukunaga, Y.; Bading, H. Extrasynaptic NMDARs oppose synaptic NMDARs by triggering CREB-shutoff and cell death pathways. *Nat. Neurosci.* **2002**, *5*, 405–414. [CrossRef]
81. Hardingham, G.E.; Bading, H. The Yin and Yang NMDA receptor signalling. *Trends Neurosci.* **2003**, *26*, 81–89. [CrossRef] [PubMed]
82. Hardingham, G.E.; Bading, H. Synaptic versus extrasynaptic NMDA receptor signalling: Implications for neurodegenerative disorders. *Nat. Rev. Neurosci.* **2010**, *11*, 682–696. [CrossRef] [PubMed]
83. Parsons, M.P.; Raymond, L.A. Extrasynaptic NMDA receptor involvement in central nervous system disorders. *Neuron* **2014**, *82*, 279–293. [CrossRef] [PubMed]
84. Matute, C.; Domercq, M.; Sanchez-Gomez, M.V. Glutamate-mediated glial injury. *Glia* **2006**, *53*, 212–224. [CrossRef] [PubMed]
85. Picaud, S.A.; Larsson, H.P.; Grant, G.B.; Lecar, H.; Werblin, F.S. Glutamate-gated chloride channel with glutamate-transporter-like properties in cone photoreceptors of the tiger salamander. *J. Neurophysiol.* **1995**, *74*, 1760–1771. [CrossRef]
86. Palmer, M.J.; Taschenberger, H.; Hull, C.; Tremere, L.; von Gersdorff, H. Synaptic activation of presynaptic glutamate transporter currents in nerve terminals. *J. Neurosci.* **2003**, *23*, 4831–4841. [CrossRef]
87. Smajda, B.R.; DeVries, S.H. Glutamate spillover between mammalian cone photoreceptors. *J. Neurosci.* **2011**, *31*, 13431–13441. [CrossRef]
88. Lee, A.; Anderson, A.R.; Barnett, N.L.; Stevens, M.G.; Pow, D.V. Alternate splicing and expression of the glutamate transporter EAAT5 in the rat retina. *Gene* **2012**, *506*, 283–288. [CrossRef]
89. Tse, D.Y.; Chung, I.; Wu, S.M. Possible roles of glutamate transporter EAAT5 in mouse cone bipolar cell light responses. *Vis. Res.* **2014**, *103*, 63–74. [CrossRef]
90. Chen, I.; Pant, S.; Wu, Q.; Cater, R.J.; Sobti, M.; Vandenberg, R.J.; Stewart, A.G.; Tajkhorshid, E.; Font, J.; Ryan, R.M. Gluta mate transporters have a chloride channel with two hydrophobic gates. *Nature* **2021**, *591*, 327–331. [CrossRef]
91. Bligard, G.W.; DeBrecht, J.; Smith, R.G.; Lukasiewicz, P.D. Light-evoked glutamate transporter EAAT5 activation coordinates with conventional feedback inhibition to control rod bipolar cell output. *J. Neurophysiol.* **2020**, *123*, 1828–1837. [CrossRef] [PubMed]
92. Tang, F.S.; Yuan, H.L.; Liu, J.B.; Zhang, G.; Chen, S.Y.; Ke, J.B. Glutamate transporters EAAT2 and EAAT5 differentially shape synaptic transmission from rod bipolar cell terminals. *eNeuro* **2022**, *9*, ENEURO.0074-22.2022. [CrossRef] [PubMed]
93. Thoreson, W.B.; Chhunchha, B. EAAT5 glutamate transporter rapidly binds glutamate with micromolar affinity in rods. *J. Gen. Physiol.* **2023**, *155*, e202313349. [CrossRef]
94. Lukasiewicz, P.D.; Bligard, G.W.; DeBrecht, J.D. EAAT5 glutamate transporter mediated inhibition in the vertebrate retina. *Front. Cell. Neurosci.* **2021**, *15*, 662859.
95. Rauen, T.; Taylor, W.R.; Kuhlbrodt, K.; Wiessner, M. High-affinity glutamate transporters in the rat retina: A major role of the glial glutamate transporter GLAST-1 in transmitter clearance. *Cell Tiss. Res.* **1998**, *291*, 19–31. [CrossRef]
96. Pow, D.V.; Barnett, N.L.; Penfold, P. Are neuronal transporters relevant for glutamate homeostasis? *Neurochem. Int.* **2000**, *37*, 191–198. [CrossRef]

MDPI AG
Grosspeteranlage 5
4052 Basel
Switzerland
Tel.: +41 61 683 77 34

Biomedicines Editorial Office
E-mail: biomedicines@mdpi.com
www.mdpi.com/journal/biomedicines

Lightning Source LLC
Chambersburg PA
CBHW062051220926
51850CB00010B/2738